DRUG
INTERACTIONS
HANDBOOK

Richard Harkness, R. Ph.

Prentice-Hall, Inc.
Englewood Cliffs, New Jersey

Prentice-Hall International, Inc., *London*
Prentice-Hall of Australia, Pty. Ltd., *Sydney*
Prentice-Hall Canada, Inc., *Toronto*
Prentice-Hall of India Private Ltd., *New Delhi*
Prentice-Hall of Japan, Inc., *Tokyo*
Prentice-Hall of Southeast Asia Pte. Ltd., *Singapore*
Whitehall Books, Ltd., *Wellington, New Zealand*
Editora Prentice-Hall do Brasil Ltda., *Rio de Janeiro*

© 1984 *by*
Richard Harkness

This book is a reference work based on research
by the author. The opinions expressed herein are
not necessarily those of or endorsed by the pub-
lisher. The directions stated in this book are in no
way to be considered a substitute for consultation
with a duly liscensed doctor.

Library of Congress Cataloging in Publication Data

Harkness, Richard.
  Drug interactions handbook.

  Includes index.
  1. Drug interactions—Dictionaries. I. Title.
[DNLM: 1. Drug interactions—Handbooks.   2. Drug therapy—
Adverse effects—Handbooks.   QV 38 H282d]
RM302.H367 1984   615′.7045   83-21167
ISBN 0-13-220954-3
ISBN 0-13-220947-0

Printed in the United States of America

Introduction

Adverse drug interactions are responsible for many thousands of hospital admissions in the United States each year. One recent year-long study conducted in drug stores found that nearly one in four of all prescription customers experienced a significant drug interaction at some time during the year. Such interactions have caused serious crises that in some instances have resulted in deaths. Fortunately, the number of interactions that have caused fatalities is a very small percentage of the total number of drug interactions that occur. Much more common are interactions that cause an increase in toxicity or a decrease in therapeutic effect of a medication with the result that the patient doesn't feel as well as he should or doesn't get well as quickly as he should. Sometimes the interaction produces no observable symptoms at all. Chronic diseases such as high blood pressure, diabetes, and heart disease may not be controlled properly. If the physician is unaware of a drug interaction, he might make faulty treatment decisions.

Today's prescription drugs are effective and potent. Interactions between them are a very real problem. It is difficult for a busy physician or pharmacist to take the time to monitor for drug interactions for each patient, even if the physician or pharmacist is on the lookout for the hundreds of possible interactions. When you combine this fact with the realization that many patients are receiving multiple drug therapy—including nonprescription medications they take on their own—and that the physician or pharmacist may be unaware of the majority of potential interactions, you begin to see the magnitude of the problem.

I monitor for drug interactions regularly in my practice of pharmacy and in my work as a nursing home consultant. When I see a potential problem, I notify the prescribing physician. Usually he/she is grateful. Often, the physician had been blaming a patient's adverse symptoms or lack of proper response to a medication on some unknown cause or on the disease/illness being treated. Suddenly comes the realization that the undetected drug interaction is more likely than not the culprit. With this knowledge, the physician adjusts the dosage or times of administration of the medications to alleviate the problem.

People are recognizing more and more the need to become active partners in their own health care. Drug interaction is an area in which everyone involved—patient, physician, pharmacist, nurse—can work together for the benefit of the patient.

The purpose of this book is to provide a reliable, easy-to-use reference guide to adverse drug interactions. It is written for the layperson, yet its comprehensiveness makes it suitable for medical practitioners as well.

The lack of an interaction listing for any two drugs should not imply that they do not interact when given together. Drug interactions can be complex and unpredictable, and new interactions are discovered regularly.

You should consult your physician for recommendations on managing a suspected interaction.

QUESTIONS AND ANSWERS ABOUT DRUG INTERACTIONS

WHAT IS A DRUG INTERACTION?

Simply stated, a drug interaction occurs whenever one drug alters the effect of another drug. The drug altered may be made less active or more active.

WHAT HAPPENS TO YOU IF YOU TAKE INTERACTING DRUGS?

There are great variations in individual reactions. Influencing factors include your genetic makeup, kidney and liver functions, age (those over fifty and infants are most susceptible), whether there are any underlying illnesses or diseases, the amount of the drugs taken, the duration of therapy, the time interval between the taking of the two drugs, and which drug is taken first. For these reasons, it is possible that the effect may be insignificant on one person and extremely hazardous on another. The important thing is to be aware that there *could* be a problem.

HOW EXACTLY DO TWO DRUGS INTERACT?

As background, here is a simplified pharmacology lesson: A drug taken by mouth goes through four basic processes in the body. It passes from the mouth into the stomach and intestinal tract. From there it is *absorbed* into the bloodstream and *distributed* throughout the body where it exerts its effects. It is then broken down or *metabolized* by the liver. Finally, this broken-down form is *excreted* (eliminated from the body) by the kidneys in the urine.

In a drug interaction, one drug modifies one or more of the above processes on the other drug. This type of interaction is called a *pharmacokinetic* interaction.

The other primary type of interaction is called a *pharmacologic* interaction. In this type, the effect of one drug "adds on" (synergism) to increase the effect of another drug; or "subtracts from" (antagonism) to decrease the effect of another drug.

DOES THIS MEAN THAT INTERACTING DRUGS CANNOT BE TAKEN TOGETHER?

Not always. Usually, the dose or time of administration of one drug can be altered to offset adverse effects. Some interactions are beneficial and are deliberately exploited for this reason. There are many cases, however, in which certain drugs should not be given together under any circumstances. The important thing—and a recurring theme of this book—is for the physician to be made *aware* of a potential interaction so that he can act knowledgeably.

Richard Harkness

How To Use
The Drug Interactions Handbook

Each chapter covers drug interactions for the medications used to treat a particular ailment or condition. If you know what you're taking a particular drug for, you can turn to the corresponding chapter and find all the interactions involving that drug; or you can look in the index to find the page numbers where it appears—page numbers shown in BOLD print indicate the chapter pages where that drug is discussed and where all of its interactions are grouped together.

A chapter is divided into three parts:

1. Discussion of the ailment or condition.
2. Brand name section.
3. Drug interactions section.

The *Brand Name* section shows the brand names according to the drug category or family they belong to. Within each category, brand names are listed alphabetically and the generic name is shown in parentheses beside the brand name.

The *Drug Interactions* section lists the drug interactions alphabetically by category name or by generic name. Each interaction paragraph tells what happens when an interaction occurs, its results, and what side effects to expect from the interaction. Brand names of interacting drugs are also provided.

Within a chapter, look in the *Brand Name* section to find the category name or the generic name of the particular drug you are interested in, then turn to the *Drug Interactions* section to find all interaction involving it.

Throughout the book, especially significant interactions are indicated by an asterisk.

Contents

1

Drug Interactions in Treatment of Acne

Acne (Acne vulgaris to be exact) is a chronic disorder caused by increased activity of the sebaceous glands, which normally produce an oily substance called *sebum* to lubricate skin and hair. Sebum and shedded skin cells plug pores and cause impactions which eventually turn to whiteheads, blackheads, and pimples. Oversecretion of sebum is triggered by a male sex hormone called *androgen* (in both males and females). Acne sufferers may be more sensitive to this hormone.

Since sebaceous glands are most common on the face, chest, neck, and back, acne predominates in these areas.

The "acne decade"—from about ages thirteen to twenty-three—is a universal phenomenon afflicting over 90 percent of the population to some degree.

Treatment of acne consists of using a variety of topically applied drying and peeling preparations. In severe cases, the physician may prescribe the antibiotic tetracycline to be taken by mouth over a long period of time. The antibiotic combats bacteria aggravating acne and changes the fatty acid composition of sebum.

All the drug interactions discussed in this chapter involve tetracycline. Accutane (retinoic acid), a derivative of vitamin A, is the latest development in oral treatment for severe acne. As yet there are no documented drug interactions involving it.

BRAND NAMES

TETRACYCLINE FAMILY:

Achromycin (tetracycline)
Aureomycin (chlortetracycline)
Bristacycline (tetracycline)
Cyclopar (tetracycline)
Declomycin (demeclocycline)
Doxy-Tabs (doxycycline)
Doxychel (doxycycline)
Minocin (minocycline)
Panmycin (tetracycline)
Retet-S (tetracycline)
Robitet (tetracycline)

Rondomycin (methacycline)
SK-Tetracycline (tetracycline)
Sumycin (tetracycline)
Terramycin (oxytetracycline)
Tetra-Bid (tetracycline)
Tetrachel (tetracycline)
Tetracyn (tetracycline)
Tetrex (tetracycline)
Vibramycin (doxycycline)
Vibratab (doxycycline)

DRUG INTERACTIONS

NOTE: "TETRACYCLINES (ALL)" refers to all the tetracyclines—tetracycline, chlortetracycline, demeclocycline, doxycycline, methacycline, minocycline, oxytetracycline.

DOXYCYCLINE....BARBITURATES

THE EFFECT OF DOXYCYCLINE MAY BE DECREASED. RESULT: The acne condition may not respond to the doxycycline treatment unless the dosage is raised. Barbiturates are prescribed as sedatives or sleeping pills. DOXYCYCLINE (Doxy-Tabs, Doxychel, Vibramycin, Vibratab). Brand names of barbiturates:

phenobarbital
Alurate
Amytal
Butisol
Buticap
Carbrital
Eskabarb
Lotusate

Luminal
Mebaral
Nembutal
Seconal
Sedadrops
Solfoton
Tuinal

DOXYCLINE....CARBAMAZEPINE (Tegretol)

THE EFFECT OF DOXYCYCLINE MAY BE DECREASED. RESULT: The acne condition may not respond to the doxycycline treatment unless the dosage is raised. Carbamezepine is prescribed to control seizures in disorders such as epilepsy.

DOXYCYCLINE....PHENYTOIN (Dilantin)

THE EFFECT OF DOXYCYCLINE MAY BE DECREASED. RESULT: The acne condition may not respond to the doxycycline treatment unless the dosage is raised. Phenytoin is prescribed to control seizures in disorders such as epilepsy.

DOXYCYCLINE....PRIMIDONE (Mysoline)

THE EFFECT OF DOXYCYCLINE MAY BE DECREASED. RESULT: The acne condition may not respond to the doxycycline treatment unless the dosage is raised. Primidone is prescribed to control seizures in disorders such as epilepsy. DOXYCYCLINE (Doxy-Tabs, Doxychel, Vibramycin, Vibratab).

TETRACYCLINES (ALL)....ANTACIDS

(AlternaGel, Delcid, Di-Gel, Gelusil, Kudrox, Maalox, Mylanta, Riopan, WinGel, etc.)

THE EFFECT OF TETRACYCLINE MAY BE DECREASED. RESULT: The acne condition may not respond to the tetracycline treatment. To prevent this interaction, do not take these medications within two hours of each other. Sodium bicarbonate antacids (e.g., Alka-Seltzer) probably do not interact with tetracycline significantly.

TETRACYCLINES (ALL)....ANTICOAGULANTS

THE EFFECT OF THE ANTICOAGULANT MAY BE INCREASED. Anticoagulants are used to thin the blood and prevent it from clotting. RESULT: Increased risk of hemorrhage. Report symptoms such as black or tarry stools, bleeding or bruising anywhere on the body. DOXYCYCLINE (Doxy-Tabs, Doxychel, Vibramycin, Vibratab) is the tetracycline most likely to cause this interaction. Coumadin is the most widely used anticoagulant drug. Anticoagulant brand names:

Athrombin-K (warfarin)	Hedulin (phenindione)
Coufarin (warfarin)	Liquamar (phenprocouman)
Coumadin (warfarin)	Miradon (anisindione)
dicumarol (various companies)	Panwarfin (warfarin)

TETRACYCLINES (ALL)
....BIRTH CONTROL PILLS (oral contraceptives)

THE EFFECT OF BIRTH CONTROL PILLS MAY BE DECREASED. RESULT: Increased risk of pregnancy unless an alternate method of contraception is used during the antibiotic treatment regimen. Breakthrough bleeding is a symptom of a possible interaction. Oral contraceptive brand names:

Brevicon	Nordette
Demulen	Norinyl
Enovid	Norlestrin
Loestrin	Ortho-Novum
Lo-Ovral	Ovcon
Micronor	Ovral
Modicon	Ovrette
Nor-Q.D.	Ovulen

TETRACYCLINES (ALL)....DIGOXIN (Lanoxin)

THE EFFECT OF DIGOXIN MAY BE INCREASED. Digoxin is used to treat congestive heart failure or to restore irregular heart beats to normal rhythm. RESULT: Possible adverse side effects caused by too much digoxin. Report symptoms such as nausea, visual disturbances, confusion, loss of energy, headache, heart irregularities.

TETRACYCLINES (ALL)....ESTROGENS (female hormones)

THE EFFECT OF ESTROGENS MAY BE DECREASED. Estrogens are prescribed for estrogen deficiency during menopause and after hysterectomy (surgical removal of the uterus), to prevent painful swelling of the breasts after pregnancy in women choosing not to nurse, and to treat amenorrhea (failure to menstruate). RESULT: The conditions may not be controlled properly during antibiotic treatment. Brand names of estrogens:

Amen	Estrovis
Aygestin	Evex
DES	Feminone
Estinyl	Menest
Estrace	Menrium
Estratab	Milprem

Norlutate   Premarin
Norlutin   Provera
Ogen   Tace
PMB

TETRACYCLINES (ALL)....IRON

THE EFFECT OF TETRACYCLINE MAY BE DE-CREASED. RESULT: The acne condition may not respond to the tetracycline treatment. To prevent this interaction, do not take within two hours of each other. IRON is listed on vitamin-mineral supplement labels as ferrous sulfate or ferrous gluconate.

TETRACYCLINES (ALL)....LAXATIVES

(only those containing magnesium:
citrate of magnesia, epsom salts, milk of magnesia)

THE EFFECT OF TETRACYCLINE MAY BE DE-CREASED. RESULT: The acne condition may not respond to the tetracycline treatment. To prevent this interaction, do not take these medications within two hours of each other.

*TETRACYCLINES (ALL)....MILK, DAIRY PRODUCTS

THE EFFECT OF TETRACYCLINE MAY BE DE-CREASED. NOTE: This interactions applies to all tetracyclines except DOXYCYCLINE and MINOCYCLINE. RESULT: The acne condition may not respond to the tetracycline treatment. To prevent this interaction, do not take within two hours of each other. Note: All food will decrease the absorption of tetracycline to a degree, so it is best to take this antibiotic between meals.

TETRACYCLINES (ALL)....PENICILLINS

THE EFFECT OF PENICILLIN MAY BE DECREASED. Penicillin is an antibiotic used to treat a wide variety of infections. RESULT: The infection may not respond properly to treatment. Penicillin brand names (generic names in parentheses):

Amcill (ampicillin)   Betapen-VK (penicillin VK)
Amoxicillin (various companies)   Cyclapen-W (cyclacillin)
Amoxil (amoxicillin)   Dynapen (dicloxacillin)
Ampicillin (various companies)   Geocillin (carbenicillin)

Larotid (amoxicillin)
Ledercillin VK (penicillin VK)
Nafcil (nafcillin)
Omnipen (ampicillin)
Pathocil (dicloxacillin)
Pen-Vee K (penicillin VK)
Penapar VK (penicillin VK)
Penbritin (ampicillin)
penicillin VK (various companies)
Pensyn (ampicillin)
Pfizerpen A (ampicillin)
Pfizerpen VK (penicillin VK)
Polycillin (ampicillin)
Polymox (amoxicillin)
Principen (ampicillin)

Prostaphlin (oxacillin)
Robamox (amoxicillin)
Robicillin VK (penicillin VK)
Spectrobid (bacampicillin)
Supen (ampicillin)
Tegopen (cloxacillin)
Totacillin (ampicillin)
Trimox (amoxicillin)
Utimox (amoxicillin)
Unipen (nafcillin)
V-Cillin K (penicillin VK)
Veracillin (dicloxacillin)
Versapen (hetacillin)
Wymox (amoxicillin)

TETRACYCLINES (ALL)....VITAMIN A

THIS COMBINATION MAY CAUSE PRESSURE WITHIN THE SKULL with symptoms such as severe headache, nausea, visual disturbances. Avoid taking a vitamin supplement containing vitamin A during extended tetracycline treatment.

TETRACYCLINES (ALL)....ZINC

THE EFFECT OF TETRACYCLINE MAY BE DE-CREASED. NOTE: This interaction applies to all tetracyclines except DOXYCYCLINE and MINOCYCLINE. RESULT: The acne condition may not respond to the tetracycline treatment. To prevent this interaction, do not take within two hours of each other. ZINC is a mineral found in many vitamin-mineral supplements.

2

Drug Interactions in Treatment of Alcoholism

DISULFIRAM (Antabuse) is the drug prescribed to deter alcohol ingestion. Its purpose is to make the experience of taking a drink so unpleasant that the alcoholic will stay "on the wagon" and avoid the urge to drink an alcoholic beverage. A person taking disulfiram should be aware of its potential to interact with several other drugs. First, let's take a look at the way it interacts with alcohol in any form. In this case, the adverse side effects of a drug interaction are deliberately exploited:

*DISULFIRAM....ALCOHOL (beer, liquor, wine, etc.)

THIS COMBINATION MAY PRODUCE THE "DIS-ULFIRAM REACTION." RESULT: Nausea, vomiting, dizziness, flushing, shortness of breath, severe headache, visual disturbances, heart palpitations, possible unconsciousness. NOTE: Alcohol-containing cough syrups and vitamin tonics and even topically applied preparations containing alcohol can also cause this reaction.

*DISULFIRAM....ANTICOAGULANTS

THE EFFECT OF THE ANTICOAGULANT MAY BE INCREASED. Anticoagulants are used to thin the blood and prevent it from clotting. RESULT :Increased risk of hemorrhage. Report symptoms such as black or tarry stools, bruising or bleeding anywhere on the body. Anticoagulant brand names:

Athrombin-K (warfarin)
Coufarin (warfarin)
Coumadin (warfarin)
dicumarol (various companies)

Hedulin (phenindione)
Liquamar (phenprocoumon)
Miradon (anisindione)
Panwarfin (warfarin)

DISULFIRAM....ISONIAZID (INH, Niconyl, Nydrazid)

THIS COMBINATION MAY CAUSE LOSS OF COORDI-
NATION, ABERRANT OR PSYCHOTIC BEHAVIOR.
Isoniazid is used to treat tuberculosis.

DISULFIRAM....METRONIDAZOLE (Flagyl, Metryl, Satric)

THIS COMBINATION MAY CAUSE CONFUSION, AB-
ERRANT OR PSYCHOTIC BEHAVIOR. Metronidazole is used
to treat *Trichomonas vaginalis*, a type of vaginitis.

DISULFIRAM....MERCAPTOPURINE (Purinethol)

THIS COMBINATION MAY CAUSE LIVER DAMAGE.
Report symptoms such as fever, headache, weakness, malaise, loss
of appetite, jaundice (yellow skin). Mercaptopurine is used in
cancer treatment.

*DISULFIRAM....PHENYTOIN (Dilantin)

THE EFFECT OF PHENYTOIN MAY BE INCREASED.
Phenytoin is used to control seizures in disorders such as epilepsy.
RESULT: Adverse side effects caused by too much phenytoin.
Report symptoms such as drowsiness, visual disturbances, loss of
coordination. Other interacting phenytoin-type drugs are etho-
toin (Peganone) and mephenytoin (Mesantoin).

3

Drug Interactions in Treatment of Allergies

Allergic reactions are usually caused by the body's release of histamine in response to invasion by an allergen. Some people are more susceptible to allergens than others.

The most common allergy syndrome is SAR (Seasonal Allergic Rhinitis), known as *hay fever* or *pollinosis*. It is caused by ragweed, grass pollen, and tree pollens, and recurs annually during the pollinating season. Individuals suffering symptoms throughout the year have what is termed *perennial allergic rhinitis*, and are susceptible to allergens in house dust, mold and fungus spores, feathers, talcum powder, and animal dander.

Symptoms include uncontrollable sneezing attacks, itching all over, runny or stuffy nose, itchy and watery eyes, sensitivity to light, headache and irritability, insomnia, and lack of appetite.

The most effective treatment is the early use of antihistamines—preventively—before histamine is released in response to an allergen's invasion. Antihistamines work by taking up some of the places where histamine normally "plugs in" to cells, thus diminishing histamine's ability to cause an allergic reaction.

Interactions in this chapter focus on the *antihistamines*, which are the most frequently used drugs for this type of allergy treatment. For some allergic reactions—skin rashes, hives, insect stings—physicians may also prescribe a corticosteroid drug. Available now are these corticosteroid nasal inhalation products for use in severe cases of seasonal or perennial allergic rhinitis: dexamethasone (Decadron Turbinaire), funisolide (Nasalide spray), and beclomethasone (Beconase inhaler, Vancenase inhaler). (See *Arthritis* chapter for corticosteroid drug interactions.)

23

BRAND NAMES

ANTIHISTAMINE PRODUCTS:

Actidil (triprolidine)
Antivert (meclizine)
Atarax (hydroxyzine)
Benadryl (diphenhydramine)
Bendectin (doxylamine)
Bonine (meclizine)
Chlor-Trimeton
   (chlorpheniramine)
Clistin (carbinoxamine)
Decapryn (doxylamine)
Dimetane (brompheniramine)
Dramamine (dimenhydrinate)
Histadyl (methapyrilene)

Inhiston (pheniramine)
Marezine (cyclizine)
Optimine (azatadine)
PBZ (tripelennamine)
Periactin (cyproheptadine)
Polaramine
   (dexchlorpheniramine)
Pyronil (pyrrobutamine)
Tavist (clemastine)
Temaril (trimeprazine)
Teldrin (chlorpheniramine)
Triten (dimethindene)
Vistaril (hydroxyzine)

DRUG INTERACTIONS

The antihistamines are center nervous system depressants. They depress or impair functions such as coordination and alertness. Excessive depression and impairment can occur when an antihistamine is taken with any other central nervous system depressant as shown by the following interactions:

ANTIHISTAMINES....ALCOHOL (beer, liquor, wine—all alcoholic drinks)

RESULT: Drowsiness, dizziness, loss of muscle coordination and mental alertness, making it hazardous to drive or do other things requiring complete alertness; in severe cases, failure of blood circulation and breathing functions causing coma and death.

ANTIHISTAMINES....ANTICHOLINERGIC DRUGS

A. THIS COMBINATION MAY CAUSE EXCESSIVE "ANTICHOLINERGIC" SIDE EFFECTS. RESULT: blurred vision, dry mouth, constipation, heart palpitations, slurred speech, difficulty in urination, stomach irritation, possible toxic psychosis (agitation, disorientation, delirium).
B. CERTAIN ANTICHOLINERGIC DRUGS CAN CAUSE EXCESSIVE DEPRESSANT SIDE EFFECTS. RESULT: Drowsi-

ness, dizziness, loss of muscle coordination and mental alertness, making it hazardous to drive or do other things requiring complete alertness; in severe cases, failure of blood circulation and breathing functions causing coma and death. The anticholinergic products causing this interaction include Akineton, Artane, Cogentin, Kemadrin, Norflex, Pagitane, Robinul, and Transderm-Scop. Brand names and uses of anticholinergic drugs (generic names in parentheses):

Those used to control tremors resulting from Parkinson's disease or from treatment with antipsychotic drugs:

Akineton (biperiden)
Artane (trihexyphenidyl)
Cogentin (benztropine)
Kemadrin (procyclidine)
Pagitane (cycrimine)

Those used in stomach, digestive tract disorders:

Bentyl (dicyclomine)
Combid (isopropamide)
Probanthine (propantheline)
Robinul (glycopyrrolate)

Others:

Norflex (orphenadrine)—a muscle relaxant
Transderm-Scop (scopolamine)—a small disc attached behind the
  ear for motion sickness

ANTIHISTAMINES....ANTICONVULSANT DRUGS

RESULT: Drowsiness, dizziness, loss of muscle coordination and mental alertness, making it hazardous to drive or do other things requiring complete alertness; in severe cases, failure of blood circulation and breathing functions causing coma and death. Anticonvulsant drugs are used to control seizures in disorders such as epilepsy. Anticonvulsant drug brand names (generic names in parentheses):

Depakene (valproic acid)   Peganone (ethotoin)
Dilantin (phenytoin)   Tegretol (carbamazepine)
Mesantoin (mephenytoin)   Tridione (trimethadione)
Mysoline (primidone)   Zarontin (ethosuximide)

ANTIHISTAMINES....ANTIDEPRESSANTS (CYCLIC TYPE)

RESULT: Drowsiness, dizziness, loss of muscle coordination and mental alertness, making it hazardous to drive or do other things requiring complete alertness; in severe cases, failure of blood circulation and breathing functions causing coma and death. Antidepressants are used to alleviate mental depression and elevate the mood. Antidepressant brand names (generic names in parentheses):

Adapin (doxepin)
Asendin (amoxapine)
Aventyl (nortriptyline)
Desyrel (trazadone)
Elavil (amitriptyline)
Endep (amitriptyline)
Etrafon (amitriptyline/
 perphenazine)
Limbitrol (amitriptyline/
 chlordiazepoxide)
Ludiomil (maprotiline)

Norpramin (desipramine)
Pamelor (nortriptyline)
Pertofrane (desipramine)
Sinequan (doxepin)
Surmontil (trimipramine)
Tofranil, Tofranil-PM
 (imipramine)
Triavil (amitriptyline/
 perphenazine)
Vivactil (protriptyline)

ANTIHISTAMINES....ANTIPSYCHOTIC DRUGS

RESULT: Drowsiness, dizziness, loss of muscle coordination and mental alertness, making it hazardous to drive or do other things requiring complete mental alertness; in severe cases, failure of blood circulation and breathing functions causing coma and death. The antipsychotic drugs are major tranquilizers used to treat severe mental disorders such as schizophrenia. Most of these agents are of the phenothiazine drug family. Antipsychotic brand names (generic names in parentheses):

PHENOTHIAZINE TYPE:
 Compazine (prochlorperazine)
 Mellaril (thioridazine)
 Proketazine (carphenazine)
 Prolixin (fluphenazine)
 Quide (piperacetazine)
 Serentil (mesoridazine)
 Sparine (promazine)
 Stelazine (trifluoperazine)
 Thorazine (chlorpromazine)

Tindal (acetophenazine)
Trilafon (perphenazine)
Vesprin (triflupromazine)

OTHERS:
Haldol (haloperidol)
Loxitane (loxapine)
Moban (molindone)
Navane (thiothixene)
Taractan (chlorprothixene)

ANTIHISTAMINES....HIGH BLOOD PRESSURE DRUGS

(only the nerve blockers clonidine, guanabenz, methyldopa, reserpine)

RESULT: Drowsiness, dizziness, loss of muscle coordination and mental alertness, making it hazardous to drive or do other things requiring complete alertness; in severe cases, failure of blood circulation and breathing functions causing coma and death. High blood pressure drugs are used to lower the blood pressure. Interacting high blood pressure drugs (brand names in parentheses):

clonidine (Catapres, Combipres)
guanabenz (Wytensin)
methyldopa (Aldoclor, Aldomet, Aldoril)
reserpine type drugs:
deserpidine (Enduronyl, Harmonyl, Oreticyl)
rauwolfia (Raudixin, Rauzide)
reserpine (Diupres, Diutensen-R, Hydropres, Rau-Sed, Regroton, Renese-R, Reserpoid, Salutensin, Sandril, Ser-Ap-Es, Serpasil, Serpasil-Apresoline, Serpasil-Esidrix)

ANTIHISTAMINES....FENFLURAMINE (Pondimin)

RESULT: Drowsiness, dizziness, loss of muscle coordination and mental alertness, making it hazardous to drive or do other things requiring complete alertness; in severe cases, failure of blood circulation and breathing functions causing coma and death. Fenfluramine is a diet pill.

ANTIHISTAMINES.... MUSCLE RELAXANTS

RESULT: Drowsiness, dizziness, loss of muscle coordination and mental alertness, making it hazardous to drive or do other things requiring complete alertness; in severe cases, failure of blood circulation and breathing functions causing coma and death. Muscle relaxants are prescribed to provide relief for acute, painful musculo-skeletal conditions. Brand names of muscle relaxants:

Dantrium	Quinamm
Flexeril	Rela
Lioresal	Robaxin
Norflex	Robaxisal
Norgesic	Skelaxin
Norgesic Forte	Soma
Paraflex	Soma Compound
Parafon Forte	Valium

ANTIHISTAMINES....NARCOTICS

RESULT: Drowiness, dizziness, loss of muscle coordination and mental alertness, making it hazardous to drive or do other things requiring complete alertness; in severe cases, failure of blood circulation and breathing functions causing coma and death. Narcotics are used to relieve moderate to severe pain. Brand names of narcotics:

Codeine products:
Ascriptin w/Codeine, Bancap w/Codeine, Bufferin w/Codeine, Empirin w/Codeine, Empracet w/Codeine, Fiorinal w/Codeine, Phenaphen w/Codeine, Tylenol w/Codeine
Other narcotic or narcotic-like products:
Demerol, Dilaudid, Dolophene, morphine, Merpergan Fortis, Norcet, Numorphan, Percocet, Percodan, Synalgos-DC, Talwin, Talwin Compound, Tylox, Vicodan, Zactane, Zactirin

ANTIHISTAMINES....PROPOXYPHENE (Darvon, Darvocet-N, Dolene)

RESULT: Drowsiness, dizziness, loss of muscle coordination and mental alertness, making it hazardous to drive or do other things requiring complete alertness; in severe cases, failure of blood circulation and breathing functions causing coma and death. Propoxyphene is a pain reliever used to alleviate mild to moderate pain.

ANTIHISTAMINES....SLEEPING PILLS

RESULT: Drowsiness, dizziness, loss of muscle coordination and mental alertness, making it hazardous to drive or do other things requiring complete alertness; in severe cases, failure of blood circulation and breathing functions causing coma and death. Sleeping pills are prescribed for insomnia. The two types of sleeping pills are *barbiturates* and *non-barbiturates*. Brand names of sleeping pills:

Barbiturate Sleeping pills:
phenobarbital, Alurate, Amytal, Butisol, Buticap, Carbrital, Eskabarb, Lotusate, Luminal, Mebaral, Nembutal, Seconal, Sedadrops, Solfoton, Tuinal

Non-Barbiturate Sleeping pills (generic names in parentheses):
Ativan (lorazepam)—also used as a tranquilizer, Dalmane (flurazepam), Doriden (glutethimide), Halcion (triazolam), Noctec (chloral hydrate), Noludar (methyprylon), Parest (methaqualone), Placidyl (ethchlorvynol), Quaalude (methaqualone), Restoril (temazepam), Somnos (chloral hydrate), Triclos (triclofos), Valmid (ethinamate)

ANTIHISTAMINES....TRANQUILIZERS

RESULT: Drowsiness, dizziness, loss of muscle coordination and mental alertness, making it hazardous to drive or do other things requiring complete alertness; in severe cases, failure of blood circulation and breathing functions causing coma and death. Tranquilizers are prescribed to alleviate nervousness and anxiety. The two major types of tranquilizers are *benzodiazepines*—the most widely used—and *non-benzodiazepines*. Tranquilizer brand names (generic names in parentheses):

Benzodiazepine Tranquilizers:
Ativan (lorazepam)
Centrax (prazepam)
Dalmane (flurazepam)—prescribed as a sleeping pill
Halcion (triazolam)—prescribed as a sleeping pill
Librium (chlordiazepoxide)
Limbitrol (chlordiazepoxide/amitriptyline)—also used as an antidepressant
Paxipam (halazepam)
Restoril (temazepam)—prescribed as a sleeping pill

Serax (oxazepam)
SK-Lygen (chlordiazepoxide)
Tranxene (clorazepate)
Valium (diazepam)
Xanax (alprazolam)
Non-Benzodiazepine Tranquilizers:
Atarax (hydroxyzine)
Equanil (meprobamate)
meprobamate (various companies)
Meprospan (meprobamate)
Meprotab (meprobamate)
Miltown (meprobamate)
Trancopal (chlormezanone)
Tybatran (tybamate)
Vistaril (hydroxyzine)

4

Drug Interactions
in Arthritis Treatment

Arthritis is a disease causing inflammation of the joints. The two major types are called osteoarthritis and rheumatoid arthritis. *Osteoarthritis* or degenerative arthritis worsens with aging as bone cartilage wears down. Pain and inflammation are aggravated by weather changes and activity. The debilitating effects of *rheumatoid arthritis* can occur at any age, causing swollen, painful joints and eventually joint deformities.

Bursitis (pain and inflammation usually in the shoulder region) and soft tissue athletic injuries such as *strains* and *sprains* also go into this chapter since they are treated with the same drugs.

Drugs used in treatment alleviate the swelling, inflammation, and pain of arthritic conditions. The two major families of drugs used are *corticosteroids* and *non-corticosteroids* (also called nonsteroidal anti-inflammatory agents).

The *corticosteroids* cause significant and varied effects on the body. Because of their high potential for causing adverse side effects, physicians prescribe them mainly for short-term treatment of arthritic conditions, such as an acute flareup.

The *non-corticosteroids* are prescribed for both short-term treatment and long-term management of arthritic conditions. The exceptions are phenylbutazone (Azolid, Butazolidin) and oxyphenbutazone (Tandearil), which are prescribed only for short-term use because of their potential for causing adverse side effects. These drugs reduce joint swelling, pain, and morning stiffness. The most widely used drug in this family is common aspirin, which remains the drug of first choice.

CORTICOSTEROIDS:

Aristocort (triamcinolone)
Celestone (betamethasone)
Cortef (hydrocortisone)
Decadron (dexamethasone)
Delta-Cortef (prednisolone)
Deltasone (prednisone)
hydrocortisone (various
    companies)

Kenacort (triamcinolone)
Medrol (methylprednisolone)
Meticorten (prednisone)
Orasone (prednisone)
prednisone (various companies)

NON-CORTICOSTEROIDS:

Aspirin
    Anacin, Ascriptin, Aspergum, Bayer, Bufferin, CAMA, Eco-
    trin, Empirin, Measurin, Momentum, Pabirin, Persistin, St.
    Joseph Aspirin; other products containing aspirin-like in-
    gredients: Arthralgen, Arthropan, Calurin, Disalcid, Dol-
    obid, Magan, Mobidin, Pabalate, Salrin, Uracel, Uromide

Anaprox (naproxen)
Butazolidin (phenylbutazone)
Clinoril (sulindac)
Feldene (piroxicam)
Indocin (indomethacin)
Meclomen (meclofenamate)
Motrin (ibuprofen)
Nalfon (fenoprofen)
Naprosyn (naproxen)
Ponstel (mefenamic acid)
Rufen (ibuprofen)
Tandearil (oxyphenbutazone)
Tolectin (tolmetin)
Zomax (zomepirac)

I. CORTICOSTEROID FAMILY INTERACTIONS
(These apply to all the corticosteroid drugs)

CORTICOSTEROID....ACETAZOLAMIDE (Diamox)

THIS COMBINATION CAN CAUSE THE BODY TO
LOSE TOO MUCH POTASSIUM AND HOLD TOO MUCH
SODIUM. Report symptoms of potassium depletion: muscular
weakness or cramps, large urine output, bradycardia (slow heart
beat) or tachycardia (rapid heart beat), cardiac arrhythmias (heart

beat irregularities), low blood pressure with dizziness, faintness. Report symptoms of too much sodium: edema (excess body fluid), thirst, scant urine output, confusion, high blood pressure, hyperexcitability. Acetazolamide is used in glaucoma and certain seizure disorders.

CORTICOSTEROID....ANTACIDS (containing MAGNESIUM)

THIS COMBINATION CAN CAUSE THE BODY TO LOSE TOO MUCH POTASSIUM AND HOLD TOO MUCH SODIUM. Report symptoms of potassium depletion: muscular weakness or cramps, large urine output, bradycardia (slow heart beat) or tachycardia (rapid heart beat), cardiac arrhythmias (heart beat irregularities), low blood pressure with dizziness, faintness. Report symptoms of too much sodium: edema (excess body fluid), thirst, scant urine output, confusion, high blood pressure, hyperexcitability. Interacting antacid brand names:

Alkets	Kudrox
Aludrox	Maalox
BiSoDol	Magnatril
Camalox	Milk of Magnesia
Creamalin	Mylanta
Delcid	Riopan
Di-Gel	Silain-Gel
Gelusil	Simeco
Kolantyl	WinGel

CORTICOSTEROID....ANTICOAGULANT DRUGS

A. THE EFFECT OF THE ANTICOAGULANT MAY BE DECREASED. Anticoagulants are used to thin the blood and prevent it from clotting. RESULT: The blood may clot despite anit-clot treatment.

B. THIS COMBINATION PARADOXICALLY MAY CAUSE EXCESS BLEEDING. RESULT: Increased risk of hemorrhage. The most widely used anticoagulant drug is Coumadin. Anticoagulant drug brand names (generic names in parentheses):

Athrombin-K (warfarin)	Hedulin (phenindione)
Coufarin (warfarin)	Liquamar (phenprocoumon)
Coumadin (warfarin)	Miradon (anisindione)
dicumarol (various companies)	Panwarfin (warfarin)

CORTICOSTEROID....ASPIRIN

(Anacin, Ascriptin, Aspergum, Bayer, Bufferin, CAMA, Ecotrin, Empirin, Measurin, Momentum, Pabirin, Persistin, St. Joseph Aspirin)

THE EFFECT OF ASPIRIN MAY BE DECREASED. Aspirin is a salicylate pain reliever that also reduces fever and inflammation. It is a mainstay drug used in treating arthritic conditions. RESULT: The symptoms may not be controlled properly unless the dose of aspirin is raised to higher than normal levels. There is also an increased risk of stomach bleeding and ulceration with this combination. Brand names of salicylate-containing pain relievers interacting similarly to aspirin: Arthralgen, Arthropan, Calurin, Disalcid, Dolobid, Magan, Mobidin, Pabalate, Salrin, Uracel, Uromide. CAUTION: When the corticosteroid-type drug is stopped, the aspirin dose should be lowered to prevent aspirin toxicity. Note: Many other products contain aspirin—check product labels.

CORTICOSTEROID....BARBITURATES

(phenobarbital, Alurate, Amytal, Butisol, Buticap, Carbrital, Eskabarb, Lotusate, Luminal, Mebaral, Nembutal, Seconal, Sedadrops, Solfoton, Tuinal)

THE EFFECT OF THE CORTICOSTEROID DRUG MAY BE DECREASED. RESULT: The arthritic condition may require larger doses of corticosteroids. Barbiturates are used for sedation or as sleeping pills.

CORTICOSTEROID ....BIRTH CONTROL PILLS (oral contraceptives)

(Brevicon, Demulen, Enovid, Loestrin, Lo-Ovral, Micronor, Modicon, Nor-Q.D., Nordette, Norinyl, Norlestrin, Ortho-Novum, Ovcon, Ovral, Ovrette, Ovulen)

THE EFFECT OF THE CORTICOSTEROID DRUG MAY BE INCREASED. RESULT: Adverse side effects caused by too much corticosteroid drug. Report symptoms such as weight gain, swelling, excessive thirst and urination, decreased ability to fight infections, loss of energy, weakness.

CORTICOSTEROID....DIABETES DRUGS

THE EFFECT OF THE DIABETES DRUG MAY BE DE-CREASED. The diabetes drugs are used to lower the blood sugar level in diabetics. RESULT: The blood sugar level may remain too high. Diabetes drug brand names (generic names in parentheses):

Diabinese (chlorpropamide)
Dymelor (acetohexamide)
Orinase (tolbutamide)
Tolinase (tolazamide)
Insulin (injection)

CORTICOSTEROID....DIGITALIS

THE EFFECT OF DIGITALIS MAY BE INCREASED. Digitalis is used to treat congestive heart failure and to restore irregular heart beats to normal rhythm. RESULT: Possible heart irregularities from too much digitalis. Lanoxin is the most widely used digitalis drug. Digitalis brand names (generic names in parentheses):

Crystodigin (digitoxin)
Digifortis (digitalis)
Lanoxin (digoxin)
Purodigin (digitoxin)

CORTICOSTEROID....DIURETIC DRUGS

THIS COMBINATION CAN CAUSE THE BODY TO LOSE TOO MUCH POTASSIUM AND HOLD TOO MUCH SODIUM. Report symptoms of potassium depletion: muscular weakness or cramps, large urine output, bradycardia (slow heart beat) or tachycardia (rapid heart beat), cardiac arrhythmias (heart beat irregularities), low blood pressure with dizziness, faintness. Report symptoms of too much sodium: edema (excess body fluid), thirst, scant urine output, confusion, high blood pressure, hyper-excitability. The diuretic drugs remove excess body fluid and are used to treat high blood pressure and congestive heart failure. Those involved in this drug interaction are termed "potassium-losing" diuretics and the brand names (generic names in parentheses) are:

Anydron (cyclothiazide)
Aquatag (bezthiazide)
Aquatensin (methyclothiazide)
Diucardin (hydroflumethiazide)
Diulo (metolazone)
Diuril (chlorothiazine)
Edecrin (ethacrynic acid)
Enduron (methyclothiazide)
Esidrix (hydrochlorothiazide)
Exna (benzthiazide)
Hydrodiuril (hydrochlorothiazide)

Hydromox (quinethazone)
Hygroton (chlorthalidone)
Lasix (furosemide)
Metahydrin (trichlormethiazide)
Naqua (trichlormethiazide)
Naturetin (bendroflumethiazide)
Oretic (hydrochlorothiazide)
Renese (polythiazide)
Saluron (hydroflumethiazide)
Zaroxolyn (metolazone)

NOTE: The combination diuretic products listed below contain a "potassium-sparing" diuretic ingredient to offset the effect of the "potassium-losing" ingredient, so these products may not interact as significantly:

Aldactazide (hydrochlorothiazide/spironolactone)
Dyazide (hydrochlorothiazide/triamterene)
Moduretic (hydrochlorothiazide/amiloride)

CORTICOSTEROID
....ESTROGENS (female hormones)

(Amen, Aygestin, DES, Estinyl, Estrace, Estratab, Estrovis, Evex, Feminone, Menest, Menrium, Milprem, Norlutate, Norlutin, Ogen, PMB, Premarin, Provera, Tace)

THE EFFECT OF THE CORTICOSTEROID DRUG MAY BE INCREASED. RESULT: Adverse side effects caused by too much corticosteroid drug. Report symptoms such as weight gain, swelling, excessive thirst and urination, decreased ability to fight infections, loss of energy, weakness. Estrogens are prescribed for estrogen deficiency during menopause and after hysterectomy (surgical removal of the uterus), to prevent painful swelling of the breasts after pregnancy in women choosing not to nurse, and to treat amenorrhea (failure to menstruate).

CORTICOSTEROID....INDOMETHACIN (Indocin)

THE ADVERSE EFFECTS OF EACH DRUG MAY BE INCREASED. Both drugs are used to treat arthritic conditions. RESULT: Increased risk of stomach bleeding and ulceration. Report symptoms such as abdominal pain (especially after eating), black or tarry stools, unusual loss of energy.

CORTICOSTEROID....LAXATIVES

THIS COMBINATION CAN CAUSE THE BODY TO LOSE TOO MUCH POTASSIUM AND HOLD TOO MUCH SODIUM. Report symptoms of potassium depletion: muscular weakness or cramps, large urine output, bradycardia (slow heart beat) or tachycardia (rapid heart beat), cardiac arrhythmias (heart beat irregularities), low blood pressure with dizziness, faintness. Report symptoms of too much sodium: edema (excess body fluid), thirst, scant urine output, confusion, high blood pressure, hyperexcitability.

CORTICOSTEROID....LEVODOPA (Dopar, Larodopa, Sinemet)

THIS COMBINATION CAN CAUSE THE BODY TO LOSE TOO MUCH POTASSIUM AND HOLD TOO MUCH SODIUM. Report symptoms of potassium depletion: muscular weakness or cramps, large urine output, bradycardia (slow heart beat) or tachycardia (rapid heart beat), cardiac arrhythmias (heart beat irregularities), low blood pressure with dizziness, faintness. Report symptoms of too much sodium: edema (excess body fluid), thirst, scant urine output, confusion, high blood pressure, hyper-excitability. Levodopa is used to control the tremors of Parkinson's disease.

CORTICOSTEROID....PHENYTOIN (Dilantin)

THE EFFECT OF THE CORTICOSTEROID DRUG MAY BE DECREASED. RESULT: The arthritic condition may not be controlled properly. Phenytoin is used to control seizures in disorders such as epilepsy. Two other phenytoin-type drugs are Mesantoin (mephenytoin) and Peganone (ethotoin).

CORTICOSTEROID....PRIMIDONE (Mysoline)

THE EFFECT OF THE CORTICOSTEROID DRUG MAY BE DECREASED. RESULT: The arthritic condition may not be controlled properly. Primidone is used to control seizures in disorders such as epilepsy.

CORTICOSTEROID....RIFAMPIN (Rifadin, Rimactane)

THE EFFECT OF THE CORTICOSTEROID DRUG MAY BE DECREASED. RESULT: The arthritic condition may not be controlled properly. Rifampin is used in tuberculosis treatment and may be given to suspected meningitis carriers.

*CORTICOSTEROID....SMALLPOX VACCINE

THIS COMBINATION MAY CAUSE INCREASED SUS-CEPTIBILITY TO INFECTION due to suppression of the body's immune system. Serious and possibly fatal infections may result. This interaction may occur also with topical corticosteroid preparations. NONPRESCRIPTION CORTICOSTEROID TOPICAL PREPARATIONS (cream, ointment, spray): Caladryl Hydrocortisone, Caldecort, ClearAid, Clinicort, Cortaid, Cortizone-5, Dermolate, Lanacort). EXAMPLES OF PRESCRIPTION-ONLY CORTICOSTEROID TOPICAL PREPARATIONS (cream, ointment, spray): Aristocort, Cort-Dome, Hytone, Kenalog, Mycolog, Valisone.

II. NON-CORTICOSTEROID INTERACTIONS

A. NON-CORTICOSTEROID FAMILY INTERACTIONS
(These apply to all the non-corticosteroid drugs)

NON-CORTICOSTEROID....BETA BLOCKER HEART DRUGS

THE EFFECT OF THE BETA BLOCKER DRUG MAY BE DECREASED. Beta blockers are used to treat angina, irregular heart beats, and high blood pressure. RESULT: The conditions may not be controlled properly. Beta blocker brand names (generic names in parentheses):

    Blocadren (timolol)
    Corgard (nadolol)
    Inderal (propranolol)
    Lopressor (metoprolol)
    Tenormin (atenolol)
    Visken (pindolol)

NON-CORTICOSTEROID....DIURETIC DRUGS

THE EFFECT OF THE DIURETIC DRUG MAY BE DECREASED. The diuretics remove excess body fluid (edema) and are used to treat high blood pressure and congestive heart failure. RESULT: The condition treated may not be controlled properly. Diuretic brand names (generic names in parentheses):

Aldactazine (hydrochlorothiazide/
  spironolactone)
Anydron (cyclothiazide)
Aquatag (benzthiazide)
Aquatensin (methyclothiazide)
Diucardin (hydroflumethiazide)
Diulo (metolazone)
Diuril (chlorothiazide)
Dyazide (hydrochlorothiazide/
  triamterene)
Endecrin (ethacrynic acid)
Enduron (methyclothiazide)
Esidrix (hydrochlorothiazide)
Exna (benzthiazide)

Hydrodiuril (hydrochlorothiazide)
Hydromox (quinethazone)
Hygroton (chlorthalidone)
Lasix (furosemide)
Metahydrin (trichlormethiazide)
Moduretic (hydrochlorothiazide/
  amiloride)
Naqua (trichlormethiazide)
Naturetin (bendroflumethiazide)
Oretic (hydrochlorothiazide)
Renese (polythiazide)
Saluron (hydroflumethiazide)
Zaroxolyn (metolazone)

NON-CORTICOSTEROID....LITHIUM

(Eskalith, Lithane, Lithobid, Lithonate, Lithotab)

THE EFFECT OF LITHIUM MAY BE INCREASED. Lithium is an antipsychotic drug used to treat manic depressive disorders. RESULT: Possible adverse side effects from too much lithium. Report symptoms such as weakness, lethargy, dry mouth, loss of appetite, abdominal pain, dizziness, nausea, confusion, lack of muscle coordination, slurred speech.

B. INDIVIDUAL NON-CORTICOSTEROID DRUG INTERACTIONS
(These apply only to the specific non-corticosteroid drug listed)

ASPIRIN....ANTACIDS

THE EFFECTS OF ASPIRIN MAY BE DECREASED. Antacid brand names:

AlternaGel
Delcid
Di-Gel
Gelusil
Kudrox

Maalox
Mylanta
Riopan
WinGel

ASPIRIN....ANTICOAGULANT DRUGS

THE EFFECT OF THE ANTICOAGULANT MAY BE INCREASED. Anticoagulants are used to thin the blood and prevent it from clotting. RESULT: Increased risk of hemorrhage. Aspirin can cause stomach irritation/ulceration, which may be worsened by this drug interaction. Report symptoms such as black or tarry stools, bleeding or bruising, abdominal pain (especially after eating), unusual loss of energy. Coumadin is the most widely used anticoagulant drug. Anticoagulant drug brand names (generic names in parentheses):

Athrombin-K (warfarin)	Hedulin (phenindione)
Coufarin (warfarin)	Liquamar (phenprocoumon)
Coumadin (warfarin)	Miradon (anisindione)
dicumarol (various companies)	Panwarfin (warfarin)

ASPIRIN....CORTICOSTEROID DRUGS

THE EFFECT OF ASPIRIN MAY BE DECREASED. RESULT: The symptoms may not be controlled properly unless the dose of aspirin is raised to higher than normal levels. There is also an increased risk of stomach bleeding and ulceration with this combination. Corticosteroid brand names (generic names in parentheses):

Aristocort (triamcinolone)	Kenacort (triamcinolone)
Celestone (betamethasone)	Medrol (methylprednisolone)
Cortef (hydrocortisone)	Meticorten (prednisone)
Decadron (dexamethasone)	Orasone (prednisone)
Delta-Cortef (prednisolone)	prednisone (various companies)
Deltasone (prednisone)	
hydrocortisone (various companies)	

ASPIRIN....METHOTREXATE (Mexate)

THE EFFECT OF METHOTREXATE MAY BE INCREASED. Methotrexate is used in cancer treatment and for psoriasis. Possible adverse side effects from too much methotrexate. Report symptoms such as nausea, diarrhea, black or tarry stools, skin rash, mouth ulcers.

ASPIRIN....PROBENECID (Benemid, ColBenemid)

THE EFFECT OF PROBENECID MAY BE DECREASED. Probenecid is used to treat gout. RESULT: The condition may not be controlled properly, especially if aspirin is taken in the larger doses required for arthritic conditions.

ASPIRIN....SULFINPYRAZONE (Anturane)

THE EFFECT OF SULFINPYRAZONE MAY BE DE-CREASED. Sulfinpyrazone is used to treat gout. RESULT: The condition may not be controlled properly, especially if aspirin is taken in the larger doses required for arthritic conditions. There is also an increased risk of stomach irritation and bleeding. In addition, the aspirin blood level may increase to toxic concentrations causing *salicylism*. Report symptoms such as tinnitus (ringing in the ears), deafness, dizziness or nausea, restlessness, delirium, rapid breathing, burning sensations.

ASPIRIN....VITAMIN C

THE EFFECT OF VITAMIN C MAY BE DECREASED. Vitamin C prevents scurvy. RESULT: Vitamin C deficiency and symptoms of scurvy: bleeding gums, tongue sores, pain in muscles or joints, weight loss, lethargy. NOTE: High doses of vitamin C (over 2000 mg a day) can raise aspirin blood levels to toxic concentrations causing *salicylism*. Be alert for symptoms such as tinnitus (ringing in the ears), deafness, dizziness or nausea, restlessness, delirium, rapid breathing, burning sensations.

INDOMETHACIN (Indocin)....ANTICOAGULANT DRUGS

THE EFFECT OF THE ANTICOAGULANT MAY BE INCREASED. Anticoagulants are used to thin the blood and prevent it from clotting. RESULT: Increased risk of hemorrhage. Indomethacin can cause stomach irritation/ulceration, which may be worsened by this drug interaction. Report symptoms such as black or tarry stools, bleeding or bruising, abdominal pain, unusual loss of energy. Coumadin is the most widely used anticoagulant drug. Anticoagulant drug brand names (generic names in parentheses):

Athrombin-K (warfarin)	Hedulin (phenindione)
Coufarin (warfarin)	Liquamar (phenprocoumon)
Coumadin (warfarin)	Miradon (anisindione)
dicumarol (various companies)	Panwarfin (warfarin)

INDOMETHACIN (Indocin)....CORTICOSTEROIDS

THIS COMBINATION MAY CAUSE STOMACH UL-CERATION AND BLEEDING. Both these drugs are used to treat arthritic conditions. Report symptoms such as abdominal pain (especially after eating), black or tarry stools, unusual loss of energy.

INDOMETHACIN (Indocin)....PHENYLPROPANOLAMINE

THE EFFECT OF PHENYLPROPANOLAMINE MAY BE INCREASED. Phenylpropanolamine, a nasal decongestant, tends to raise the blood pressure. RESULT: The blood pressure may rise too high and cause headache and other adverse side effects. Phenylpropanolamine is the most widely used decongestant drug in cold and cold/cough products (see *Cold* chapter) and is the primary active ingredient in nonprescription weight loss products ("diet pills") because of its appetite suppression effect (see *Obesity* chapter). Read label list of ingredients to see whether the product contains phenylpropanolamine, often referred to as PPA.

INDOMETHACIN (Indocin)....PROBENECID (Benemid, ColBenemid)

THE EFFECT OF INDOMETHACIN MAY BE IN-CREASED. RESULT: Possible adverse side effects from too much indomethacin. Toxic symptoms include stomach irritation and bleeding, dizziness, headache, blurred vision, ringing in the ears (tinnitus), deafness, weakness, sore throat. Probenecid is used in gout treatment.

MEFENAMIC ACID (Ponstel)....ANTICOAGULANT DRUGS

THE EFFECT OF THE ANTICOAGULANT MAY BE INCREASED. Anticoagulants are used to thin the blood and prevent it from clotting. RESULT: Increased risk of hemorrhage. Mefenamic acid can cause stomach irritation/ulceration, which may be worsened by this drug interaction. Report symptoms such as black or tarry stools, bleeding or bruising, abdominal pain, unusual loss of energy. Coumadin is the most widely used anticoagulant drug. Anticoagulant drug brand names (generic names in parentheses):

Athrombin-K (warfarin)	Hedulin (phenindione)
Coufarin (warfarin)	Liquamar (phenprocoumon)
Coumadin (warfarin)	Miradon (anisindione)
dicumarol (various companies)	Panwarfin (warfarin)

*OXYPHENBUTAZONE (Tandearil)....ANTICOAGULANT DRUGS

THE EFFECT OF THE ANTICOAGULANT MAY BE INCREASED. Anticoagulants are used to thin the blood and prevent it from clotting. RESULT: Increased risk of hemorrhage; also increased risk of oxyphenbutazone-caused stomach bleeding and ulceration. This is a dangerous interaction and the physician should avoid prescribing this combination. Coumadin the is the most widely used anticoagulant drug. Anticoagulant drug brand names (generic names in parentheses):

Athrombin-K (warfarin)   Hedulin (phenindione)
Coufarin (warfarin)   Liquamar (phenprocoumon)
Coumadin (warfarin)   Miradon (anisindione)
dicumarol (various companies)   Panwarfin (warfarin)

OXYPHENBUTAZONE (Tandearil) ....DIABETES DRUGS

THE EFFECT OF THE DIABETES DRUG MAY BE INCREASED. Diabetes drugs lower the blood sugar level. RESULT: The blood sugar level may fall too low. Report symptoms such as dizziness, weakness, faintness, sweating, headache, confusion, visual disturbances, heart palpitations or tachycardia (rapid heart beat). Diabetes drug brand names (generic names in parentheses):

Diabinese (chlorpropamide)
Dymelor (acetohexamide)
Orinase (tolbutamide)
Tolinase (tolazamide)

OXYPHENBUTAZONE (Tandearil) ....METHANDROSTENOLONE (Dianabol)

THE EFFECT OF OXYPHENBUTAZONE MAY BE INCREASED. RESULT: Possible adverse side effects from too much oxyphenbutazone. Report symptoms such as swelling of feet or lower legs, weight gain, black or tarry stools, bruising or bleeding. Methandrostenolone is a male hormone.

OXYPHENBUTAZONE Tandearil)....PHENYTOIN(Dilantin)

THE EFFECT OF PHENYTOIN MAY BE INCREASED. Phenytoin is an anticonvulsant drug used to control seizures in epilepsy. RESULT: Increased risk of adverse side effects from too much phenytoin. Report symptoms such as dizziness, drowsiness, lack of muscle coordination, double vision or any other unusual visual disturbances. Two other phenytoin-type drugs are Mesantoin (mephenytoin) and Peganone (ethotoin).

*PHENYLBUTAZONE (Azolid, Butazolidin)
....ANTICOAGULANT DRUGS

THE EFFECT OF THE ANTICOAGULANT MAY BE INCREASED. Anticoagulants are used to thin the blood and prevent it from clotting. RESULT: Increased risk of hemorrhage; also increased risk of phenylbutazone-caused stomach bleeding and ulceration. This is a dangerous interaction and the physician should avoid prescribing this combination. Coumadin is the most widely used anticoagulant drug. Anticoagulant drug brand names (generic names in parentheses):

Athrombin-K (warfarin)	Hedulin (phenindione)
Coufarin (warfarin)	Liquamar (phenprocoumon)
Coumadin (warfarin)	Miradon (anisindione)
dicumarol (various companies)	Panwarfin (warfarin)

PHENYLBUTAZONE (Azolid, Butazolidin)
....DIABETES DRUGS

THE EFFECT OF THE DIABETES DRUG MAY BE INCREASED. Diabetes drugs lower the blood sugar level. RESULT: The blood sugar level may fall too low. Report symptoms such as dizziness, weakness, faintness, sweating, headache, confusion, visual disturbances, heart palpitations or tachycardia (rapid heart beat). Diabetes drug brand names (generic names in parentheses):

Diabinese (chlorpropamide)
Dymelor (acetohexamide)
Orinase (tolbutamide)
Tolinase (tolazamide)

PHENYLBUTAZONE (Azolid, Butazolidin)
....METHOTREXATE (Mexate)

THE EFFECT OF METHOTREXATE MAY BE INCREASED. Methotrexate is an antineoplastic drug used to treat cancer and psoriasis. RESULT: Possible adverse side effects from too much methotrexate. Report symptoms such as diarrhea, nausea, skin rash, skin and mouth ulcers, loss of hair.

PHENYLBUTAZONE (Azolid, Butazolidin)
....PHENYTOIN (Dilantin)

THE EFFECT OF PHENYTOIN MAY BE INCREASED. Phenytoin is an anticonvulsant drug used to control seizures in epilepsy. RESULT: Increased risk of adverse side effects from too much phenytoin. Report symptoms such as dizziness, drowsiness, lack of muscle coordination, double vision or any other unusual visual disturbances. Two other phenytoin-type drugs are Mesantoin (mephenytoin) and Peganone (ethotoin).

SULINDAC (Clinoril)....ANTICOAGULANT DRUGS

THE EFFECT OF THE ANTICOAGULANT MAY BE INCREASED. Anticoagulants are used to thin the blood and prevent it from clotting. RESULT: Increased risk of hemorrhage. Report symptoms such as black or tarry stools, bleeding or bruising, unusual loss of energy. Coumadin is the most widely used anticoagulant drug. Anticoagulant drug brand names (generic names in parentheses):

Athrombin-K (warfarin)	Hedulin (phenindione)
Coufrin (warfarin)	Liquamar (phenprocoumon)
Coumadin (warfarin)	Miradon (anisindione)
dicumarol (various companies)	Panwarfin (warfarin)

5

Asthma (Bronchial)

Bronchial asthma causes difficulty in breathing due to contriction of airways and bronchioles in the lungs. The asthmatic reaction, depending on the sufferer, may be associated with certain drugs, foods and food preservatives, stress, exercise, respiratory tract infections, or inhaled pollutants such as pollen, mold, or dust.

Three primary types of drugs are used to treat asthma: *Epinephrine Family* (albuterol, ephedrine, epinephrine, isoproterenol, metaproterenol, terbutaline); *Theophylline Family* (aminophylline, dyphylline, oxtriphylline, theophylline); and *Corticosteroid* products for inhalation (beclomethasone, dexamethasone). *Corticosteroid Oral* products (tablet, capsule, liquid) are listed in the *Arthritis* chapter.

Epinephrine and theophylline are bronchodilators which open up constricted air passages to allow easier breathing. Corticosteroids counter the allergic or inflammatory reaction causing the constricted air passages.

(NOTE: Many nonprescription asthma products contain antihistamines, ephedrine, and phenobarbital. For antihistamine interactions, see *Allergy* chapter, for phenobarbital interactions, see *Insomnia* chapter . Examples of nonprescription theophylline-ephedrine combination products, some of which also contain a small amount of phenobarbital, are: Bronitin, Bronkaid, Bronkotabs, Primatene M, Primatene P, Tedral.)

BRAND NAMES

I. EPINEPHRINE FAMILY PRODUCTS
(tablet, liquid, inhalant):

Aerolone (isoproterenol)   AsthmaNefrin (epinephrine)
Alupent (metaproterenol)   Brethine (terbutaline)

Bricanyl (terbutaline)
Bronitin (epinephrine)
Bronkaid (epinephrine)
Dispos-a-Med (isoproterenol)
Duo-Medihaler (isoproterenol)
Ephedrine (various companies)
Isuprel (isoproterenol)
Medihaler-Epi (epinephrine)

Medihaler-Iso (isoproterenol)
Metaprel (metaproterenol)
Norisodrine (isoproterenol)
Primatene (epinephrine)
Proventil (albuterol)
Vapo-Iso-Solution (isoproterenol)
Ventolin (albuterol)

II. THEOPHYLLINE FAMILY PRODUCTS
(tablet, capsule, liquid):

Accurbron (theophylline)
Bronkodyl (theophylline)
Choledyl (oxtriphylline)
Dilor (dyphylline)
Elixicon (theophylline)
Elixophyllin (theophylline)
LaBID (theophylline)
Lufyllin (dyphylline)
Quibron-T (theophylline)
Respbid (theophylline)
Slo-Phyllin (theophylline)
Somophyllin (aminophylline)

Somophyllin-T (theophylline)
Sustaire (theophylline)
Theobid (theophylline)
Theodur (theophylline)
Theolair (theophylline)
Theophyl (theophylline)
Theovent (theophylline)
   Multi-ingredient products
   containing theophylline:
   Amesec, Asbron G, Brondecon,
   Marax, Mudrane, Quibron,
   Tedral SA

III. CORTICOSTEROID FAMILY PRODUCTS FOR INHALATION:

Beclovent (beclomethasone)
Decadron Respihaler (dexamethasone)
Vanceril (beclomethasone)

NOTE: For interactions involving the corticosterid-type products your physician prescribes for asthma, see the *Arthritis* chapter—all *corticosteroid* interactions discussed there apply to these.

DRUG INTERACTIONS

The most commonly used drugs for asthma are those of the epinephrine and theophylline families. Both are central nervous system stimulants. Excessive stimulation can occur when an asthma drug of this type is taken with any other central nervous system stimulant. Therefore, in addition to the other interactions, be aware of this general interaction:

ASTHMA DRUG (EPINEPHRINE/THEOPHYLLINE)....
OTHER STIMULANT DRUGS

(This interaction applies to *all* the epinephrine and theophylline family drugs listed in the *Brand Names* section). RESULT: Excessive central nervous system stimulation with nervousness, agitation, tremors, tachycardia (rapid heart beat), heart palpitations, fever, loss of muscle coordination, rapid, shallow breathing, insomnia; in severe cases, a dangerous rise in blood pressure can occur, indicated by headache, visual disturbances, or confusion. The physician faced with this combination should monitor the patient carefully and adjust the dosages to minimize the additive stimulant effects. Here are the interacting stimulant categories and brand names:

AMPHETAMINES—Used as diet pills (this use is now in disfavor); for behavior problems in children; and for narcolepsy (uncontrollable desire to sleep). Brand names: Benzedrine, Biphetamine, Delcobese, Desoxyn, Dexedrine, Didrex, Obetrol.

ANTIDEPRESSANTS (MAOI type)—The MAOI antidepressants, prescribed for mental depression, are not used as much now that the safer cyclic antidepressants such as Elavil and Sinequan are available. Brand names of the MAOI type: Marplan, Nardil, Eutonyl, Parnate.

CAFFEINE—The stimulant in coffee, tea, cola beverages, in some nonprescription diet pills, products for cold and cough, pain, and menstrual discomfort.

COLD/COUGH PRODUCTS CONTAINING DECONGESTANT DRUGS—Decongestant drugs listed on nonprescription product labels (the same drugs are used in prescription-only products): (a) ORAL drugs (tablet, capsule, liquid)—ephedrine, methoxyphenamine, phenylephrine, phenylpropanolamine, pseudoephedrine; NASAL drugs (drops, spray, inhaler)—oxymetazoline, phenylephrine, propylhexedrine, xylometazoline

DEANOL (Deaner)—Used in hyperkinetic behavior and learning disorders.

DIET PILLS (nonprescription) containing phenylpropanolamine—Brand names: Anorexin, Appedrine, Appress, Ayds (capsule, droplets), Coffee-Break, Control, Dex-A-Diet II, Dexatrim, Diadax, Diet Gard, Dietac, E-Z Trim, P.P.A., P.V.M., Permathene-12, Pro Dax 21, Prolamine, Resolution, Super Odrinex, Ultra-Lean, Vita-Slim

DIET PILLS (prescription-only) containing non-amphetamines. Brand names: Adipex, Fastin, Ionamin, Mazanor, Melfiat, Plegine, Pre-Sate, Preludin, Sanorex, Tenuate, Tenuate Dospan, Tepanil, Tepanil Ten-Tab, Unifast, Voranil

METHYLPHENIDATE (Ritalin)—Used in hyperkinetic behavior and learning disorders in children; narcolepsy (uncontrollable desire to sleep); mild depression; apathetic or withdrawn senile behavior.

PEMOLINE (Cylert)—Used in hyperkinetic behavior and learning disorders in children.

PENTYLENETETRAZOL (Metrazol)—Used to enhance mental and physical activity in the elderly.

*EPINEPHRINE FAMILY
....ANTIDEPRESSANTS (CYCLIC TYPE)

THE EFFECT OF THE EPINEPHRINE-TYPE DRUG MAY BE INCREASED. RESULT: Possible cardiac arrhythmias (irregularities in heart beat) or dangerous increase in blood pressure. Report symptoms such as heart irregularities, headache, fever, visual disturbances. Antidepressants are used to alleviate mental depression and elevate the mood. NOTE: The antidepressant Desyrel (trazadone) may not interact. Antidepressant brand names (generic names in parentheses):

Adapin (doxepin)
Asendin (amoxapine)
Aventyl (nortriptyline)
Desyrel (trazadone)
Elavil (amitriptyline)
Endep (amitriptyline)
Etrafon (amitriptyline/
   perphenazine)
Limbitrol (amitriptyline/
   chlordiazepoxide)
Ludiomil (maprotiline)

Norpramin (desipramine)
Pamelor (nortriptyline)
Pertofrane (desipramine)
Sinequan (doxepin)
Surmontil (trimipramine)
Tofranil, Tofranil-PM
   (imipramine)
Triavil (amitriptyline/
   perphenazine)
Vivactil (protriptyline)

EPINEPHRINE....ANTIPSYCHOTIC DRUGS

THIS COMBINATION CAN CAUSE A DANGEROUS DROP IN BLOOD PRESSURE. RESULT: dizziness, weakness, faintness; possible seizures or shock. Antipsychotics or "major" tranquilizers are used to treat severe mental disorders such as schizophrenia. Most antipsychotics are of the phenothiazine family. Antipsychotic brand names (generic names in parentheses):

> PHENOTHIAZINES: Compazine (prochlorperazine), Mellaril (thioridazine), Proketazine (carphenazine), Prolixin (fluphenazine), Quide (piperacetazine), Serentil (mesoridazine), Sparine (promazine), Stelazine (trifluoperazine), Thorazine (chlorpromazine), Tindal (acetophenazine), Trilafon (perphenazine), Vesprin (triflupromazine)
> OTHERS: Haldol (haloperidol), Loxitane (loxapine), Moban (molindone), Navane (thiothixene), Taractan (chlorprothixene)

EPINEPHRINE FAMILY....BETA BLOCKER HEART DRUGS

THE EFFECT OF THE EPINEPHRINE-TYPE DRUG ON ASTHMA MAY BE ANTAGONIZED. RESULT: Lung bronchial tubes may not be opened enough to relieve the asthmatic episode. NOTE: Beta blocker drugs which minimally antagonize epinephrine's effect on the lungs are Lopressor (metoprolol) and Tenormin (atenolol). This combination can also cause a paradoxical dangerous increase in blood pressure with symptoms such as fever, headache, visual disturbances. Also, epinephrine antagonizes the effects of the beta blocker. Beta blockers are used to prevent angina, to restore irregular heart beats to normal rhythm, and to lower high blood pressure. Beta blocker brand names (generic names in parentheses):

> Blocadren (timolol)
> Corgard (nadolol)
> Inderal (propranolol)
> Lopressor (metoprolol)
> Tenormin (atenolol)
> Visken (pindolol)

EPINEPHRINE FAMILY....DIABETES DRUGS

THE EFFECT OF THE DIABETES DRUG MAY BE DECREASED. Diabetes drugs are used to lower the blood sugar level in diabetics. RESULT: The blood sugar level may remain too high. Report symptoms such as excessive thirst and hunger, unusually large urine output, drowsiness, fatigue, loss of coordination, weight loss. Diabetes drug brand names (generic names in parentheses):

Diabinese (chlorpropamide)
Dymelor (acetohexamide)
Orinase (tolbutamide)
Tolinase (tolazamide)
Insulin (several brands)

EPINEPHRINE FAMILY....DIGITALIS HEART DRUGS

THIS COMBINATION MAY OVERSTIMULATE THE HEART. Digitalis is used to treat congestive heart failure and to restore irregular heart beats to normal rhythm. RESULT: Possible cardiac arrhythmias (irregularities in heart beat). Digitalis brand names (generic names in parentheses):

Crystodigin (digitoxin)
Digifortis (digitalis)
Lanoxin (digoxin)
Purodigin (digitoxin)

EPINEPHRINE FAMILY....HIGH BLOOD PRESSURE DRUGS

THE EFFECT OF THE HIGH BLOOD PRESSURE DRUG MAY BE ANTAGONIZED. RESULT: The high blood pressure may not be controlled properly. Interacting high blood pressure drugs (brand names in parentheses):

captopril (Capoten)
clonidine (Catapres, Combipres)
guanabenz (Wytensin)
guanethidine (Esimil, Ismelin)
hydralazine (Apresazide, Apresoline-Esidrix, Apresoline, Dralserp, Dralzine, Ser-Ap-Es, Serpasil-Apresoline, Unipres)
methyldopa (Aldoclor, Aldomet, Aldoril)
minoxidil (Loniten)
reserpine-type drugs:
    deserpidine (Enduronyl, Harmonyl, Oreticyl)
    rauwolfia (Raudixin, Rauzide)
    reserpine (Diupres, Diutensen-R, Hydropres, Rau-Sed, Regroton, Renese-R, Reserpoid, Salutensin, Sandril, Ser-Ap-Es, Serpasil, Serpasil-Apresoline, Serpasil-Esidrix)

THEOPHYLLINE FAMILY....ALCOHOL (beer, liquor, wine, etc.)

THE EFFECT OF THE THEOPHYLLINE-TYPE DRUG MAY BE DECREASED. RESULT: The asthma may not be controlled properly. NOTE: The theophylline drug diphylline (Dilor, Lufyllin) may not interact.

THEOPHYLLINE FAMILY....ALLOPURINOL (Zyloprim)

THE EFFECT OF THE THEOPHYLLINE-TYPE DRUG MAY BE INCREASED. RESULT: Adverse side effects from too much theophylline. Report symptoms such as nausea, dizziness, headache, irritability, tremors, insomnia, tachycardia (rapid heart beat), cardiac arrhythmias (irregularities in heart beat); seizures may occur. NOTE: The theophylline drug diphylline (Dilor, Lufyllin) may not interact.

THEOPHYLLINE FAMILY....BARBITURATES

THE EFFECT OF THE THEOPHYLLINE-TYPE DRUG MAY BE DECREASED. RESULT: The asthma may not be controlled properly. NOTE: The theophylline drug diphylline (Dilor, Lufyllin) may not interact. Barbiturates are used as sedatives or sleeping pills. Barbiturate brand names:

phenobarbital	Luminal
Alurate	Mebaral
Amytal	Nembutal
Butisol	Seconal
Buticap	Sedadrops
Carbrital	Solfoton
Eskabarb	Tuinal
Lotusate	

THEOPHYLLINEE FAMILY....BETA BLOCKER HEART DRUGS

THE EFFECTS OF THE THEOPHYLLINE-TYPE DRUG ON ASTHMA MAY BE ANTAGONIZED. RESULT: Lung bronchial tubes may not be opened enough to relieve the asthmatic episode. NOTE: Beta blocker drugs which minimally antagonize theophylline's effect on the lungs are Lopressor (metoprolol) and

Tenormin (atenolol). Beta blocker drugs are used to prevent angina, to restore irregular heart beats to normal rhythm, and to lower high blood pressure. Beta blocker brand names (generic names in parentheses):

Blocadren (timolol)
Corgard (nadolol)
Inderal (propranolol)
Lopressor (metoprolol)
Tenormin (atenolol)
Visken (pindolol)

THEOPHYLLINE FAMILY....CIGARETTE SMOKING

THE EFFECT OF THEOPHYLLINE MAY BE DE-CREASED. RESULT: The asthma may not be controlled properly. Smokers may require an increase in theophylline dosage of 50% to 100%. A person stabilized on theophylline should not start or stop smoking without notifying the physician.

THEOPHYLLINE FAMILY....CIMETIDINE (Tagamet)

THE EFFECT OF THE THEOPHYLLINE-TYPE DRUG MAY BE INCREASED. RESULT: Adverse side effects from too much theophylline. Report symptoms such as nausea, dizziness, headache, irritabity, tremors, insomnia, tachycardia (rapid heart beat), cardiac arrhythmias (irregularities in heart beat); seizures may occur. NOTE: The theophylline drug diphylline (Dilor, Lufyllin) may not interact. Cimetidine is used to treat stomach and duodenal ulcers.

THEOPHYLLINE FAMILY
....ERYTHROMYCIN ANTIBIOTICS

THE EFFECT OF THE THEOPHYLLINE-TYPE DRUG MAY BE INCREASED. RESULT: Adverse side effects from too much theophylline. Report symptoms such as nausea, dizziness, headache, irritability, tremors, insomnia, tachycardia (rapid heart beat), cardiac arrhythmias (irregularities in heart beat); seizures may occur. NOTE: The theophylline drug diphylline (Dilor, Lufyllin) does not interact. Erythromycin is an antibiotic prescribed to combat infection. Erythromycin brand names:

Bristamycin   Ethril
E.E.S.   Ilosone
E-Mycin   Ilotycin
Ery-Tab   Pediamycin
Eryc   Robimycin
Erypar   Wyamycin S
EryPed

*THEOPHYLLINE FAMILY....INFLUENZA VACCINE

THE EFFECT OF THE THEOPHYLLINE-TYPE DRUG MAY BE INCREASED. RESULT: Adverse side effects from too much theophylline. Report symptoms such as nausea, dizziness, headache, irritability, tremors, insomnia, tachycardia (rapid heart beat), cardiac arrhythmias (irregularities in heart beat); seizures may occur. The physician should continue to monitor theophylline blood levels for several weeks after the flu shot, especially in the elderly. NOTE: The theophylline drug diphylline (Dilor, Lufyllin) may not interact.

THEOPHYLLINE FAMILY....LITHIUM (Eskalith, Lithane, Lithobid, Lithonate, Lithotab)

THE EFFECT OF LITHIUM MAY BE DECREASED. Lithium is an antipsychotic drug used to treat manic depressive disorders. RESULT: The condition treated may not be controlled properly.

THEOPHYLLINE FAMILY....PHENYTOIN (Dilantin)

THE EFFECT OF PHENYTOIN MAY BE DECREASED. Phenytoin is an anticonvulsant drug used to control seizures in disorders such as epilepsy. RESULT: The seizure disorder may not be controlled properly.

THEOPHYLLINE FAMILY....TRANQUILIZERS

THE EFFECT OF THE THEOPHYLLINE-TYPE DRUG MAY BE DECREASED. RESULT: The asthma may not be controlled properly. NOTE: The theophylline drug diphylline (Dilor, Lufyllin) may not interact. Tranquilizers are used to relieve nervousness and anxiety. The tranquilizers involved in this interaction belong to the benzodiazepine family. Tranquilizer brand names (generic names in parentheses):

Ativan (lorazepam)
Centrax (prazepam)
Dalmane (flurazepam)—
   prescribed as a sleeping pill
Halcion (triazolam)—prescribed
   as a sleeping pill
Librium (chlordiazepoxide)
Limbitrol (chlordiazepoxide/
   amitriptyline)

Paxipam (halezepam)
Restoril (temazepam)—prescribed
   as a sleeping pill
Serax (oxazepam)
SK-Lygen (chlordiazepoxide)
Tranxene (clorazepate)
Valium (diazepam)
Xanax (alprazolam).

THEOPHYLLINE FAMILY....TROLEANDOMYCIN (TAO)

THE EFFECT OF THE THEOPHYLLINE-TYPE DRUG MAY BE INCREASED. RESULT: Adverse side effects from too much theophylline. Report symptoms such as nausea, dizziness, headache, irritability, tremors, insomnia, tachycardia (rapid heart beat), cardiac arrhythmias (irregularities in heart beat); seizures may occur. NOTE: The theophylline drug diphylline (Dilor, Lufyllin) may not interact. Troleandomycin is an antibiotic used to combat infection.

6

Birth Control Pill
Drug Interactions

Ease, convenience, and effectiveness make the birth control pill the most popular contraceptive method. The "pill" works by preventing ovulation (release of an egg from the ovary).

BRAND NAMES

BIRTH CONTROL PILL (ORAL CONTRACEPTIVE) BRAND NAMES:

Brevicon	Nordette
Demulen	Norinyl
Enovid	Norlestrin
Loestrin	Ortho-Novum
Lo-Ovral	Ovcon
Micronor	Ovral
Modicon	Ovrette
Nor-Q.D.	Ovulen

Ever hear of women becoming pregnant even though they vow that they've never missed a pill? It could have been a result of a drug interaction which diminished the effectiveness of the birth control pill. The female hormones used in the pill have the potential to interact with a multitude of other drugs. The drug families that interact with birth control pills are: antibiotics, anticoagulants, anticonvulsants, antidepressants, barbiturates, corticosteroids, and tranquilizers. Other interactions, which are discussed following the drug family interactions, involve these individual drugs: caffeine, folic acid (vitamin B_9), pyridoxine (vitamin B_6), troleandomycin (TAO), and vitamin C.

DRUG INTERACTIONS

BIRTH CONTROL PILL....ANTIBIOTICS

THE EFFECT OF THE BIRTH CONTROL PILL MAY BE DECREASED. Antibiotics are prescribed to fight infection. The antibiotic types listed below either lessen the body's absorption of the birth control pill's hormonal ingredients or cause the body to eliminate the ingredients faster. RESULT: Increased risk of pregnancy unless an alternate method of contraception is used during the antibiotic treatment regimen. Breakthrough bleeding is a symptom of a possible interaction.

A. Penicillin-type Antibiotics

These are prescribed for upper respiratory tract (nose and throat) infections such as strep throat; ear infections; chronic bronchitis; pneumonia; urinary tract (bladder and kidney) infections; and gonorrhea. Penicillin brand names (generic names in parentheses):

Amcill (ampicillin)
amoxicillin (various companies)
Amoxil (amoxicillin)
ampicillin (various companies)
Betapen-VK (penicillin VK)
Cyclapen-W (cyclacillin)
Dynapen (dicloxacillin)
Geocillin (carbenicillin)
Larotid (amoxicillin)
Ledercillin VK (penicillin VK)
Nafcil (nafcillin)
Omnipen (ampicillin)
Pathocil (dicloxacillin)
Pen-Vee-K (penicillin VK)
Penapar VK (penicillin VK)
Penbritin (ampicillin)
penicillin VK (various companies)
Pensyn (ampicillin)
Pfizerpen A (ampicillin)

Pfizerpen VK (penicillin VK)
Polycillin (ampicillin)
Polymox (amoxicillin)
Principen (ampicillin)
Prostaphlin (oxacillin)
Robamox (amoxicillin)
Robicillin VK (penicillin VK)
Spectrobid (bacampicillin)
Supen (ampicillin)
Tegopen (cloxacillin)
Totacillin (ampicillin)
Trimox (amoxicillin)
Utimox (amoxicillin)
Unipen (nafcillin)
V-Cillin K (penicillin VK)
Veracillin (dicloxacillin)
Versapen (hetacillin)
Wymox (amoxicillin)

B. Tetracycline-type Antibiotics

These are prescribed for some of the same kinds of infections as penicillin and also for other infections such as cholera, Rocky

Mountain Spotted Fever, chancre sores, conjunctivitis of the eye, and intestinal amebiasis. Dermatologists often prescribe it for severe acne. Tetracycline brand names (generic names in parentheses):

Achromycin (tetracycline)   Rondomycin (methacycline)
Aureomycin (chlortetracycline)   Sumycin (tetracycline)
Bristacycline (tetracycline)   Terramycin (oxytetracycline)
Cyclopar (tetracycline)   Tetra-Bid (tetracycline)
Declomycin (demeclocycline)   Tetrachel (tetracycline)
Doxychel (doxycycline)   tetracycline (various companies)
Minocin (minocycline)   Tetracyn (tetracycline)
Panmycin (tetracycline)   Tetrex (tetracycline)
Retet-S (tetracycline)   Vibramycin (doxycycline)
Robitet (tetracycline)   Vibratab (doxycycline)

C. Sulfonamide-type Antibiotics

These are prescribed primarily for cystitis or urinary tract (bladder and kidney) infections. Sulfonamide brand names (generic names in parentheses):

Azulfidine (sulfasalazine)—   Renoquid (sulfacytine)
  prescribed for ulcerative colitis   SK-Soxazole (sulfisoxazole)
Bactrim (sulfamethoxazole)   Septra (sulfamethoxazole)
Bactrim DS (sulfamethoxazole/   Septra DS (sulfamethoxazole/
  trimethoprim)   trimethoprim)
Gantanol (sulfamethoxazole)   Sulla (sulfameter)
Gantrisin (sulfisoxazole)   Thiosulfil (sulfamethizole)

D. Individual Antibiotics

Chloramphenicol (Chloromycetin, Mychel) is an antibiotic prescribed only for serious infections for which less potentially dangerous antibiotics are ineffective.

Neomycin (Mycifradin, Neobiotic) is an antibiotic prescribed for certain types of diarrhea and other highly specific conditions.

Nitrofurantoin (Furadantin, Macrodantin) is an antibiotic prescribed for urinary tract (bladder and kidney) infections.

Rifampin (Rifadin, Rimactane) is a specialized antibiotic used to treat tuberculosis and may also be given to suspected meningitis carriers.

BIRTH CONTROL PILL....ANTICOAGULANT DRUGS

THE EFFECT OF THE ANTICOAGULANT DRUG MAY BE DECREASED. Anticoagulants are prescribed to thin the blood and prevent it from clotting. RESULT: The blood may clot despite anticoagulant treatment. Coumadin is the most widely used anticoagulant. Anticoagulant brand names (generic names in parentheses):

Athrombin-K (warfarin)
Coufarin (warfarin)
Coumadin (warfarin)
dicumarol (various companies)

Hedulin (phenindione)
Miradon (anisindione)
Panwarfin (warfarin)

BIRTH CONTROL PILL
....ANTICONVULSANT DRUGS

A. THE EFFECT OF THE BIRTH CONTROL PILL MAY BE DECREASED. RESULT: Approximately twenty-five times increased risk of pregnancy unless an alternate method of contraception is used. Breakthrough bleeding is a symptom of a possible interaction.

B. THE EFFECT OF THE ANTICONVULSANT MAY BE DECREASED. Anticonvulsants are prescribed to control seizures in disorders such as epilepsy. RESULT: The seizure disorder may not be controlled properly. Dilantin is the most widely used anticonvulsant. Anticonvulsant brand names (generic names in parentheses):

Depakene (valproic acid)
Dilantin (phenytoin)
Mesantoin (mephenytoin)
Mysoline (primidone)

Peganone (ethotoin)
Tegretol (carbamazepine)
Tridione (trimethadione)
Zarontin (ethosuximide)

BIRTH CONTROL PILL
....ANTIDEPRESSANTS (CYCLIC TYPE)

THE EFFECT OF THE ANTIDEPRESSANT DRUG MAY BE INCREASED OR DECREASED. Antidepressants are prescribed to alleviate mental depression and elevate the mood. RESULT: If increased antidepressant effect, possible adverse side effects caused by too much antidepressant drug. Report symptoms such as blurred vision, dry mouth, difficult urination, constipation, tachycardia (rapid heart beat), symptoms of toxic psychosis (agitation, disorientation, delirium), cardiac arrhythmias (heart beat irregularities), loss of coordination, possible convulsions. If decreased antidepressant effect, the depression may not be controlled properly. Elavil and Sinequan are the most frequently prescribed antidepressants. NOTE: The antidepressant trazadone (Desyrel) may not interact. Antidepressant brand names (generic names in parentheses):

Adapin (doxepin)

Asendin (amoxapine)

Aventyl (nortriptyline)

Desyrel (trazadone)

Elavil (amitriptyline)

Endep (amitriptyline)

Etrafon (amitriptyline/ perphenazine)—also a tranquilizer

Limbitrol (amitriptyline/ chlordiazepoxide)—also a tranquilizer

Ludiomil (maprotiline)

Norpramin (desipramine)

Pamelor (nortriptyline)

Pertofrane (desipramine)

Sinequan (doxepin)

Surmontil (trimipramine)

Tofranil, Tofranil-PM (imipramine)

Triavil (amitriptyline/ perphenazine)—also a tranquilizer

Vivactil (protriptyline)

BIRTH CONTROL PILL....BARBITURATES

THE EFFECT OF THE BIRTH CONTROL PILL MAY BE DECREASED. RESULT: Approximately twenty-five times increased risk of pregnancy unless an alternate method of contraception is used. Breakthrough bleeding is a symptom of a possible interaction. Barbiturates are prescribed as sedatives or as sleeping pills. Brand names of barbiturates:

phenobarbital

Alurate

Amytal

Butisol

Buticap

Carbrital

Eskabarb

Lotusate

Luminal

Mebaral

Nembutal

Seconal

Sedadrops

Solfoton

Tuinal

BIRTH CONTROL PILL....CORTICOSTEROIDS

THE EFFECT OF THE CORTICOSTEROID DRUG MAY BE INCREASED. Corticosteroids are prescribed for arthritis, severe allergies, asthma, endocrine disorders, leukemia, colitis, and enteritis (inflammation of the intestinal tract), and various skin, lung, and eye diseases. RESULT: Adverse side effects caused by too much corticosteroid drug. Report symptoms such as weight gain, swelling, excessive thirst and urination, internal pain, decreased ability to fight infections, unusual loss of energy. Corticosteroid brand names (generic names in parentheses):

Aristocort (triamcinolone)	Kenacort (triamcinolone)
Celestone (betamethasone)	Medrol (methylprednisolone)
Cortef (hydrocortisone)	Meticorten (prednisone)
Decadron (dexamethasone)	Orasone (prednisone)
Delta-Cortef (prednisolone)	prednisone (various companies)
Deltasone (prednisone)	
hydrocortisone (various companies)	

BIRTH CONTROL PILL....TRANQUILIZERS

A. THE EFFECT OF THE BIRTH CONTROL PILL MAY BE DECREASED. RESULT: Possible increased risk of pregnancy unless an alternate method of contraception is used. Breakthrough bleeding is a symptom of a possible interaction.

B. THE EFFECT OF CERTAIN TRANQUILIZERS MAY BE INCREASED (Librium, Limbitrol, SK-Lygen, Valium); THE EFFECT OF OTHER TRANQUILIZERS MAY BE DECREASED. (See following tranquilizer list.) Tranquilizers are prescribed to alleviate nervousness and anxiety. They may also be prescribed for insomnia. The tranquilizers involved in this interaction are of the benzodiazepine family. Valium is the most frequently used tranquilizer. Tranquilizer brand names (generic names in parentheses):

Ativan (lorazepam)	Paxipam (halazepam)
Centrax (prazepam)	Restoril (temazepam)—prescribed as a sleeping pill
Dalmane (flurazepam)—prescribed as a sleeping pill	Serax (oxazepam)
Halcion (triazolam)—prescribed as a sleeping pill	SK-Lygen (chlordiazepoxide)
Librium (chlordiazepoxide)	Tranxene (clorazepate)
Limbitrol (chlordiazepoxide/amitriptyline)—also an antidepressant	Valium (diazepam)
	Xanax (alprazolam)

OTHER BIRTH CONTROL PILL INTERACTIONS

BIRTH CONTROL PILL....CAFFEINE

THE EFFECT OF CAFFEINE MAY BE INCREASED. Caffeine is the stimulant found in coffee, tea, cola beverages, and in nonprescription diet pills, products for cold/cough, pain, and menstrual discomfort—read product label list of ingredients.

RESULT: Possible adverse side effects from "caffeinism." Symptoms are nervousness, agitation, irritability, insomnia, headache.

BIRTH CONTROL PILL....FOLIC ACID (Vitamin B₉)

THE EFFECT OF FOLIC ACID MAY BE DECREASED. Folic acid is one of the B-complex vitamins. RESULT: Possible folic acid deficiency. Be alert for symptoms such as loss of energy, uncommon memory lapses, pale complexion, nervousness and irritability, digestive tract symptoms. To counter the effects of this interaction, take a vitamin supplement containing folic acid or eat a fresh fruit and a green leafy vegetable daily.

BIRTH CONTROL PILL....PYRIDOXINE (Vitamin B₆)

THE EFFECT OF PYRIDOXINE MAY BE DECREASED. Pyridoxine is one of the B-complex vitamins. RESULT: Possible pyridoxine deficiency. Watch for symptoms such as numbness or tingling of the feet or lower legs, tenderness, weakness, skin lesions, anemia. To counter the effects of this interaction, take a vitamin supplement containing pyridoxine. Foods containing pyridoxine include whole grain cereals and legumes (peas, beans, etc.).

BIRTH CONTROL PILL....TROLEANDOMYCIN (TAO)

THIS COMBINATION CAN CAUSE CHOLESTATIC JAUNDICE. Jaundice symptoms include a yellow discoloration of the skin and eyes. Troleandomycin is an antibiotic. The physician should avoid prescribing this antibiotic to women taking birth control pills.

BIRTH CONTROL PILL....VITAMIN C

THE EFFECT OF THE BIRTH CONTROL PILL MAY BE INCREASED. If the vitamin is taken intermittently, the risk of pregnancy is increased during the time it is *not* taken due to a "rebound" effect from the lowering of the blood level of the birth control pill's hormonal ingredients. Breakthrough bleeding is a sign of a possible interaction. This interaction occurs with larger doses of vitamin C—1000 milligrams or more daily. Taking vitamin C in the 250-500 milligrams range will probably prevent this interaction.

7

Drug Interactions in the Prevention of Blood Clots

The leg veins are very susceptible to blood clots following surgery or a heart attack or during any extended period of inactivity such as recuperating in bed. The danger is that a leg clot will break free and move to the heart or lungs.

Anticoagulant drugs are prescribed to thin the blood and prevent it from clotting.

BRAND NAMES

ANTICOAGULANT DRUGS

Athrombin-K (warfarin)   Hedulin (phenindione)
Coufarin (warfarin)   Liquamar (phenprocoumon)
Coumadin (warfarin)   Miradon (anisindione)
dicumarol (various companies)   Panwarfin (warfarin)

The most widely used anticoagulant drug is warfarin in the Coumadin brand name.

The interactions are divided into two categories: drugs that *increase* the effect of the anticoagulant and drugs that *decrease* the effect of the anticoagulant.

ANTICOAGULANTS ARE SUBJECT TO MORE CLINICALLY SIGNIFICANT DRUG INTERACTIONS THAN ANY OTHER DRUG. For this reason, I've provided a quick brand name reference list of interacting drugs after each part of the *Drug Interactions* section.

DRUG INTERACTIONS

I. INTERACTIONS IN WHICH THE EFFECT OF THE ANTICOAGULANT MAY BE INCREASED

When prescribing any of the following drugs to a patient stabilized on anticoagulant therapy, the physician should monitor blood clotting time frequently, usually lowering the dosage of the anticoagulant when starting the other drug and raising it again after the patient finishes the other drug.

ANTICOAGULANT....ALLOPURINOL (Zyloprim)

THE EFFECT OF THE ANTICOAGULANT MAY BE INCREASED. RESULT: Increased risk of hemorrhage. Report symptoms such as bruising or bleeding anywhere on the body, black or tarry stools. Allopurinol is used to treat gout.

*ANTICOAGULANT....ASPIRIN

(Anacin, Ascriptin, Aspergum, Bayer, Bufferin, CAMA, Ecotrin, Empirin, Measurin, Momentum, Pabirin, Persistin, St. Joseph Aspirin)

THE EFFECT OF THE ANTICOAGULANT MAY BE INCREASED. RESULT: Increased risk of hemorrhage. Report symptoms such as bruising or bleeding anywhere on the body, black or tarry stools. Aspirin is used to alleviate mild to moderate pain in toothache and headache, and for arthritic and muscular aches and pain. Brand names of salicylate-containing pain relievers interacting similarly to aspirin:

Arthralgen	Mobidin
Arthropan	Pabalate
Calurin	Salrin
Disalcid	Uracel
Dolobid	Uromide
Magan	

ANTICOAGULANT....CHLORAL HYDRATE (Noctec, Somnos)

THE EFFECT OF THE ANTICOAGULANT MAY BE INCREASED. RESULT: Increased risk of hemorrhage. Report symptoms such as bruising or bleeding anywhere on the body, black or tarry stools. Chloral hydrate is a sleeping pill, used for insomnia.

ANTICOAGULANT....CHLORAMPHENICOL
(Chloromycetin, Mychel)

THE EFFECT OF THE ANTICOAGULANT MAY BE INCREASED. RESULT: Increased risk of hemorrhage. Report symptoms such as bruising or bleeding anywhere on the body, black or tarry stools. Chloramphenicol is an antibiotic prescribed for serious infections when less potentially dangerous antibiotics are ineffective.

ANTICOAGULANT....CIMETIDINE (Tagamet)

THE EFFECT OF THE ANTICOAGULANT MAY BE INCREASED. RESULT: Increased risk of hemorrhage. Report symptoms such as bruising or bleeding anywhere on the body,. black or tarry stools. Cimetidine is used to treat stomach and duodenal ulcers. NOTE: This interaction probably does not occur with the anticoagulant anisindione (Miradon) and phenindione (Hedulin).

*ANTICOAGULANT... .CLOFIBRATE (Atromid-S)

THE EFFECT OF THE ANTICOAGULANT MAY BE INCREASED. RESULT: Increased risk of hemorrhage. Report symptoms such as bruising or bleeding anywhere on the body, black or tarry stools. Clofibrate is prescribed to lower elevated blood cholesterol levels.

ANTICOAGULANT....DIABETES DRUGS

A. THE EFFECT OF THE ANTICOAGULANT MAY BE INCREASED. RESULT: Increased risk of hemorrhage. Report symptoms such as bruising or bleeding anywhere on the body, black or tarry stools.

B. THE EFFECT OF THE DIABETES DRUG MAY BE INCREASED. Diabetes drugs are used to lower the blood sugar level in diabetics. RESULT: The blood sugar level may fall too low. Report symptoms of hypoglycemia (low blood sugar): nervousness, faintness, weakness, sweating, confusion, cardiac arrhythmias (heart beat irregularities), tachyycardia (rapid heart beat), loss of coordination, visual disturbances. Diabetes drug brand names (generic names in parentheses):

Diabinese (chlorpropamide)
Dymelor (acetohexamide)
Orinase (tolbutamide)
Tolinase (tolazamide)

*ANTICOAGULANT....DISULFIRAM (Antabuse)

THE EFFECT OF THE ANTICOAGULANT MAY BE INCREASED. RESULT: Increased risk of hemorrhage. Report symptoms such as bruising or bleeding anywhere on the body, black or tarry stools. Disulfiram is prescribed in the treatment of alcoholism.

ANTICOAGULANT....ETHACRYNIC ACID (Edecrin)

THE EFFECT OF THE ANTICOAGULANT MAY BE INCREASED. RESULT: Increased risk of hemorrhage. Report symptoms such as bruising or bleeding anywhere on the body, black or tarry stools. Ethacrynic acid is a potent diuretic used to remove edema (excess body fluid) in the treatment of high blood pressure and congestive heart failure.

ANTICOAGULANT....INDOMETHACIN (Indocin)

THE EFFECT OF THE ANTICOAGULANT MAY BE INCREASED. RESULT: Increased risk of hemorrhage. Report symptoms such as bruising or bleeding anywhere on the body, black or tarry stools. Indomethacin is a non-corticosteroid agent used to relieve pain and inflammation in conditions such as arthritis.

ANTICOAGULANT....INFLUENZA VACCINE

THE EFFECT OF THE ANTICOAGULANT MAY BE INCREASED. RESULT: Increased risk of hemorrhage. Report symptoms such as bruising or bleeding anywhere on the body, black or tarry stools. NOTE: This interaction probably does not occur with the anticoagulants anisindione (Miradon) and phenindione (Hedulin).

*ANTICOAGULANT... .MALE HORMONES (androgens)

THE EFFECT OF THE ANTICOAGULANT MAY BE INCREASED. RESULT: Increased risk of hemorrhage. Report symptoms such as bruising or bleeding anywhere on the body, black or tarry stools. Male hormones are prescribed for osteoporosis (brittleness or softness of bones often seen in elderly or in debilitated patients); for some forms of anemia. Male hormone brand names (generic names in parentheses):

Adroyd (oxymetholone)
Anadrol (oxymetholone)
Anavar (oxandrolone)
Danocrine (danazol)
Dianabol (methandrostenolone)

Durabolin (nandrolone)
Maxibolin (ethylestrenol)
Nandrolin (nandrolone)
Winstrol (stanozolol)

ANTICOAGULANT....MEFENAMIC ACID (Ponstel)

THE EFFECT OF THE ANTICOAGULANT MAY BE INCREASED. RESULT: Increased risk of hemorrhage. Report symptoms such as bruising or bleeding anywhere on the body, black or tarry stools. Mefenamic acid is a non-corticosteroid pain reliever for short-term use.

ANTICOAGULANT....METHIMAZOLE (Tapazole)

THE EFFECT OF THE ANTICOAGULANT MAY BE INCREASED. RESULT: Increased risk of hemorrhage. Report symptoms such as bruising or bleeding anywhere on the body, black or tarry stools. Methimazole is prescribed for hyperthyroidism.

*ANTICOAGULANT....METRONIDAZOLE (Flagyl, Metryl, Satric)

THE EFFECT OF THE ANTICOAGULANT MAY BE INCREASED. RESULT: Increased risk of hemorrhage. Report symptoms such as bruising or bleeding anywhere on the body, black or tarry stools. Metronidazole is prescribed for vaginitis (trichomoniasis).

ANTICOAGULANT....NALIDIXIC ACID (NegGram)

THE EFFECT OF THE ANTICOAGULANT MAY BE INCREASED. RESULT: Increased risk of hemorrhage. Report symptoms such as bruising or bleeding anywhere on the body, black or tarry stools. Nalidixic acid is prescribed for cystitis or urinary tract (bladder, kidney) infections.

*ANTICOAGULANT....OXYPHENBUTAZONE (Tandearil)

THE EFFECT OF THE ANTICOAGULANT MAY BE INCREASED. RESULT: Increased risk of hemorrhage. Report symptoms such as bruising or bleeding anywhere on the body, black or tarry stools. Oxyphenbutazone is prescribed for short-term use in acute inflammatory conditions such as arthritis and bursitis.

*ANTICOAGULANT....PEPTO BISMOL

THE EFFECT OF THE ANTICOAGULANT MAY BE INCREASED. RESULT: Increased risk of hemorrhage. Report symptoms such as bruising or bleeding anywhere on the body, black or tarry stools. Pepto Bismol, used for diarrhea, contains a salicylate ingredient which interacts similarly to aspirin.

*ANTICOAGULANT....PHENYLBUTAZONE (Azolid A, Butazolidin)

THE EFFECT OF THE ANTICOAGULANT MAY BE INCREASED. RESULT: Increased risk of hemorrhage. Report symptoms such as bruising or bleeding anywhere on the body, black or tarry stools. Phenylbutazone is prescribed for short-term use in acute inflammatory conditions such as arthritis and bursitis.

ANTICOAGULANT....PROPYLTHIOURACIL (various companies)

THE EFFECT OF THE ANTICOAGULANT MAY BE INCREASED. RESULT: Increased risk of hemorrhage. Report symptoms such as bruising or bleeding anywhere on the body, black or tarry stools. Propylthiouracil is used to treat hyperthyroidism.

ANTICOAGULANT....QUINIDINE

THE EFFECT OF THE ANTICOAGULANT MAY BE INCREASED. RESULT: Increased risk of hemorrhage. Report symptoms such as bruising or bleeding anywhere on the body, black or tarry stools. Quinidine is used to restore irregular heart beats to normal rhythm. Quinidine brand names:

Cardioquin, Duraquin, Quinaglute Dura-Tabs, Quinidex Extentabs, Quinora.

ANTICOAGULANT....QUININE (Coco-Quinine, Quinamm, Quine)

THE EFFECT OF THE ANTICOAGULANT MAY BE INCREASED. RESULT: Increased risk of hemorrhage. Report symptoms such as bruising or bleeding anywhere on the body, black or tarry stools. Quinine is a nonprescription drug used for malaria and nighttime leg cramps.

*ANTICOAGULANT....SULFINPYRAZONE (Anturane)

THE EFFECT OF THE ANTICOAGULANT MAY BE INCREASED. RESULT: Increased risk of hemorrhage. Report symptoms such as bruising or bleeding anywhere on the body, black or tarry stools. Sulfinpyrazone is prescribed for gouty arthritis.

ANTICOAGULANT....SULINDAC (Clinoril)

THE EFFECT OF THE ANTICOAGULANT MAY BE INCREASED. RESULT: Increased risk of hemorrhage. Report symptoms such as bruising or bleeding anywhere on the body, black or tarry stools. Sulindac is a non-corticosteroid agent prescribed for arthritic conditions and for mild to moderate pain in general.

*ANTICOAGULANT....SULFONAMIDE ANTIBIOTICS

THE EFFECT OF THE ANTICOAGULANT MAY BE INCREASED. RESULT: Increased risk of hemorrhage. Report symptoms such as bruising or bleeding anywhere on the body, black or tarry stools. Sulfonamides are antibiotics prescribed to combat infection, especially cystitis or urinary tract (bladder and kidney) infections. Sulfonamide antibiotic brand names:

Azulfidine (sulfasalazine)—   Gantanol (sulfamethoxazole)
  prescribed for ulcerative colitis   Gantrisin (sulfisoxazole)
Bactrim (sulfamethoxazole)   Renoquid (sulfacytine)
Bactrim DS (sulfamethoxazole)   SK-Soxazole (sulfisoxazole)

Septra (sulfamethoxazole)   Sulla (sulfameter)
Septra DS (sulfamethoxazole)   Thiosulfil (sulfamethizole)

ANTICOAGULANT....TETRACYCLINE ANTIBIOTICS

THE EFFECT OF THE ANTICOAGULANT MAY BE INCREASED. RESULT: Increased risk of hemorrhage. Report symptoms such as bruising or bleeding anywhere on the body, black or tarry stools. Tetracycline is an antibiotic prescribed to combat infection. This interaction occurs primarily with doxycycline (Doxychel, Vibramycin, Vibratab), but can occur with other members of the tetracycline family in high doses of the tetracycline.

*ANTICOAGULANT....THYROID

THE EFFECT OF THE ANTICOAGULANT MAY BE INCREASED. RESULT: Increased risk of hemorrhage. Report symptoms such as bruising or bleeding anywhere on the body, black or tarry stools. This interaction occurs only in cases in which patients already stabilized on anticoagulants are given thyroid. If the patient has been taking thyroid before anticoagulant therapy is begun, this interaction has not been found to occur. Thyroid is prescribed to correct hypothyroidism (insufficient function of the thyroid gland) and goiter (enlargement of the thyroid gland). Thyroid brand names:

Armour Thyroid (thyroid)   Proloid (thyroglobulin)
Cytomel (liothyronine)   Synthroid (levothyroxine)
Euthroid (liotrix)   Thyrar (thyroid)
Levothroid (levothyroxine)   Thyrolar (liotrix).

QUICK REFERENCE LIST BY BRAND NAME OF PRODUCTS WHICH MAY INCREASE THE EFFECT OF ANTICOAGULANTS (generic names in parentheses):

*Adroyd (oxymetholone)   Arthralgen (salicylate)
*Anacin (aspirin)   *Arthropan (salicylate)
 Anadrol (oxymetholone)   *Ascriptin (aspirin)
 Anavar (oxandrolone)   *Aspergum (aspirin)
*Antabuse (disulfiram)   *aspirin
*Anturane (sulfinpyrazone)   *Atromid-S (clofibrate)
*Armour Thyroid (thyroid)   *Azolid (phenylbutazone)

*Azulfidine (sulfasalazine)
*Bactrim (sulfamethoxazole/
  trimethoprim)
*Bactrim DS (sulfamethoxazole/
  trimethoprim)
*Bayer (aspirin)
*Bufferin (aspirin)
*Butazolidin (phenylbutazone)
*Calurin (salicylate)
*CAMA (aspirin)
Chloromycetin
  (chloramphenicol)
Clinoril (sulindac)
*Cytomel (liothyronine)
*Danocrine (danazol)
*Dianabol (methandrostenolone)
*Disalcid (salicylate)
*Dolobid (salicylate)
Doxychel (doxycycline)
*Durabolin (nandrolone)
*Ecotrin (aspirin)
Edecrin (ethacrynic acid)
*Empirin (aspirin)
*Euthroid (liotrix)
*Flagyl (metronidazole)
*Gantanol (sulfamethoxazole)
*Gantrisin (sulfisoxazole)
Indocin (indomethacin)
influenza vaccine
*Levothroid (levothyroxine)
*Magan (salicylate)
*Maxibolin (ethylestrenol)
*Measurin (aspirin)
*Mobidin (salicylate)
*Momentum (aspirin)

Mychel (chloramphenicol)
*Nandrolin (nandrolone)
NegGram (nalidixic acid)
*Pabalate (salicylate)
*Pabirin (aspirin)
*Pepto Bismol
*Persistin (aspirin)
Ponstel (mefenamic acid)
*Proloid (thyroglobulin)
Propacil (propylthiouracil)
Propylthiouracil (various
  companies)
*Renoquid (sulfacytine)
*Salrin (salicylate)
*Septra (sulfamethoxazole/
  trimethoprim)
*Septra DS (sulfamethoxazole/
  trimethoprim)
*SK-Soxazole (sulfisoxazole)
*St. Joseph Aspirin
*Sulla (sulfameter)
*Synthroid (levothyroxine)
Tagamet (cimetidine)
*Tandearil (oxyphenbutazone)
Tapazole (methimazole)
*Thiosulfil (sulfamethizole)
*Thyrar (thyroid)
*thyroid (various companies)
*Thyrolar (liotrix)
*uracel (salicylate)
*Uromide (salicylate)
Vibramycin (doxycycline)
Vibratab (doxycycline)
*Winstrol (stanozolol)
Zyloprim (allopurinol).

II. INTERACTIONS IN WHICH THE EFFECT OF THE ANTICOAGULANT MAY BE DECREASED

When prescribing any of the following drugs to a patient stabilized on anticoagulant therapy, the physician should monitor blood clotting time frequently, usually raising the dosage of the anticoagulant when starting the other drug and lowering it again (to prevent hemorrhage) after the patient finishes the other drug.

ANTICOAGULANT....ALCOHOL (beer, liquor, wine, etc.)

THE EFFECT OF THE ANTICOAGULANT MAY BE DECREASED. RESULT: The blood may clot despite anticoagulant treatment.

*ANTICOAGULANT... .BARBITURATES

THE EFFECT OF THE ANTICOAGULANT MAY BE DECREASED. RESULT: The blood may clot despite anticoagulant treatment. Barbiturates are used as sedatives or sleeping pills. Brand names of barbiturates:

phenobarbital	Luminal
Alurate	Mebaral
Amytal	Nembutal
Butisol	Seconal
Buticap	Sedadrops
Carbrital	Solfoton
Eskabarb	Tuinal
Lotusate	

ANTICOAGULANT
....BIRTH CONTROL PILLS (oral contraceptives)

(Brevicon, Demulen, Enovid, Loestrin, Lo-Ovral, Micronor, Modicon, Nor-Q.D., Nordette, Norinyl, Norlestrin, Ortho-Novum, Ovcon, Ovral, Ovrette, Ovulen)

THE EFFECT OF THE ANTICOAGULANT MAY BE DECREASED. RESULT: The blood may clot despite anticoagulant treatment.

*ANTICOAGULANT... .CARBAMAZEPINE (Tegretol)

THE EFFECT OF THE ANTICOAGULANT MAY BE DECREASED. RESULT: The blood may clot despite anticoagulant treatment. Carbamazepine is used to control seizures in disorders such as epilepsy.

ANTICOAGULANT....CHOLESTYRAMINE (Cuemid, Questran)

THE EFFECT OF THE ANTICOAGULANT MAY BE DECREASED. RESULT: The blood may clot despite anticoagulant treatment. Cholestyramine is used in some patients with elevated cholesterol levels.

ANTICOAGULANT....CORTICOSTEROIDS:

THE EFFECT OF THE ANTICOAGULANT MAY BE DECREASED. RESULT: The blood may clot despite anticoagulant treatment. Corticosteroids are prescribed for arthritis, severe allergies, asthma, endocrine disorders, leukemia, colitis and enteritis (inflammation of the intestinal tract), and various skin, lung, and eye diseases. Corticosteroid brand names:

Aristocort (triamcinolone)
Celestone (betamethasone)
Cortef (hydrocortisone)
Decadron (dexamethasone)
Delta-Cortef (prednisolone)
Deltasone (prednisone)
hydrocortisone (various
  companies)

Kenacort (triamcinolone)
Medrol (methylprednisolone)
Meticorten (prednisone)
Orasone (prednisone)
prednisone (various companies).

ANTICOAGULANT....ESTROGENS (female hormones)

THE EFFECT OF THE ANTICOAGULANT MAY BE DECREASED. RESULT: The blood may clot despite anticoagulant treatment. Estrogen brand names:

Amen
Aygestin
DES
Estinyl
Estrace
Estratab
Estrovis
Evex
Feminone
Menest

Menrium
Milprem
Norlutate
Norlutin
Ogen
PMB
Premarin
Provera
Tace

ANTICOAGULANT....ETHCHLORVYNOL (Placidyl)

THE EFFECT OF THE ANTICOAGULANT MAY BE DECREASED. RESULT: The blood may clot despite anticoagulant treatment. Ethchlorvynol is used as a sleeping pill.

*ANTICOAGULANT....GLUTETHIMIDE (Doriden)

THE EFFECT OF THE ANTICOAGULANT MAY BE DECREASED. RESULT: The blood may clot despite anticoagulant treatment. Glutethimide is used as a sleeping pill.

*ANTICOAGULANT....GRISEOFULVIN

THE EFFECT OF THE ANTICOAGULANT MAY BE DECREASED. RESULT: The blood may clot despite anticoagulant treatment. Griseofulvin is given by mouth to combat a variety of fungal infections, especially ringworm of the nails. Griseofulvin brand names:

Fulvicin P/G
Fulvicin-U/F
Grifulvin V
Grisactin
Gris-PEG

*ANTICOAGULANT....PHENYTOIN (Dilantin)

A. THE EFFECT OF THE ANTICOAGULANT MAY BE DECREASED. RESULT: The blood may clot despite anticoagulant treatment. B. THE EFFECT OF PHENYTOIN MAY BE INCREASED. Phenytoin is used to control seizures in disorders such as epilepsy. RESULT: Possible adverse side effects from too much phenytoin. Report symptoms such as visual disturbances, loss of coordination. This interaction occurs primarily with the anticoagulant dicumarol. Other interacting phenytoin-like drugs are Mesantoin (mephenytoin) and Peganone (ethotoin).

*ANTICOAGULANT....PRIMIDONE (Mysoline)

THE EFFECT OF THE ANTICOAGULANT MAY BE DECREASED. RESULT: The blood may clot despite anticoagulant treatment. Primidone is used to control seizures in disorders such as epilepsy.

*ANTICOAGULANT....RIFAMPIN (Rifadin, Rifamate, Rimactane)

THE EFFECT OF THE ANTICOAGULANT MAY BE DECREASED. RESULT: The blood may clot despite anticoagulant treatment. Rifampin is used to treat tuberculosis and may be given to suspected meningitis carriers.

ANTICOAGULANT....VITAMIN K

THE EFFECT OF THE ANTICOAGULANT MAY BE DECREASED. RESULT: The blood may clot despite anticoagulant treatment. Vitamin K causes the blood to clot. Brand names of vitamin K:

AquaMEPHYTON
Konakion
Mephyton
Synkayvite.

QUICK REFERENCE LIST BY BRAND NAME OF PRODUCTS THAT MAY DECREASE THE EFFECT OF ANTICOAGULANTS (generic names in parentheses):

*Alurate (barbiturate)
Amen (estrogen)
*Amytal (barbiturate)
Aristocort (triamcinolone)
Aygestin (estrogen)
Birth control pills
Brevicon (birth control pill)
*Buticap (barbiturate)
*Butisol (barbiturate)
*Carbrital (barbiturate)
Celestone (betamethasone)
Cortef (hydrocortisone)
Cuemid (cholestyramine)
Decadron (dexamethasone)
Delta-Cortef (prednisolone)
Deltasone (prednisone)
DES (estrogen)
Demulen (birth control pill)
*Dilantin (phenytoin)
*Doriden (glutethimide)
Enovid (birth control pill)

*Eskabarb (barbiturate)
Estrace (estrogen)
Estratab (estrogen)
Estrovis (estrogen)
Evex (estrogen)
Feminone (estrogen)
*Fulvicin (griseofulvin)
*Grifulvin (griseofulvin)
*Grisactin (griseofulvin)
*Gris-Peg (griseofulvin)
hydrocortisone (various companies)
Kenacort (triamcinolone)
Loestrin (birth control pill)
Lo-Ovral (birth control pill)
*Lotusate (barbiturate)
*Luminal (barbiturate)
*Mebaral (barbiturate)
Medrol (methylprednisolone)
Menest (estrogen)
Menrium (estrogen)

Mephyton (vitamin K)
*Mesantoin (mephenytoin)
Meticorten (prednisone)
Micronor (birth control pill)
Milprem (estrogen)
Modicon (birth control pill)
*Mysoline (primidone)
*Nembutal (barbiturate)
Nor-Q.D. (birth control pill)
Nordette (birth control pill)
Norinyl (birth control pill)
Norlestrin (birth control pill)
Norlutate (estrogen)
Norlutin (estrogen)
Ogen (estrogen)
Orasone (prednisone)
Ortho-Novum (birth control pill)
Ovcon (birth control pill)
Ovral (birth control pill)
Ovrette (birth control pill)
Ovulen (birth control pill)

PMB (estrogen)
*Peganone (ethotoin)
*phenobarbital (various
  companies)
Placidyl (ethchlorvynol)
prednisone (various companies)
Premarin (estrogen)
Provera (estrogen)
Questran (cholestyramine)
*Rifadin (rifampin)
*Rifamate (rifampin)
*Rimactane (rifampin)
*Sedadrops (barbiturate)
*Seconal (barbiturate)
*Solfoton (barbiturate)
Synkayvite (vitamin K)
*Tegretol (carbamazepine)
Tace (estrogen)
*Tuinal (barbiturate)
vitamin K

8

Drug Interactions in Treatment of Cancer

A cancer or malignant tumor occurs when the growth of normal body cells goes wild, overrunning nearby normal cells. To complicate an already serious problem, a tumor may *metastasize,* or spread to other parts of the body. Heredity, environmental carcinogens, and viruses may all play a role in the development of this dreaded disease. Treatment, aimed at remission or cure, includes surgery, radiation, and chemical therapy.

The drugs used to treat cancer are called *antineoplastics.* Depending on the type of cancer, other drugs may also be used, including antibiotics, hormones, and corticosteroids. In this chapter the focus is on drug interactions of primary cancer drugs.

BRAND NAMES

CANCER DRUGS

Adriamycin (doxorubicin)
Adrucil (fluorouracil)
Alkeran (melphalan)
BCNU (carmustine)
Cosmegen (actinomycin)
Cytoxan (cyclophosphamide)
Efudex (fluorouracil)
Elspar (asparaginase)
Imuran (azathioprine)

Leukeran (chlorambacil)
Mexate (methotrexate)
Mutamycin (mitomycin)
Myleran (bisulfan)
Oncovin (vincristine)
Platinol (cisplatin)
Purinethol (mercaptopurine)
Velban (vinblastine)
5-FU (fluorouracil).

DRUG INTERACTIONS

I. CANCER DRUG FAMILY INTERACTIONS
(These apply to all the cancer drugs)

CANCER DRUG....CHLORAMPHENICOL (Chloromycetin, Mychel)

THIS COMBINATION MAY CAUSE INCREASED RISK OF BONE MARROW DEPRESSION. Chloramphenicol is an antibiotic used to combat infection. Symptoms include sore throat, fever, chills, bleeding anywhere on the body, black or tarry stools, fever, mouth sores, loss of energy.

*CANCER DRUG....SMALLPOX VACCINE (AND OTHER LIVE VACCINES)

THIS COMBINATION MAY CAUSE INCREASED SUS-CEPTIBILITY TO INFECTION by suppressing the body's immune system. Serious and possibly fatal infections can result.

II. INDIVIDUAL CANCER DRUG INTERACTIONS
(These apply only to the specific cancer drug listed)

*AZATHIOPRINE (Imuran)....ALLOPURINOL (Zyloprim)

THE EFFECT OF AZATHIOPRINE MAY BE IN-CREASED. RESULT: Possible adverse side effects from too much azathioprine. Report symptoms such as nausea, jaundice (yellow skin), sore throat, fever, chills, bleeding anywhere on the body, black or tarry stools, fever, mouth sores, loss of energy. Allopurinol is used to treat gout.

CISPLATIN (Platinol)
....AMINOGLYCOSIDE ANTIBIOTICS

THIS COMBINATION CAN CAUSE HEARING LOSS AND KIDNEY DAMAGE. RESULT: These adverse effects may be permanent. Report symptoms such as nausea, hearing loss, dizziness, vertigo, tinnitus (ringing in the ears); excessive thirst, marked decrease in urine output, loss of appetite, shortness of breath, weakness, drowsiness. Aminoglycosides are specialized antibiotics used to combat certain types of infections. Aminoglycoside brand names (generic names in parentheses):

Kantrex (kanamycin)
Klebcil (kanamycin)
Mycifradin (neomycin)
neomycin (various companies)

CYCLOPHOSPHAMIDE (Cytoxan)....ALLOPURINOL (Zyloprim)

THE EFFECT OF CYCLOPHOSPHAMIDE MAY BE IN-CREASED. RESULT: Adverse side effects from too much cyclophosphamide. Report symptoms such as nausea, loss of hair, pain or frequency of urination; sore throat, fever, chills, bleeding anywhere on the body, black or tarry stools, fever, mouth sores, loss of energy. Allopurinol is used to treat gout.

MERCAPTOPURINE (Purinethol)....ALLOPURINOL (Zyloprim)

THE EFFECT OF MERCAPTOPURINE MAY BE IN-CREASED. RESULT: Adverse side effects from too much mercaptopurine. Report symptoms such as nausea, jaundice (yellow skin), sore throat, fever, chills, bleeding anywhere on the body, black or tarry stools, fever, mouth sores, loss of energy. Allopurinol is used to treat gout.

MERCAPTOPURINE (Purinethol)....DISULFIRAM (Antabuse)

THIS COMBINATION MAY CAUSE LIVER DAMAGE. Report symptoms such as fever, headache, weakness, malaise, loss of appetite, jaundice (yellow skin). Disulfiram is used in alcoholism treatment.

*METHOTREXATE (Mexate)....ASPIRIN

(Anacin, Ascriptin, Aspergum, Bayer, Bufferin, CAMA, Ecotrin, Empirin, Measurin, Momentum, Pabirin, Persistin, St. Joseph Aspirin)

THE EFFECT OF METHOTREXATE MAY BE IN-CREASED. RESULT: Adverse side effects from too much methotrexate. Symptoms include nausea, bleeding anywhere on the body, black or tarry stools, diarrhea, skin rash, skin or mouth ulcers, hair loss, sore throat, fever, chills, loss of energy.

Brand names of salicylate-containing pain relievers interacting similarly to aspirin: Arthralgen, Arthropan, Calurin, Disalcid, Dolobid, Magan, Mobidin, Pabalate, Salrin, Uracel, Uromide.

METHOTREXATE (Mexate)....PEPTO BISMOL

(Contains aspirin-like salicylate)

THE EFFECT OF METHOTREXATE MAY BE INCREASED. RESULT: Adverse side effects from too much methotrexate. Symptoms include nausea, bleeding anywhere on the body, black or tarry stools, diarrhea, skin rash, skin or mouth ulcers, hair loss, sore throat, fever, chills, loss of energy.

METHOTREXATE (Mexate)....PHENYLBUTAZONE (Butazolidin)

THE EFFECT OF METHOTREXATE MAY BE INCREASED. RESULT: Adverse side effects from too much methotrexate. Symptoms include nausea, bleeding anywhere on the body, black or tarry stools, diarrhea, skin rash, skin or mouth ulcers, hair loss, sore throat, fever, chills, loss of energy. Phenylbutazone is used to treat acute inflammatory conditions such as arthritis, bursitis, and muscle sprains.

METHOTREXATE (Mexate)....PROBENECID (Benemid, ColBenemid)

THE EFFECT OF METHOTREXATE MAY BE INCREASED. RESULT: Adverse side effects from too much methotrexate. Symptoms include nausea, bleeding anywhere on the body, black or tarry stools, diarrhea, skin rash, skin or mouth ulcers, hair loss, sore throat, fever, chills, loss of energy. Probenecid is used to treat gout.

METHOTREXATE (Mexate) ....SULFONAMIDE ANTIBIOTICS

THE EFFECT OF METHOTREXATE MAY BE INCREASED. RESULT: Adverse side effects from too much methotrexate. Symptoms include nausea, bleeding anywhere on the body, black or tarry stools, diarrhea, skin rash, skin or mouth ulcers, hair loss, sore throat, fever, chills, loss of energy. Sulfonamides are antibiotics used to combat infections, especially urinary tract infections. Sulfonamide brand names (generic names in parenthesis):

Azulfidine (sulfasalazine)—
  prescribed for ulcerative colitis
Bactrim (sulfamethoxazole)
Bactrim DS (sulfamethoxazole)
Gantanol (sulfamethoxazole)
Gantrisin (sulfisoxazole)

Renoquid (sulfacytine)
SK-Soxazole (sulfisoxazole)
Septra (sulfamethoxazole)
Septra DS (sulfamethoxazole)
Sulla (sulfameter)
Thiosulfil (sulfamethizole)

9

Drug Interactions in the Treatment of Cold and Cough

The most widespread human ailment is the common cold, which hits each person an average of twice a year. Most colds are contracted during times of temperature change—in early fall, just after midwinter, and in early spring.

The vast majority of colds are caused by viruses—called rhinoviruses and coronaviruses. These viruses are spread through the air by sneezing and coughing or by physical contact.

The onset of a cold is abrupt. Initial symptoms may be a dry, itchy throat and nose, headache or body aches, or a cough. Children usually have a fever. Secretions increase, the nose runs and becomes congested, the eyes water, and nasal irritation causes sneezing. Prompting these symptoms is a substance called *histamine,* which the body releases in response to viral invasion.

Currently there is no cure for the cold. Interferon holds some promise due to its antiviral activity.

The body's natural defenses will restore normalcy within a few days. Sufferers desiring relief in the meantime can choose from products containing two types of drugs: *decongestants* and *antihistamines.*

Decongestants reverse nasal congestion by shrinking swollen blood vessels in the nasal mucosa, allowing easier breathing and better nasal and sinus drainage.

Antihistamines have a drying effect, which counters symptoms caused by hypersecretion, such as runny nose and watery, itchy eyes. The earlier an antihistamine is taken during a cold, the more effective it is.

DECONGESTANT DRUGS

ORAL:
  ephedrine
  methoxyphenamine
  phenylephrine
  phenylpropanolamine
  pseudoephedrine
NASAL SPRAY, DROPS, INHALER:
  oxymetazoline
  phenylephrine
  propylhexedrine
  xylometazoline

ANTIHISTAMINES

azatadine
bromodiphenhydramine
brompheniramine
carbinoxamine
chlorpheniramine
clemastine
cyproheptadine
dexbrompheniramine
dexchlorpheniramine
dimethidene
doxylamine

methapyrilene
phenindamine
pheniramine
phenyltoloxamine
pyrilamine
pyrrobutamine
thenyldiamine
thenylpyramine
tripelennamine
triprolidine

BRAND NAMES

There are dozens of products—both prescription and non-prescription—used to alleviate symptoms of the common cold. *All* of them contain decongestants and/or antihistamines. No attempt is made in this chapter to comprehensively list product names as in the other chapters—the modern consumer is pretty much familiar with them. Besides, nonprescription product labels list ingredients on the label. Use the list of decongestants and antihistamines provided to determine whether a particular product has a decongestant or antihistamine or a combination of both (most are combination products). Many also contain either aspirin or acetaminophen (the ingredient in Tylenol and other "non-aspirin" pain relievers); be sure and consult the *Pain* chapter for interactions involving these two auxiliary ingredients. A few remedies contain caffeine. If you take a prescription-only medication, chances are you know whether it is prescribed for your cold symptoms. Ask your pharmacist what ingredients it contains.

Multi-ingredient products are the rule rather than the exception. Many nonprescription products you might think are only for cold symptoms also contain the cough ingredient dextromethorphan, so read product labels carefully and consult the *Cough* section for interactions involving it.

Be aware that nasal sprays, drops, and inhalers contain decongestants that can be absorbed systemically—and therefore can become involved in drug interactions just as the oral tablets, capsules, and liquids can.

REPRESENTATIVE PRODUCTS FOR COLD

NONPRESCRIPTION

Antihistamine only:
  Chlor-Trimeton
  Coricidin
  Dimetane
  Teldrin
Decongestant only:
  Afrinol
  Novafed
  Ornex
  Sudafed
  Sine-Aid
Decongestant/Antihistamine combination:
  Actifed
  Chlor-Trimeton Decongestant
  Contac
  Demazin
  Drixoral
  Novafed A
  Triaminic syrup
  Trind syrup
Nasal spray, drops, inhaler (decongestant only):
  Afrin
  Duration
  Neo-Synephrine
  Sine-Off
  Sinex

PRESCRIPTION-ONLY

(Some of these may become nonprescription):

Deconamine
Dimetapp
Entex
Naldecon
Ornade

DRUG INTERACTIONS

I. DECONGESTANT DRUG INTERACTIONS

Decongestants are central nervous system stimulants. Excessive stimulation can occur when a decongestant drug is taken with any other central nervous system stimulant. Therefore, in addition to the other decongestant drug interactions, be aware of this general interaction:

DECONGESTANT....OTHER STIMULANT DRUGS

RESULT: Excessive central nervous system stimulants with nervousness, agitation, tremors, tachycardia (rapid heart beat), heart palpitations, fever, loss of muscle coordination, rapid, shallow breathing, insomnia; in severe cases, a dangerous rise in blood pressure can occur, indicated by headache, visual disturbances, or confusion. The physician faced with this combination should monitor the patient carefully and adjust the dosages to minimize the excessive stimulant effects. Interacting stimulant categories and brand names:

AMPHETAMINES—Used as diet pills (this use is now in disfavor); for behavior problems in children; and for narcolepsy (uncontrollable desire to sleep). Brand names: Benzedrine, Biphetamine, Delcobese, Desoxyn, Dexedrine, Didrex, Obetrol.

ANTIDEPRESSANTS (MAOI type)—The MAOI antidepressants, prescribed for mental depression, are not used as much now that the safer tricyclic antidepressants such as Elavil and Sinequan are available. Brand names of the MAOI type: Marplan, Nardil, Eutonyl, Parnate

ASTHMA DRUGS (EPINEPHRINE FAMILY)—Used to open air passages and make breathing easier in asthmatics. Brand names: Aerolone, Alupent, AsthmaNefrin, Brethine, Bricanyl, Bronitin,

Bronkaid, Dispos-a-Med, Duo-Medihaler, Ephedrine, Isuprel, Medihaler-Epi, Medihaler-Iso, Metaprel, Norisodrine, Primatene Proventil, Vapo-Iso-Solution, Ventolin

ASTHMA DRUGS (THEOPHYLLINE FAMILY)—Used to open air passages and make breathing easier in asthmatics. Brand names: Accurbron, Amesec, Asbron G, Brondecon, Bronkodyl, Choledyl, Dilor, Elixicon, Elixophyllin, LaBID, Lufyllin, Marax, Mudrane, Quibron, Quibron-T, Quinamm, Respbid, Slo-Phyllin, Somophyllin, Somophyllin-T, Sustaire, Tedral SA, Theobid, Theodur, Theolair, Theophyl, Theovent

CAFFEINE—The stimulant in coffee, tea, cola beverages, in some nonprescription diet pills, products for cold/cough, pain, and menstrual discomfort.

DEANOL (Deaner)—Used in hyperkinetic behavior and learning disorders.

DIET PILLS (nonprescription) containing phenylpropanolamine—Brand names: Anorexin, Appedrine, Appress, Ayds (capsule, droplets), Coffee-Break, Control, Dex-A-Diet II, Dexatrim, Diadax, Diet Gard, Dietac, E-Z Trim, P.P.A., P.V.M., Permathene-12, Pro Dax 21, Prolamine, Resolution, Super Odrinex, Ultra-Lean, Vita-Slim

DIET PILLS (prescription-only) containing non-amphetamines—Brand names: Adipex, Fastin, Ionamin, Mazanor, Melfiat, Plegine, Pre-Sate, Preludin, Sanorex, Tenuate, Tenuate Dospan, Tepanil, Tepanil Ten-Tab, Unifast, Voranil

METHYLPHENIDATE (Ritalin)—used in hyperkinetic behavior and learning disorders in children; narcolepsy (uncontrollable desire to sleep); mild depression; apathetic or withdrawn senile behavior.

PEMOLINE (Cylert)—Used in hyperkinetic learning and behavior disorders in children.

PENTYLENETETRAZOL (Metrazol)—used to enhance mental and physical activity in the elderly.

DECONGESTANT....ANTIDEPRESSANTS (CYCLIC TYPE)

THE ADVERSE SIDE EFFECTS OF EACH DRUG MAY BE INCREASED. RESULT: Possible cardiac arrhythmias (heart beat irregularities) or a dangerous rise in blood pressure. Report heart irregularities, fever, headache, visual disturbances. NOTE: Pseudoephedrine is a decongestant which does not interact. The antidepressant Desyrel (trazadone) may not interact. Antidepressant drugs are used to alleviate mental depression and elevate the mood. Antidepressant brand names (generic names in parentheses):

Adapin (doxepin)
Asendin (amoxapine)
Aventyl (nortriptyline)
Desyrel (trazadone)
Elavil (amitriptyline)
Endep (amitriptyline)
Etrafon (amitriptyline/
  perphenazine)
Limbitrol (amitriptyline/
  chlordiazepoxide)
Ludiomil (maprotiline)

Norpramin (desipramine)
Pamelor (nortriptyline)
Pertofrane (desipramine)
Sinequan (doxepin)
Surmontil (trimipramine)
Tofranil, Tofranil-PM
  (imipramine)
Triavil (amitriptyline/
  perphenazine)
Vivactil (protriptyline)

DECONGESTANT....DIABETES DRUGS

THE EFFECT OF THE DIABETES DRUG MAY BE ANTAGONIZED. Diabetes drugs are used to lower the blood sugar level in diabetics. RESULT: The blood sugar level may remain too high. Report symptoms such as excessive thirst and hunger, unusually large urine output, drowsiness, fatigue, loss of coordination, weight loss. Diabetes drug brand names (generic names in parentheses):

Diabinese (chlorpropamide)
Dymelor (acetohexamide)
Orinase (tolbutamide)
Tolinase (tolazamide)
Insulin (several brands)

DECONGESTANT....BETA BLOCKER HEART DRUGS

THE EFFECT OF THE BETA BLOCKER MAY BE ANTAGONIZED. Beta blockers are used to prevent angina, to restore irregular heart beats to normal rhythm, and to lower blood pressure. RESULT: The conditions may not be controlled properly. This combination can also cause a paradoxical dangerous rise in blood pressure with symptoms such as fever, headache, visual disturbances. Beta blocker brand names:

Blocadren (timolol)
Corgard (nadolol)
Inderal (propranolol)
Lopressor (metoprolol)

Tenormin (atenolol)
Visken (pindolol)

DECONGESTANT....DIGITALIS HEART DRUGS

THIS COMBINATION MAY OVERSTIMULATE THE HEART. Digitalis is used to treat congestive heart failure and to restore irregular heart beats to normal rhythm. RESULT: Possible cardiac arrhythmias (heart beat irrgularities). Digitalis brand names (generic names in parentheses):

Crystodigin (digitoxin)
Digifortis (digitalis)
Lanoxin (digoxin)
Purodigin (digitoxin)

DECONGESTANT....HIGH BLOOD PRESSURE DRUGS

THE EFFECT OF THE HIGH BLOOD PRESSURE DRUG MAY BE ANTAGONIZED. RESULT: The high blood pressure may not be controlled properly. The high blood pressure drug guanethidine can sometimes cause a paradoxical dangerous rise in blood pressure with symptoms such as fever, headache, visual disturbances. High blood pressure drugs (brand names in parentheses):

captopril (Capoten)
clonidine (Catapres, Combipres)
guanabenz (Wytensin)
guanethidine (Esimil, Ismelin)
hydralazine (Apresazide, Apresoline-Esidrix, Apresoline, Dralserp, Dralzine, Ser-Ap-Es, Serpasil-Apresoline, Unipres)
methyldopa (Aldoclor, Aldomet, Aldoril)
minoxidil (Loniten)
reserpine-type drugs:
  rauwolfia (Raudixin, Rauzide)
  deserpidine (Enduronyl, Harmonyl, Oreticyl)
  reserpine (Diupres, Diutensen-R, Hydropres, Rau-Sed, Regroton, Renese-R, Reserpoid, Salutensin, Sandril, Ser-Ap-Es, Serpasil, Serpasil-Apresoline, Serpasil-Esidrix)

DECONGESTANT....INDOMETHACIN (Indocin)

THIS COMBINATION CAN CAUSE THE BLOOD PRESSURE TO RISE TOO HIGH. Report symptoms such as headache, visual disturbances. Indomethacin is used to alleviate pain and inflammation in arthritic conditions.

II. ANTIHISTAMINE DRUG INTERACTIONS

Antihistamines are central nervous system depressants. They depress or impair functions such as coordination and alertness. Excessive depression and impairment can occur when an antihistamine is taken with any other central system depressant as shown by the following interactions:

ANTIHISTAMINES....ALCOHOL (beer, liquor, wine—all alcoholic drinks)

RESULT: Drowsiness, dizziness, loss of muscle coordination and mental alertness making it hazardous to drive or do other things requiring complete alertness; in severe cases, failure of blood circulation and breathing functions causing coma and death.

ANTIHISTAMINES....ANTICHOLINERGIC DRUGS

A. THIS COMBINATION MAY CAUSE EXCESSIVE "ANTICHOLINERGIC" SIDE EFFECTS. RESULT: Blurred vision, dry mouth, constipation, heart palpitations, slurred speech, difficulty in urination, stomach irritation, possible toxic psychosis (agitation, disorientation, delirium).

B. SOME ANTICHOLINERGIC DRUGS CAN CAUSE EXCESSIVE DEPRESSANT SIDE EFFECTS. RESULT: Drowsiness, dizziness, loss of muscle coordination and mental alertness, making it hazardous to drive or do other activities requiring complete alertness; in severe cases, failure of blood circulation and breathing functions causing coma and death. The anticholinergic products causing this interaction include Akineton, Artane, Cogentin, Kemadrin, Norflex, Pagitane, Robinul, and Transderm-Scop. Brand names and uses of anticholinergic drugs (generic names in parentheses):

> Used to control tremors resulting from Parkinson's disease or from treatment with antipsychotic drugs.
> Akineton (biperiden)
> Artane (trihexyphenidyl)
> Cogentin (benztropine)

Kemadrin (procyclidine)
Pagitane (cycrimine)
Used in stomach, digestive tract disorders.
Bentyl (dicyclomine)
Combid (isopropamide)
Probanthine (propantheline)
Robinul (glycopyrrolate)
Others.
Norflex (orphenadrine)—Used as a muscle relaxant. Transderm-Scop (scopolamine)—A small disc attached behind the ear for motion sickness.

ANTIHISTAMINES....ANTICONVULSANT DRUGS

RESULT: Drowsiness, dizziness, loss of muscle coordination and mental alertness, making it hazardous to drive or do other things requiring complete alertness; in severe cases, failure of blood circulation and breathing functions causing coma and death. Anticonvulsant drugs are used to control seizures in disorders such as epilepsy. Anticonvulsant drug brand names (generic names in parentheses):

Depakene (valproic acid)
Dilantin (phenytoin)
Mesantoin (mephenytoin)
Mysoline (primidone)

Peganone (ethotoin)
Tegretol (carbamazepine)
Tridione (trimethadione)
Zarontin (ethosuximide)

ANTIHISTAMINES
....ANTIDEPRESSANTS (CYCLIC TYPE)

RESULT: Drowsiness, dizziness, loss of muscle coordination and mental alertness, making it hazardous to drive or do other activities requiring complete alertness; in severe cases, failure of blood circulation and breathing functions causing coma and death. Antidepressants are used to alleviate mental depression and elevate the mood. Antidepressant brand names (generic names in parentheses):

Adapin (doxepin)
Asendin (amoxapine)
Aventyl (nortriptyline)
Desyrel (trazadone)
Elavil (amitriptyline)

Endep (amitriptyline)
Etrafon (amitriptyline/
  perphenazine)
Limbitrol (amitriptyline/
  chlordiazepoxide)

Ludiomil (maprotiline)
Norpramin (desipramine)
Pamelor (nortriptyline)
Pertofrane (desipramine)
Sinequan (doxepin)
Surmontil (trimipramine)

Tofranil, Tofranil-PM
  (imipramine)
Triavil (amitriptyline/
  perphenazine)
Vivactil (protriptyline)

ANTIHISTAMINES....ANTIPSYCHOTIC DRUGS

RESULT: Drowsiness, dizziness, loss of muscle coordination and mental alertness, making it hazardous to drive or do other activities requiring complete alertness; in severe cases, failure of blood circulation and breathing functions causing coma and death. The antipsychotic drugs are used to treat mental disorders. These drugs are sometimes referred to as "major" tranquilizers, as opposed to "minor" tranquilizers such as Valium. Most of these agents are of the phenothiazine drug family. Antipsychotic brand names (generic names in parentheses):

PHENOTHIAZINE TYPE:
  Compazine (prochlorperazine)
  Mellaril (thioridazine)
  Proketazine (carphenazine)
  Prolixin (fluphenazine)
  Quide (piperacetazine)
  Serentil (mesoridazine)
  Sparine (promazine)
  Stelazine (trifluoperazine)
  Thorazine (chlorpromazine)
  Tindal (acetophenazine)
  Trilafon (perphenazine)
  Vesprin (triflupromazine)
OTHERS:
  Haldol (haloperidol)
  Loxitane (loxapine)
  Moban (molindone)
  Navane (thiothixene)
  Taractan (chlorprothixene).

ANTIHISTAMINES....HIGH BLOOD PRESSURE DRUGS

(only the nerve blockers clonidine, guanabenz, methyldopa, reserpine)

RESULT: Drowsiness, dizziness, loss of muscle coordination and mental alertness, making it hazardous to drive or do other things requiring complete alertness; in severe cases, failure of blood circulation and breathing functions causing coma and death. High blood pressure drugs are used to lower the blood pressure. Interacting high blood pressure drugs (brand names in parentheses):

clonidine (Catapres, Combipres)
guanabenz (Wytensin)
methyldopa (Aldoclor, Aldomet, Aldoril)
reserpine-type drugs:
 rauwolfia (Raudixin, Rauzide)
 deserpidine (Enduronyl, Harmonyl, Oreticyl)
 reserpine (Diupres, Diutensen-R, Hydropres, Rau-Sed, Regroton, Renese-R, Reserpoid, Salutensin, Sandril, Ser-Ap-Es, Serpasil, Serpasil-Apresoline, Serpasil-Esidrix)

ANTIHISTAMINES....FENFLURAMINE (Pondimin)

RESULT: Drowsiness, dizziness, loss of muscle coordination and mental alertness, making it hazardous to drive or do other activities requiring complete alertness; in severe cases, failure of blood circulation and breathing functions causing coma and death. Fenfluramine is a diet pill.

ANTIHISTAMINES....MUSCLE RELAXANTS

RESULT: Drowsiness, dizziness, loss of muscle coordination and mental alertness, making it hazardous to drive or do other things requiring complete alertness; in severe cases, failure of blood circulation and breathing functions causing coma and death. Muscle relaxants are prescribed to provide relief for acute, painful musculo-skeletal conditions. Brand names of muscle relaxants:

Dantrium	Quinamm
Flexeril	Rela
Lioresal	Robaxin
Norflex	Robaxisal
Norgesic	Skelaxin
Norgesic Forte	Soma
Paraflex	Soma Compound
Parafon Forte	Valium

ANTIHISTAMINES....NARCOTICS

RESULT: Drowsiness, dizziness, loss of muscle coordination and mental alertness, making it hazardous to drive or do other activities requiring complete alertness; in severe cases, failure of blood circulation and breathing functions causing coma and death. Narcotics are used to relieve moderate to severe pain. Brand names of narcotics:

Codeine products:
Ascriptin w/Codeine, Bancap w/Coedine, Bufferin w/Codeine, Empirin w/Codeine, Empracet w/Codeine, Fiorinal w/Codeine, Phenaphen w/Codeine, Tylenol w/Codeine
Other narcotic or narcotic-like products:
Demerol, Dilaudid, Dolophene, morphine, Merpergan Fortis, Norcet, Numorphan, Percocet, Percodan, Synalgos-DC, Talwin, Talwin Compound, Tylox, Vicodan, Zactane, Zactirin

ANTIHISTAMINES....PROPOXYPHENE (Darvon, Darvocet-N, Dolene)

RESULT: Drowsiness, dizziness, loss of muscle coordination and mental alertness, making it hazardous to drive or do other things requiring complete alertness; in severe cases, failure of blood circulation and breathing functions causing coma and death. Propoxyphene is a pain reliever used to alleviate mild to moderate pain.

ANTIHISTAMINES....SLEEPING PILLS

RESULT: Drowsiness, dizziness, loss of muscle coordination and mental alertness, making it hazardous to drive or do other activities requiring complete alertness; in severe cases, failure of blood circulation and breathing functions causing coma and death. Sleeping pills are prescribed for insomnia. The two types of sleeping pills are *barbiturates* and *non-barbiturates*. Brand names of sleeping pills:

BARBITURATE sleeping pills:
phenobarbital, Alurate, Amytal, Butisol, Buticap, Carbrital, Eskabarb, Lotusate, Luminal, Mebaral, Nembutal, Seconal, Sedadrops, Solfoton, Tuinal
NON-BARBITURATE sleeping pills (generic names in parentheses):

Ativan (lorazepam)—also a tranquilizer, Dalmane (flurazepam),Doriden (glutethimide), Halcion (triazolam), Noctec (chloral hydrate), Noludar (methyprylon), Parest (methaqualone), Placidyl (ethchlorvynol), Quaalude (methaqualone), Restoril (temazepam), Somnos (chloral hydrate), Triclos (triclofos), Valmid (ethinamate)

ANTIHISTAMINES....TRANQUILIZERS

RESULT: Drowsiness, dizziness, loss of muscle coordination and mental alertness, making it hazardous to drive or do other activities requiring complete alertness; in severe cases, failure of blood circulation and breathing functions causing coma and death. Tranquilizers are used to alleviate nervousness or anxiety. The two major types of tranquilizers are *benzodiazepines*—the most widely used—and *non-benzodiazepines*. Tranquilizer brand names (generic names in parentheses):

BENZODIAZEPINE tranquilizers:
    Ativan (lorazepam)
    Centrax (prazepam)
    Dalmane (flurazepam)—prescribed as a sleeping pill
    Halcion (triazolam)—prescribed as a sleeping pill
    Librium (chlordiazepoxide)
    Limbitrol (chlordiazepoxide/amitriptyline)—also an
        antidepressant
    Paxipam (halazepam)
    Restoril (temazepam)—prescribed as a sleeping pill
    Serax (oxazepam)
    SK-Lygen (chlordiazepoxide)
    Tranxene (chlorazepate)
    Valium (diazepam)
    Xanax (alprazolam)
NON-BENZODIAZEPINE tranquilizers:
    Atarax (hydroxyzine)
    Equanil (meprobamate)
    meprobamate (various companies)
    Meprospan (meprobamate)
    Meprotab (meprobamate)
    Miltown (meprobamate)
    Trancopal (chlormezanone)
    Tybatran (tybamate)
    Vistaril (hydroxyzine)

Cough Products

The cough is an essential reflex that clears the throat and bronchial passages of phlegm, which often accumulates during a cold. A productive cough is beneficial in that it causes expectoration (spitting up of mucus and phlegm). A nonproductive cough is bothersome and can further irritate the air passages. This second type of cough is treated with antitussives—cough preparations.

The two kinds of cough ingredients are called *expectorants* and *cough suppressants.*

Expectorants thin or liquefy phlegm in the throat and bronchial passages, thereby easing the irritation causing the cough. The expectorant used most often in cough products is guaifenesin. The expectorant for which we have a documented drug interaction is potassium iodide.

Cough suppressants act directly on the "cough center" in the brain to depress the cough reflex. Codeine and dextromethorphan are the cough suppressants used in cough preparations. Codeine is an addictive narcotic, and cough syrups containing it can be purchased only after signing your name in a narcotics registry book. Dextromethorphan is the cough suppressant used in off-the-shelf nonprescription cough products. The antihistamine diphenhydramine (Benadryl, Benylin) is now approved for use as a cough suppressant; see the antihistamine interactions in the *Cold* section.

DRUG INTERACTIONS

CODEINE....DIGOXIN

THE EFFECT OF DIGOXIN IS INCREASED. Digoxin is used to treat congestive heart failure or to restore irregular heart beats to normal rhythm. RESULT: Possible adverse side effects from too much digoxin. Report symptoms such as irregularities in heart beat, nausea, visual disturbances, headache, loss of appetite, loss of energy. This interaction occurs only with slowly dissolving digoxin products, not with the Lanoxin brand.

DEXTROMETHORPHAN....ANTIDEPRESSANTS (MAOI TYPE)

THIS COMBINATION MAY CAUSE LOW BLOOD PRESSURE, NAUSEA, FEVER, AND COMA. Antidepressants are used to alleviate mental depression and to elevate the mood. MAOI antidepressants are not used much now that the safer tricyclic antidepressants such as Elavil and Sinequan are available. MAOI antidepressant brand names:

   Eutonyl
   Marplan
   Nardil
   Parnate

POTASSIUM IODIDE....LITHIUM

   (Eskalith, Lithane, Lithobid, Lithonate, Lithotab)

   THIS COMBINATION MAY CAUSE HYPOTHYROID-ISM. RESULT: Insufficient function of the thyroid gland. Lithium is an antipsychotic drug used to treat certain severe mental disorders. POTASSIUM IODIDE brand names:

   Iodo-Niacin
   Pima
   SSKI (saturated solution of potassium iodide)

10

Drug Interactions in Treatment of Depression

Millions of people suffer from the debilitating effects of mental depression. "Mental" is a misnomer, really, as we are coming more and more to realize the likelihood of biological causes or predispositions—physical or chemical—for many so-called emotional and mental disorders.

Sufferers of depressive illness have feelings—beyond their conscious control—of hopelessness, worthlessness, and despair.

The most successful treatment has been with the use of antidepressant drugs. These drugs are believed to work by increasing the amounts of brain neurotransmitter chemicals such as serotonin or norepinephrine, and in many cases they alleviate the adverse symptoms of depression.

The two general types of antidepressant drugs are tricyclic antidepressants and MAOI (monoamine oxidase inhibitor) antidepressants. The tricyclic type are the most widely used because they are safer and less apt to cause adverse side effects. Ludiomil (maprotiline) is actually a "tetracyclic" antidepressant, but has similar side effects and interacts the same as the tricyclic drugs. Desyrel (trazadone), the newest development, is not a "cyclic" agent at all, and supposedly has fewer adverse side effects and less potential for interaction than the other types of antidepressants.

PART I—ANTIDEPRESSANTS (CYCLIC TYPE)

BRAND NAMES

Adapin (doxepin)
Asendin (amoxapine))

Aventyl (nortriptyline)
Elavil (amitriptyline)

Endep (amitriptyline)
Etrafon (amitriptyline/
   perphenazine)
Limbitrol (amitriptyline/
   chlordiazepoxide)
Ludiomil (maprotiline)
Norpramin (desipramine)
Pamelor (nortriptyline)
Pertofrane (desipramine)

Sinequan (doxepin)
Surmontil (trimipramine)
Tofranil, Tofranil-PM
   (imipramine)
Triavil (amitriptyline/
   perphenazine)
Vivactil (protriptyline)
   Other: Desyrel (trazadone)

DRUG INTERACTIONS
ANTIDEPRESSANT....OTHER DEPRESSANT DRUGS

The cyclic antidepressants and trazadone (Desyrel) are central nervous system depressants. They depress or impair functions such as coordination and alertness. Excessive *physical* depression or impairment can occur when an antidepressant is taken with any other central nervous system depressant. NOTE: This is the only documented antidepressant interaction also involving trazadone (Desyrel). RESULT: Drowsiness, dizziness, loss of muscle coordination and mental alertness; in severe cases, failure of blood circulation and breathing functions causing coma and death. The physician should monitor the patient carefully and adjust the dosages to minimize the excessive depressant effects. Interacting depressant categories and brand names:

ALCOHOL (beer, liquor, wine, etc.)
ANTIHISTAMINES (Used for allergies, colds). Brand names:
   Actidil, Antivert, Atarax, Benadryl, Bendectin, Bonine, Chlor-
   Trimeton, Clistin, Decapryn, Dimetane, Dramamine, Histadyl,
   Inhiston, Marezine, Optimine, PBZ, Periactin, Polaramine,
   Pyronil, Tavist, Teldrin, Triten, Vistaril
ANTIPSYCHOTICS (Used for severe mental disorders).
   Antipsychotic brand names: Compazine, Haldol, Loxitane,
   Mellaril, Moban, Navane, Proketazine, Prolixin, Quide, Serentil,
   Sparine, Stelazine, Taractan, Thorazine, Tindal, Trilafon,
   Vesprin
HIGH BLOOD PRESSURE DRUGS—brand names in
parentheses:
   clonidine (Catapres, Combipres)
   guanabenz (Wytensin)
   methyldopa (Aldoclor, Aldomet, Aldoril)
   reserpine-type drugs:

deserpidine (Enduronyl, Harmonyl, Oreticyl)
rauwolfia (Raudixin, Rauzide)
reserpine (Diupres, Diutensen-R, Hydropres, Rau-Sed, Regroton, Renese-R, Reserpoid, Salutensin, Sandril, Ser-Ap-Es, Serpasil, Serpasil-Apresoline, Serpasil-Esidrix)

MUSCLE RELAXANTS
Dantrium, Flexeril, Lioresal, Norflex, Norgesic, Norgesic Forte, Paraflex, Parafon Forte, Quinamm, Rela, Robaxin, Robaxisal, Skelaxin, Soma, Soma Compound, Valium

NARCOTICS
Codeine products: Ascriptin w/Codeine, Bancap w/Codeine, Bufferin w/Codeine, Empirin w/Codeine, Empracet w/Codeine, Fiorinal w/Codeine, Phenaphen w/Codeine, Tylenol w/Codeine
Other narcotic or narcotic-like products:
Demerol, Dilaudid, Dolophene, morphine, Merpergan Fortis, Norcet, Numorphan, Percocet, Percodan, Synalgos-DC, Talwin, Talwin Compound, Tylox, Vicodan, Zactane, Zactirin

PROPOXYPHENE (pain reliever):
Darvocet-N, Darvon, Dolene, Wygeric

SLEEPING PILLS
Barbiturate sleeping pills: phenobarbital, Alurate, Amytal, Butisol, Buticap, Carbrital, Eskabarb, Lotusate, Luminal, Mebaral, Nembutal, Seconal, Sedadrops, Solfoton, Tuinal
Non-Barbiturate sleeping pills: Ativan (also used as a tranquilizer), Dalmane, Doriden, Halcion, Noctec, Noludar, Parest, Placidyl, Quaalude, Restoril, Somnos, Triclos, Valmid

TRANQUILIZERS
Benzodiazepine tranquilizers (the most widely used): Ativan, Centrax, Librium, Limbitrol (also an antidepressant), Paxipam, Serax, SK-Lygen, Tranxene, Valium, Xanax
Non-Benzodiazepine Tranquilizers: Atarax, Equanil, meprobamate, Meprospan, Meprotab, Miltown, Trancopal, Tybatran, Vistaril

ANTIDEPRESSANT....AMPHETAMINES

THIS COMBINATION MAY CAUSE INCREASED CENTRAL NERVOUS SYSTEM STIMULATION. RESULT: Possible adverse side effects such as nervousness and agitation; insomnia; loss of coordination; cardiac arrhythmias (heart beat irregularities); tachycardia (rapid heart beat); tremors; slurred speech; rapid, shallow breathing. Amphetamines are used as diet pills (this use is in disfavor), for behavior problems in children, and for narcolepsy (uncontrollable desire to sleep). Amphetamine brand names:

Benzedrine   Dexedrine
Biphetamine   Didrex
Delcobese   Obetrol
Desoxyn

ANTIDEPRESSANT....ANTICONVULSANTS

THIS COMBINATION IS MUTUALLY ANTAGONISTIC. Anticonvulsants are used to control seizures in disorders such as epilepsy. RESULT: Antidepressants can aggravate seizures and therefore decrease the effect of anticonvulsants; and anticonvulsants can lessen the effect of antidepressants in controlling mental depression. Also, since these types of drugs are both central nervous system depressants, excessive *physical* depression can occur with symptoms such as drowsiness, dizziness, loss of coordination and mental alertness. Anticonvulsant brand names (generic names in parentheses):

Depakene (valproic acid)   Peganone (ethotoin)
Dilantin (phenytoin)   Tegretol (carbamazepine)
Mesantoin (mephenytoin)   Tridione (trimethadione)
Mysoline (primidone)   Zarontin (ethosuximide)

ANTIDEPRESSANT (CYCLIC TYPE) ....ANTIDEPRESSANTS (MAOI TYPE)

THIS COMBINATION CAN CAUSE SEVERE EXCITATION, FEVER, HEADACHE, CONVULSIONS. The MAOI antidepressants are not used as much now that the safer cyclic antidepressants such as Elavil and Sinequan are available. MAOI antidepressant brand names (generic names in parentheses):

Marplan (isocarboxazid)
Nardil (phenelzine)
Eutonyl (pargyline)
Parnate (tranylcypromine)

*ANTIDEPRESSANT....ASTHMA DRUGS (EPINEPHRINE FAMILY)

THIS COMBINATION CAN CAUSE EXCESSIVE STIMULATION. RESULT: Adverse side effects such as nervousness and agitation; insomnia; loss of coordination; cardiac arrhythmias (irregularities in heart beat); tachycardia (rapid heart beat); tremors; slurred speech; rapid, shallow breathing. A dangerous rise in blood pressure, indicated by severe headache, fever, visual disturbances, or confusion can occur. The asthma drugs open lung air passages to make breathing easier in bronchial asthma. Epinephrine family asthma drug brand names (generic names in parentheses):

Aerolone (isoproterenol)
Alupent (metaproterenol)
AsthmaNeferin (epinephrine)
Brethine (terbutaline)
Bricanyl (terbutaline)
Bronitin (epinephrine)
Bronkaid (epinephrine)
Dispos-a-Med (isoproterenol)
Duo-Medihaler (isoproterenol)
Ephedrine (various companies)

Isuprel (isoproterenol)
Medihaler-Epi (epinephrine)
Medihaler-Iso (isoproterenol)
Metaprel (metaproterenol)
Norisodrine (isoproterenol)
Primatene (epinephrine)
Proventil (albuterol)
Vapo-Iso-Solution (isoproterenol)
Ventolin (albuterol)

ANTIDEPRESSANT....BARBITURATES

THE EFFECT OF THE ANTIDEPRESSANT MAY BE DECREASED. RESULT: The depression may not be controlled properly. Also, since these types of drugs are both central nervous system depressants, excessive *physical* depression can occur with symptoms such as drowsiness, dizziness, loss of coordination and mental alertness. Barbiturates are used as sedatives or sleeping pills. Barbiturate drug brand names:

phenobarbital
Alurate
Amytal
Butisol
Buticap
Carbrital
Eskabarb
Lotusate

Luminal
Mebaral
Nembutal
Seconal
Sedadrops
Solfoton
Tuinal

ANTIDEPRESSANT....BENZTROPINE (Cogentin)

THIS COMBINATION MAY CAUSE EXCESSIVE "ANTI-CHOLINERGIC" SIDE EFFECTS. Report symptoms such as dry mouth, constipation, blurry vision, loss of coordination, dizziness, slurred speech, tachycardia (rapid heart beat), toxic psychosis (disorientation, agitation, delirium); also, possible excessive central nervous system depressant effect with symptoms such as drowsiness, dizziness, loss of muscle coordination and mental alertness. Benztropine is used to control tremors resulting from Parkinson's disease or from treatment with antipsychotic drugs.

ANTIDEPRESSANT....BETA BLOCKER HEART DRUGS

THE EFFECT OF THE BETA BLOCKER MAY BE DECREASED. Beta blockers are prescribed for angina, to restore irregular heart beats to normal rhythm, and to help lower high blood pressure. RESULT: The conditions treated may not be controlled properly. Beta blocker brand names (generic names in parentheses):

Blocadren (timolol)
Corgard (nadolol)
Inderal (propranolol)
Lopressor (metoprolol)
Tenormin (atenolol)
Visken (pindolol)

ANTIDEPRESSANT....BIPERIDEN (Akineton)

THIS COMBINATION MAY CAUSE EXCESSIVE "ANTICHOLINERGIC" SIDE EFFECTS. Report symptoms such as dry mouth, constipation, blurry vision, loss of coordination, dizziness, slurred speech, tachycardia (rapid heart beat), toxic psychosis (disorientation, agitation, delerium); also, possible excessive central nervous system depressant effect with symptoms such as drowsiness, dizziness, loss of muscle coordination and mental alertness. Biperiden is used to control tremors resulting from Parkinson's disease or from treatment with antipsychotic drugs.

ANTIDEPRESSANT....BIRTH CONTROL PILLS

THE EFFECT OF THE ANTIDEPRESSANT MAY BE INCREASED OR DECREASED. RESULT: If increased antidepressant effect, possible adverse side effects from too much antidepressant drug. Report symptoms such as dry mouth, constipation, blurry vision, difficulty in urination, loss of coordination, tachycardia (rapid heart beat), toxic psychosis (disorientation, agitation, delirium), fever, convulsions. If decreased antidepressant effect, the depression may not be controlled properly. Birth control pill brand names:

Brevicon	Nordette
Demulen	Norinyl
Enovid	Norlestrin
Loestrin	Ortho-Novum
Lo-Ovral	Ovcon
Micronor	Ovral
Modicon	Ovrette
Nor-Q.D.	Ovulen

ANTIDEPRESSANT....CLONIDINE (Catapres, Combipres)

THE EFFECT OF CLONIDINE MAY BE DECREASED. Clonidine is used to lower high blood pressure. RESULT: The high blood pressure may not be controlled properly. Also, possible excessive central nervous system depressant effects with symptoms such as drowsiness, dizziness, loss of muscle coordination and mental alertness.

ANTIDEPRESSANT....COLD/COUGH PRODUCTS CONTAINING DECONGESTANT DRUGS

THIS COMBINATION CAN CAUSE EXCESSIVE STIMULATION. RESULT: Adverse side effects such as nervousness and agitation; insomnia; loss of coordination; cardiac arrhythmias (irregularities in heart beat); tachycardia (rapid heart beat); tremors; slurred speech; rapid, shallow breathing. A dangerous rise in blood pressure, indicated by severe headache, fever, visual disturbances, or confusion can occur. Be aware that nasal products can be absorbed into the bloodstream and may cause an interaction. Decongestant drugs listed on nonprescription cold/cough product labels (the same drugs are used in prescription-only cold/cough products);

ORAL (tablet, capsule, liquid):
  ephedrine
  methoxyphenamine
  phenylephrine
  phenylpropanolamine
  pseudoephedrine

NASAL (drops, spray, inhaler):
oxymetazoline
phenylephrine
propylhexedrine
xylometazoline

ANTIDEPRESSANT....CYCRIMINE (Pagitane)

THIS COMBINATION MAY CAUSE EXCESSIVE "ANTI-CHOLINERGIC" SIDE EFFECTS. Report symptoms such as dry mouth, constipation, blurry vision, loss of coordination, dizziness, slurred speech, tachycardia (rapid heart beat), toxic psychosis (disorientation, agitation, delirium); also, possible excessive central nervous system depressant effect with symptoms such as drowsiness, dizziness, loss of muscle coordination and mental alertness. Cycrimine is used to control tremors resulting from Parkinson's disease or from treatment with antipsychotic drugs.

ANTIDEPRESSANT....DICYCLOMINE (Bentyl)

THIS COMBINATION MAY CAUSE EXCESSIVE "ANTI-CHOLINERGIC" SIDE EFFECTS. Report symptoms such as dry mouth, constipation, blurry vision, loss of coordination, dizziness, slurred speech, tachycardia (rapid heart beat), toxic psychosis (disorientation, agitation, delirium). Dicyclomine is used to treat stomach and digestive tract disorders.

ANTIDEPRESSANT....DIET PILLS (NONPRESCRIPTION) CONTAINING PHENYLPROPANOLAMINE

THIS COMBINATION CAN CAUSE EXCESSIVE STIMULATION. RESULT: Adverse side effects such as nervousness and agitation; insomnia; loss of coordination; cardiac arrhythmias (irregularities in heart beat); tachycardia (rapid heart beat); tremors; slurred speech; rapid, shallow breathing. A dangerous rise in blood pressure, indicated by severe headache, fever, visual disturbances, or confusion can occur. Phenylpropanolamine is a nasal decongestant drug used as the primary ingredient in the nonprescription diet pills because of its side effect of suppressing the appetite. NOTE: Many of these diet products also contain caffeine. Nonprescription diet pill brand names:

Anorexin	E-Z Trim
Appedrine	P.P.A.
Appress	P.V.M.
Ayds (capsule, droplets)	Permathene-12
Coffee-Break	Pro Dax 21
Control	Prolamine
Dex-A-Diet II	Resolution
Dexatrim	Super Odrinex
Diadax	Ultra-Lean
Diet Gard	Vita-Slim
Dietac	

ANTIDEPRESSANT.... DIPHENHYDRAMINE (Benadryl)

THIS COMBINATION MAY CAUSE EXCESSIVE "ANTI-CHOLINERGIC" SIDE EFFECTS. Report symptoms such as dry mouth, constipation, visual disturbances, loss of coordination, dizziness, slurred speech, heart palpitations, toxic psychosis (disorientation, agitation, delirium); also, possible excessive central nervous system depressant effect with symptoms such as drowsiness, dizziness, loss of muscle coordination and mental alertness. Diphenhydramine is an antihistamine used in products for allergy, cold and cough, and in nonprescription sleeping pills.

ANTIDEPRESSANT.... DISOPYRAMIDE (Norpace)

THE EFFECTS OF EACH DRUG ON THE HEART MAY BE INCREASED. Disopyramide is used to restore irregular heart beats to normal rhythm. RESULT: Possible adverse side effects such as an increase in cardiac arrhythmias (heart beat irregularities).

ANTIDEPRESSANT.... ESTROGENS (female hormones)

THE EFFECT OF THE ANTIDEPRESSANT MAY BE INCREASED OR DECREASED. RESULT: If increased antidepressant effect, possible adverse side effects from too much antidepressant drug. Report symptoms such as dry mouth, constipation, blurry vision, difficulty in urination, loss of coordination, tachycardia (rapid heart beat), toxic psychosis (disorientation, agitation, delirium), fever, convulsions. If decreased antidepressant effect, the depression may not be controlled properly. Estrogens are prescribed for estrogen deficiency during menopause and after hysterectomy (surgical removal of the uterus), to prevent painful swelling of the breasts after pregnancy in women choosing not to nurse, and to treat amenorrhea (failure to menstruate). Estrogen brand names:

Amen	Menrium
Aygestin	Milprem
DES	Norulate
Estinyl	Norlutin
Estrace	Ogen
Estratab	PMB
Estrovis	Premarin
Evex	Provera
Feminone	Tace
Menest	

ANTIDEPRESSANT....FENFLURAMINE (Pondimin)

THE EFFECT OF FENFLURAMINE MAY BE INCREASED. Fenfluramine is an appetite suppressant, or diet pill, which has sedative side effects. RESULT: Excessive sedation from too much fenfluramine. Report symptoms such as drowsiness, loss of muscle coordination and mental alertness.

ANTIDEPRESSANT....GLYCOPYRROLATE (Robinul)

THIS COMBINATION MAY CAUSE EXCESSIVE "ANTICHOLINERGIC" SIDE EFFECTS. Report symptoms such as dry mouth, constipation, visual disturbances, loss of coordination, dizziness, slurred speech, heart palpitations, toxic psychosis (disorientation, agitation, delirium); also, possible excessive central nervous system depressant effect with symptoms such as drowsiness, dizziness, loss of muscle coordination and mental alertness. Glycopyrrolate is used in stomach and digestive tract disorders.

*ANTIDEPRESSANT....GUANETHIDINE (Esimil, Ismelin)

THE EFFECT OF GUANETHIDINE MAY BE DECREASED. Guanethidine is used to treat high blood pressure. RESULT: The blood pressure may not be controlled properly. NOTE: The antidepressant doxepin (Adapin, Sinequan), in lower doses, may not interact.

ANTIDEPRESSANT....ISOPROPAMIDE (Combid)

THIS COMBINATION MAY CAUSE EXCESSIVE "ANTI-CHOLINERGIC" SIDE EFFECTS. Report symptoms such as dry mouth, constipation, blurry vision, loss of coordination, dizziness, slurred speech, tachycardia (rapid heart beat), toxic psychosis (disorientation, agitation, delirium). Isopropamide is used to treat stomach and digestive tract disorders.

ANTIDEPRESSANT....LEVODOPA (Dopar, Larodopa, Sinemet)

THE EFFECT OF LEVODOPA MAY BE DECREASED. Levodopa is used to control the tremors of Parkinson's disease. RESULT: The condition may not be controlled properly. This interaction is prevented by not giving the two drugs within two hours of each other.

ANTIDEPRESSANT....ORPHENADRINE (Norflex)

THIS COMBINATION MAY CAUSE EXCESSIVE "ANTI-CHOLINERGIC" SIDE EFFECTS. Report symptoms such as dry mouth, constipation, visual disturbances, loss of coordination, dizziness, slurred speech, heart palpitations, toxic psychosis (disorientation, agitation, delirium); also, possible excessive central nervous system depressant effect with symptoms such as drowsiness, dizziness, loss of muscle coordination and mental alertness. Orphenadrine is a muscle relaxant.

ANTIDEPRESSANT....PROCAINAMIDE (Procan, Procan SR, Pronestyl)

THE EFFECTS OF EACH DRUG ON THE HEART MAY BE INCREASED. Procainamide is used to restore irregular heart beats to normal rhythm. RESULT: Possible adverse side effects such as an increase in arrhythmias (heart beat irregularities).

ANTIDEPRESSANT....PROCYCLIDINE (Kemadrin)

THIS COMBINATION MAY CAUSE EXCESSIVE "ANTI-CHOLINERGIC" SIDE EFFECTS. Report symptoms such as dry mouth, constipation, blurry vision, loss of coordination, dizziness, slurred speech, tachycardia (rapid heart beat), toxic psychosis (disorientation, agitation, delirium); also, possible excessive central nervous system depressant effect with symptoms such as drowsiness, dizziness, loss of muscle coordination and mental alertness. Procyclidine is used to control tremors resulting from Parkinson's disease or from treatment with antipsychotic drugs.

ANTIDEPRESSANT....PROPANTHELINE (Probanthine)

THIS COMBINATION MAY CAUSE EXCESSIVE "ANTI-CHOLINERGIC" SIDE EFFECTS. Report symptoms such as dry mouth, constipation, blurry vision, loss of coordination, dizziness, slurred speech, tachycardia (rapid heart beat), toxic psychosis (disorientation, agitation, delirium). Propantheline is used to treat stomach and digestive tract disorders.

ANTIDEPRESSANT....QUINIDINE

THE EFFECTS OF EACH DRUG ON THE HEART MAY BE INCREASED. Quinidine is used to restore irregular heart beats to normal rhythm. RESULT: Possible adverse side effects such as an increase in arrhythmias (heart beat irregularities). Quinidine brand names:

Cardioquin
Duraquin
Quinaglute Dura-Tabs
Quinidex Extentabs
Quinora

ANTIDEPRESSANT....QUININE (Coco-Quinine, Quine)

THE EFFECTS OF EACH DRUG ON THE HEART MAY BE INCREASED. RESULT: Possible adverse side effects such as an increase in arrhythmias (heart beat irregularities). Quinine is a nonprescription drug used to treat malaria and nighttime leg cramps.

ANTIDEPRESSANT....RESERPINE TYPE DRUGS

THIS COMBINATION MAY CAUSE EXCESSIVE CENTRAL NERVOUS SYSTEM STIMULATION. RESULT: Severe excitation, jitteriness, and bizarre behavior.. Reserpine is used to treat high blood pressure. Reserpine type drugs (brand names in parentheses):

deserpidine (Enduronyl, Harmonyl, Oreticyl)
rauwolfia (Raudixin, Rauzide)
reserpine (Diupres, Diutensen-R, Hydropres, Rau-Sed, Regroton, Renese-R, Reserpoid, Salutensin, Sandril, Ser-Ap-Es, Serpasil, Serpasil-Apresoline, Serpasil-Esidrix)

ANTIDEPRESSANT....RIFAMPIN (Rifadin, Rimactane)

THE EFFECT OF THE ANTIDEPRESSANT MAY BE DECREASED. RESULT: The depression may not be controlled properly. Rifampin is used to treat tuberculosis and may be given to suspected meningitis carriers.

ANTIDEPRESSANT....SCOPOLAMINE (Transderm-Scop)

THIS COMBINATION MAY CAUSE EXCESSIVE "ANTICHOLINERGIC" SIDE EFFECTS. Report symptoms such as dry mouth, constipation, visual disturbances, loss of coordination, dizziness, slurred speech, heart palpitations, toxic psychosis (disorientation, agitation, delirium); also, possible excessive central nervous system depressant effect with symptoms such as drowsiness, dizziness, loss of coordination and mental alertness. Scopolamine is used for motion sickness.

ANTIDEPRESSANT....TRIHEXYPHENIDYL (Artane)

THIS COMBINATION MAY CAUSE EXCESSIVE "ANTICHOLINERGIC" SIDE EFFECTS. Report symptoms such as dry mouth, constipation, visual disturbances, loss of coordination, dizziness, slurred speech, heart palpitations, toxic psychosis (disorientation, agitation, delirium); also, possible excessive central nervous system depressant effect with symptoms such as drowsiness, dizziness, loss of muscle coordination and mental alertness. Trihexyphenidyl is used to control tremors resulting from Parkinson's disease or from treatment with antipsychotic drugs.

PART II—ANTIDEPRESSANTS (MAOI TYPE)

BRAND NAMES

Marplan (isocarboxazid)
Nardil (phenelzine)
Eutonyl (pargyline)
Parnate (tranylcypromine)

DRUG INTERACTIONS

*ANTIDEPRESSANT (MAOI TYPE)....AMPHETAMINES

THIS COMBINATION MAY CAUSE EXCESSIVE CEN-TRAL NERVOUS SYSTEM STIMULATION. RESULT: Adverse side effects such as nervousness and agitation; insomnia; loss of coordination; cardiac arrhythmias (irregularities in heart beat); tachycardia (rapid heart beat); tremors; slurred speech; rapid, shallow breathing. A dangerous rise in blood pressure, indicated by severe headache, fever, visual disturbances, or confusion, can occur. Amphetamines are used as diet pills (this use is in disfavor) for behavior problems in children, and for narcolepsy (uncontrollable desire to sleep). Amphetamine brand names:

Benzedrine
Biphetamine
Delcobese
Desoxyn
Dexedrine
Didrex
Obetrol

ANTIDEPRESSANT (MAOI TYPE) ....ANTIDEPRESSANTS (CYCLIC TYPE)

THIS COMBINATION CAN CAUSE SEVERE EXCITA-TION, FEVER, HEADACHE, CONVULSIONS. The MAOI antidepressants are not used as much now that the safer cyclic antidepressants are available. Tricyclic antidepressant brand names (generic names in parentheses):

Adapin (doxepin)
Asendin (amoxapine)
Aventyl (nortriptyline)
Elavil (amitriptyline)
Endep (amitriptyline)
Etrafon (amitriptyline/
   perphenazine)
Limbitrol (amitriptyline/
   chlordiazepoxide)
Ludiomil (maprotiline)

Norpramin (desipramine)
Pamelor (nortriptyline)
Pertofrane (desipramine)
Sinequan (doxepin)
Surmontil (trimipramine)
Tofranil, Tofranil-PM
   (imipramine)
Triavil (amitriptyline/
   perphenazine)
Vivactil (protriptyline)

ANTIDEPRESSANT (MAOI TYPE)
....ASTHMA DRUGS (EPINEPHRINE FAMILY)

THIS COMBINATION MAY CAUSE EXTRA CENTRAL NERVOUS SYSTEM STIMULATION. RESULT: Possible adverse side effects such as nervousness and agitation; insomnia; tachycardia (rapid heart beat). Asthma drugs open lung air passages to make breathing easier in asthmatic conditions. Epinephrine family asthma drug brand names (generic names in parentheses):

Aerolone (isoproterenol)
Alupent (metaproterenol)
AsthmaNefrin (epenepherine)
  Brethine (terbutaline)
Bricanyl (terbutaline)
Bronitin (epinephrine)
Bronkaid (epinephrine)
Dispos-a-Med (isoproterenol)
Duo-Medihaler (isoproterenol)

Ephedrine (various companies)
Isuprel (isoproterenol)
Medihaler-Epi (epinephrine)
Medihaler-Iso (isoproterenol)
Metaprel (metaproterenol)
Norisodrine (isoproterenol)
Primatene (epinephrine)
Proventil (albuterol)
Vapo-Iso-Solution (isoproterenol)
Ventolin (albuterol)

ANTIDEPRESSANT (MAOI TYPE)
....ASTHMA DRUGS (THEOPHYLLINE FAMILY)

THIS COMBINATION MAY CAUSE EXTRA CENTRAL NERVOUS SYSTEM STIMULATION. RESULT: Possible adverse side effects such as nervousness and agitation; insomnia; tachycardia (rapid heart beat). Asthma drugs open lung air passages to make breathing easier in asthmatic conditions. Theophylline family asthma drug brand names (generic names in parentheses):

Accurbron (theophylline)
Bronkodyl (theophylline)
Choledyl (oxtriphylline)
Dilor (dyphylline)
Elixicon (theophylline)
Elixophyllin (theophylline)
LaBID (theophylline)
Lufyllin (dyphylline)
Quibron-T (theophylline)

Respbid (theophylline)
Slo-Phyllin (theophylline)
Somophyllin (aminophylline)
Somophyllin-T (theophylline)
Sustaire (theophylline)
Theobid (theophylline)
Theodur (theophylline)
Theolair (theophylline)
Theophyl (theophylline)

Theovent (theophylline)   Amesec, Asbron G,
  Multi-ingredient products   Brondecon, Marax, Mudrane,
  containing theophylline: Quibron, Tedral SA

ANTIDEPRESSANT (MAOI TYPE)....BETA BLOCKER HEART DRUGS

THIS COMBINATION MAY CAUSE A MARKED IN-CREASE IN BLOOD PRESSURE. Beta blockers are prescribed for angina, to restore irregular heart beats to normal rhythm, and to help lower high blood pressure. Beta blocker brand names (generic names in parentheses):

Blocadren (timolol)
Corgard (nadolol)
Inderal (propranolol)
Lopressor (metoprolol)
Tenormin (atenolol)
Visken (pindolol)

ANTIDEPRESSANT (MAOI TYPE)....CAFFEINE

THIS COMBINATION MAY CAUSE EXCESSIVE CEN-TRAL NERVOUS SYSTEM STIMULATION. RESULT: Adverse side effects such as nervousness and agitation; insomnia; loss of coordination; cardiac arrhythmias (irregularities in heart beat); tachycardia (rapid heart beat); tremors; slurred speech; rapid, shallow breathing. A dangerous rise in blood pressure, indicated by severe headache, fever, visual disturbances, or con-fusion, can occur. Caffeine is the stimulant found in coffee, tea, cola beverages, and in such nonprescription products as diet pills and headache, cold/cough, menstrual, and daytime stimulant products.

*ANTIDEPRESSANT (MAOI TYPE)....COLD/COUGH PRODUCTS CONTAINING DECONGESTANT DRUGS

THIS COMBINATION MAY CAUSE EXCESSIVE CEN-TRAL NERVOUS SYSTEM STIMULATION. RESULT: Adverse side effects such as nervousness and agitation; insomnia; loss of coordination; cardiac arrhythmias (irregularities in heart beat); tachycardia (rapid heart beat); tremors; slurred speech;

rapid, shallow breathing. A dangerous rise in blood pressure, indicated by severe headache, fever, visual disturbances, or confusion can occur. Be aware that nasal products can be absorbed into the blood stream and may cause an interaction. Decongestant drugs listed on nonprescription cold/cough products labels (the same drugs are used in prescription-only cold/cough products):

ORAL (tablet, capsule, liquid):
ephedrine
methoxyphenamine
phenylephrine
phenylpropanolamine
pseudoephedrine.

NASAL (drops, spray, inhaler):
oxymetazoline
phenylephrine
propylh exedrine
xylometazoline.

ANTIDEPRESSANT (MAOI TYPE) ....DEXTROMETHORPHAN

THIS COMBINATION MAY CAUSE EXCESSIVE CENTRAL NERVOUS SYSTEM STIMULATION OR DEPRESSION. RESULT: If stimulation, symptoms are nervousness and agitation; insomnia; loss of coordination; cardiac arrhythmias (irregularities in heart beat); tachycardia (rapid heart beat); tremors; slurred speech; rapid, shallow breathing. If depression, symptoms are drowsiness, loss of muscle coordination and mental alertness. Dextromethorphan is the cough suppressant found in nonprescription cough preparations.

*ANTIDEPRESSANT (MAOI TYPE)....DIABETES DRUGS

THE EFFECT OF THE DIABETES DRUG MAY BE INCREASED. Diabetes drugs are used to lower the blood sugar level in diabetics. RESULT: The blood sugar may fall too low. Report symptoms of hypoglycemia (low blood sugar): weakness, faintness, sweating, cardiac arrythmias (heart beat irregularities), tachycardia (rapid heart beat), visual disturbances, loss of coordination, confusion, headache. Diabetes drug brand names (generic names in parentheses):

Diabinese (chlorpropamide)
Dymelor (acetohexamide)
Orinase (tolbutamide)
Tolinase (tolazamide)
Insulin (various companies)

*ANTIDEPRESSANT (MAOI TYPE)
....DIET PILLS (NONPRESCRIPTION)
CONTAINING PHENYLPROPANOLAMINE

THIS COMBINATION MAY CAUSE EXCESSIVE CEN-
TRAL NERVOUS SYSTEM STIMULATION. RESULT:
Adverse side effects such as nervousness and agitation; insomnia;
loss of coordination; cardiac arrythmias (irregularities in heart
beat); tachycardia (rapid heart beat); tremors; slurred speech;
rapid, shallow breathing. A dangerous rise in blood pressure,
indicated by severe headache, fever, visual disturbances, or confusion, can occur. Phenylopropanolamine is a nasal decongestant
drug used as the primary ingredient in the nonprescription diet
pills because of its side effect of suppressing the appetite. NOTE:
Many of these diet products also contain caffeine. Nonprescription diet pill brand names:

Anorexin	E-Z Trim
Appedrine	P.P.A.
Appress	P.V.M.
Ayds (capsule, droplets)	Permathene-12
Coffee-Break	Pro Dax 21
Control	Prolamine
Dex-A-Diet II	Resolution
Dexatrim	Super Odrinex
Diadax	Ultra-Lean
Diet Gard	Vita-Slim
Dietac	

ANTIDEPRESSANT (MAOI TYPE)....DIURETICS

THIS COMBINATION MAY CAUSE THE BLOOD PRES-
SURE TO DROP TOO LOW. RESULT: Postural hypotension (a
sudden drop in blood pressure when changing positions, especially when rising after lying or sitting). Symptoms are dizziness, weakness, faintness. Diuretics are used to lower high blood

pressure by removing excess body fluid. Diuretic drug brand names (generic names in parentheses):

Aldactazide (spironolactone, hydrochlorothiazide)
Aldactone (spironolactone)
Anhydron (cyclothiazide)
Aquatag (benzthiazide)
Aquatensin (methyclothiazide)
Diucardin (hydroflumethiazide)
Diulo (metolazone)
Diuril (chlorothiazide)
Dyazide (triamterene, hydrochlorothiazide)
Dyrenium (triamterene)
Edecrin (ethacrynic acid)
Enduron (methyclothiazide)
Esidrix (hydrochlorothiazide)

Exna (benzthiazide)
Hydrodiuril (hydrochlorothiazide)
Hydromox (quinethazone)
Hygroton (chlorthalidone)
Lasix (furosemide)
Metahydrin (trichlormethiazide)
Midamor (amiloride)
Moduretic (amiloride, hydrochlorothiazide)
Naqua (trichlormethiazide)
Naturetin (bendroflumethiazide)
Oretic (hydrochlorothiazide)
Renese (polythiazide)
Saluron (hydroflumethiazide)
Zaroxolyn (metolazone)

ANTIDEPRESSANT (MAOI TYPE) ....GUANETHIDINE (Esimil, Ismelin)

THIS COMBINATION MAY RESULT IN A MARKED RISE IN BLOOD PRESSURE indicated by severe headache, fever, visual disturbances, or confusion. Guanethidine is used to treat high blood pressure.

ANTIDEPRESSANT (MAOI TYPE)....HIGH BLOOD PRESSURE DRUGS

THIS COMBINATION MAY CAUSE THE BLOOD PRESSURE TO DROP TOO LOW. RESULT: Postural hypotension (a sudden drop in blood pressure when changing positions, especially when rising after lying or sitting). Symptoms are dizziness, weakness, faintness. High blood pressure drugs (brand names in parentheses):

captopril (Capoten)
clonidine (Catapres, Combipres)
guanabenz (Wytensin)
guanethidine (Esimil, Ismelin)
hydralazine (Apresoline, Ser-Ap-Es, Serpasil-Apresoline)

methyldopa (Aldoclor, Aldomet, Aldoril)
minoxidil (Loniten)
prazosin (Minipress)

ANTIDEPRESSANT (MAOI TYPE)
....LEVODOPA (Dopar, Larodopa, Sinemet)

THIS COMBINATION MAY CAUSE A DANGEROUS RISE IN BLOOD PRESSURE with symptoms such as headache, fever, visual disturbances, or confusion. Levodopa is used to control the tremors of Parkinson's disease.

ANTIDEPRESSANT (MAOI TYPE)
....MEPERIDINE (Demerol, Mepergan Fortis)

THIS COMBINATION CAN CAUSE EXTREME AD-VERSE SIDE EFFECTS with symptoms such as excitation, fever, low blood pressure, sweating, loss of consciousness, breathing difficulties. Meperidine is a narcotic pain reliever.

ANTIDEPRESSANT (MAOI TYPE)
....METHYLDOPA (Aldoclor, Aldomet, Aldoril)

THE EFFECT OF METHYLDOPA MAY BE DECREASED. Methyldopa is used to treat high blood pressure. RESULT: The blood pressure may not be controlled properly.

ANTIDEPRESSANT (MAOI TYPE)
....METHYLPHENIDATE (Ritalin)

THIS COMBINATION MAY CAUSE EXCESSIVE CEN-TRAL NERVOUS SYSTEM STIMULATION. RESULT: Adverse side effects such as nervousness and agitation; insomnia; loss of coordination; cardiac arrhythmias (irregularities in heart beat); tachycardia (rapid heart beat); tremors; slurred speech; rapid, shallow breathing. A dangerous rise in blood pressure, indicated by severe headache, fever, visual disturbances, or con-fusion, can occur. Methylphenidate is used in hyperkinetic be-havior disorders in children, narcolepsy (uncontrollable desire to sleep), mild depression, and apathetic or withdrawn senile behavior.

ANTIDEPRESSANT (MAOI TYPE)....RESERPINE-TYPE BLOOD PRESSURE DRUGS

THIS COMBINATION CAN CAUSE EXCESSIVE CEN-TRAL NERVOUS SYSTEM STIMULATION. RESULT: Jitteriness, marked rise in blood pressure with headache, fever, visual disturbances, confusion. Reserpine is used to treat high blood pressure. Reserpine-type drugs (brand names in parentheses):

deserpidine (Enduronyl, Harmonyl, Oreticyl)
rauwolfia (Raudixin, Rauzide)
reserpine (Diupres, Diutensen-R, Hydropres, Rau-Sed, Regroton, Renese-R, Reserpoid, Salutensin, Sandril, Ser-Ap-Es, Serpasil, Serpasil-Apresoline, Serpasil-Esidrix).

11

Drug Interactions
in Diabetes Treatment

Diabetes mellitus is a disease in which the pancreas gland fails to produce enough insulin or the body cannot use insulin properly. Insulin is a hormone which transports sugar from the blood into body cells needing it for energy. Sugar remains in the bloodstream (and appears in the urine) instead of being taken in and used by body cells. Denied sugar, the cells must burn more than ordinary amounts of fats and protein for fuel. This excessive breakdown of fats and proteins releases acid waste products into the blood.

Untreated or poorly controlled diabetes causes long-term adverse effects and may result in a metabolic crisis and diabetic coma.

Symptoms of diabetes are excessive appetite (the body recognizes its increased need for fuel); large urine output; excessive thirst (the body must replace fluid lost through urination); weakness, lethargy, drowsiness; weight loss.

The diabetic usually shows a fasting blood sugar level over 130mg/100cc and, after eating, a level over 170 mg/100cc.

Many diabetics can be treated by diet and weight control alone. Some will require oral medication. Those with juvenile-onset diabetes and adults whose diabetes is not amenable to diet and oral medication require daily insulin injections. Both pills and insulin cause a lowering of the blood sugar level. The pills work either by stimulating the pancreas to produce more insulin or by enhancing the body's ability to use insulin. Insulin injection is a direct replacement for the body's own lack of insulin.

BRAND NAME SECTION

ORAL:

Diabinese (chlorpropamide)
Dymelor (acetohexamide)
Orinase (tolbutamide)
Tolinase (tolazamide)

INJECTABLE:

Insulin

The patient and physician should monitor urine and blood sugar levels carefully during a course of treatment with any drug which interacts with a patient's diabetes drug. To maintain stable blood sugar levels, the dosage of the diabetes drug usually needs adjusting when an interacting drug is started and then readjusting when the interacting drug is stopped.

Diabetic patients, especially those taking interacting drugs, should carry a candy bar or glucose preparation such as Monojel or Glutose for emergency use to treat a sudden drop in the blood sugar level.

DRUG INTERACTIONS

I. INTERACTIONS WHICH MAY INCREASE THE EFFECT OF DIABETES DRUGS

*DIABETES DRUGS (ORAL AND INSULIN)....ALCOHOL (beer, liquor, wine, etc.)

THE EFFECT OF THE DIABETES DRUG MAY BE INCREASED. RESULT: Alcohol may cause unpredictable changes in the blood sugar level with the most serious effect being a dangerous *fall* in the blood sugar level. Report symptoms of hypoglycemia (low blood sugar): nervousness, faintness, weakness, sweating, confusion, cardiac arrhythmias (heart beat irregularities), tachycardia (rapid heart beat), loss of coordination, visual disturbances; also, an acute reaction may occur such as when an alcoholic on the antialcoholic drug disulfiram (Antabuse) ingests alcohol: dizziness, flushing, shortness of breath, severe headache, heart palpitations. *Alcohol:* beer, wine, liquor, etc; some cough syrups and vitamin "tonics." NOTE: Limiting intake of alcohol to small amounts (especially if taken with food) will probably prevent this interaction.

DIABETES DRUGS (ORAL)....ALLOPURINOL (Zyloprim)

THE EFFECT OF THE DIABETES DRUG MAY BE IN- CREASED. RESULT: The blood sugar level may fall too low. Report symptoms of hypoglycemia (low blood sugar): nervous- ness, faintness, weakness, sweating, confusion, cardiac ar- rhythmias (heart beat irregularities), tachycardia (rapid heart beat), loss of coordination, visual disturbances. Allopurinol is used to treat gout.

DIABETES DRUGS (ORAL)....ANTICOAGULANTS

A. THE EFFECT OF THE DIABETES DRUG MAY BE INCREASED. RESULT: The blood sugar level may fall too low. Report symptoms of hypoglycemia (low blood sugar): nervous- ness, faintness, weakness, sweating, confusion, cardiac ar- rhythmias (heart beat irregularities), tachycardia (rapid heart beat), loss of coordination, visual disturbances.

B. THE EFFECT OF THE ANTICOAGULANT MAY BE INCREASED. Anticoagulants are used to thin the blood and prevent it from clotting. RESULT: Increased risk of hemorrhage. Report symptoms such as bruising or bleeding anywhere on the body, black or tarry stools. Anticoagulant drug brand names (generic names in parentheses):

Athrombin-K (warfarin)	Hedulin (phenindione)
Coufarin (warfarin)	Liquamar (phenprocoumon)
Coumadin (warfarin)	Miradon (anisindione)
dicumarol (various companies)	Panwarfarin (warfarin)

*DIABETES DRUGS (ORAL) ....ANTIDEPRESSANTS (MAOI FAMILY)

THE EFFECT OF THE DIABETES DRUG MAY BE IN- CREASED. RESULT: The blood sugar level may fall too low. Report symptoms of hypoglycemia (low blood sugar): nervous- ness, faintness, weakness, sweating, confusion, cardiac arrhythmias (heart beat irregularities), tachycardia (rapid heart beat), loss of coordination, visual disturbances. The MAOI antidepressants, used to alleviate mental depression, are not used as much now that safer tricyclic antidepressants like Elavil and Sinequan are available. MAOI Antidepressant brand names (generic names in parentheses):

Marplan (isocarboxazid)
Nardil (phenelzine)
Eutonyl (pargyline)
Parnate (tranylcypromine)

DIABETES DRUGS (ORAL)....ASPIRIN

THE EFFECT OF THE DIABETES DRUG MAY BE INCREASED. RESULT: The blood sugar level may fall too low. Report symptoms of hypoglycemia (low blood sugar): nervousness, faintness, weakness, sweating, confusion, cardiac arrhythmias (heart beat irregularities), tachycardia (rapid heart beat), loss of coordination, visual disturbances. Aspirin brand names:

Anacin
Ascriptin
Aspergum
Bayer
Bufferin
CAMA
Ecotrin

Empirin
Measurin
Momentum
Pabirin
Persistin
St. Joseph Aspirin

NOTE: Here are brand names of salicylate-containing pain relievers which may interact similarly to aspirin:

Arthralgen
Arthropan
Calurin
Dolobid
Disalcid
Magan

Mobidin
Pabalate
Salrin
Uracel
Uromide

*DIABETES DRUGS (ORAL AND INSULIN)....BETA BLOCKER HEART DRUGS

THIS COMBINATION CAN EITHER INCREASE OR DECREASE THE EFFECT OF THE DIABETES DRUG. RE-

SULT: If *increased* diabetes drug effect, the blood sugar level may fall too low. Report symptoms of hypoglycemia (low blood sugar), which will be even more pronounced with physical exertion or exercise: sweating, nervousness, faintness, weakness, confusion, cardiac arrhythmias (heart beat irregularities), tachycardia (rapid heart beat), loss of coordination, visual disturbances—be aware that taking the beta blocker drug can *hide* these warning symptoms. If *decreased* diabetes drug effect, the blood sugar level may remain too high. Report symptoms of hyperglycemia (high blood sugar); excessive thirst, large urine output, weight loss, hunger, lethargy, drowsiness, loss of coordination. Beta blocker heart drugs are prescribed for angina, to restore irregular heart beats to normal rhythm, and to help lower high blood pressure. Beta blocker brand names (generic names in parentheses):

Blocadren (timolol)
Corgard (nadolol)
Inderal (propranolol)
Lopressor (metoprolol)
Tenormin (atenolol)
Visken (pindolol)

DIABETES DRUGS (ORAL)
....CHLORAMPHENICOL (Chloromycetin, Mychel)

THE EFFECT OF THE DIABETES DRUG MAY BE IN-CREASED. RESULT: The blood sugar level may fall too low. Report symptoms of hypoglycemia (low blood sugar): nervousness, faintness, weakness, sweating, confusion, cardiac arrhythmias (heart beat irregularities), tachycardia (rapid heart beat), loss of coordination, visual disturbances. This combination can also cause bone marrow depression—report symptoms such as sore throat, fever, mouth sores, bleeding anywhere on the body, unusual loss of energy. Chloramphenicol is an antibiotic prescribed to combat infection.

DIABETES DRUGS (ORAL)....CLOFIBRATE (Atromid-S)

THE EFFECT OF THE DIABETES DRUG MAY BE IN-CREASED. RESULT: The blood sugar level may fall too low. Report symptoms of hypoglycemia (low blood sugar); nervousness, faintness, weakness, sweating, confusion, cardiac arrhythmias (heart beat irregularities), tachycardia (rapid heart beat), loss of coordination, visual disturbances. Clofibrate is used to lower elevated blood cholesterol and triglycerides.

DIABETES DRUGS (ORAL)....GUANETHIDINE (Esimil, Ismelin)

THE EFFECT OF THE DIABETES DRUG MAY BE IN-CREASED. RESULT: The blood sugar level may fall too low. Report symptoms of hypoglycemia (low blood sugar): nervousness, faintness, weakness, sweating, confusion, cardiac arrhythmias (heart beat irregularities), tachycardia (rapid heart beat), loss of coordination, visual disturbances. Guanethidine is prescribed for severe high blood pressure.

DIABETES DRUGS (ORAL)....INSULIN

THE EFFECT OF BOTH DRUGS MAY BE INCREASED. RESULT: Additive hypoglycemia (low blood sugar). This interaction may occur during "crossover" periods when switching from an oral diabetes drug to insulin and vice-versa. Be aware of the low blood sugar symptoms: nervousness, faintness, weakness, sweating, confusion, cardiac arrhythmias (heart beat irregularities), tachycardia (rapid heart beat), loss of coordination, visual disturbances.

DIABETES DRUGS (ORAL AND INSULIN)....MALE HORMONES (androgens)

THE EFFECT OF THE DIABETES DRUG MAY BE IN-CREASED. RESULT: The blood sugar level may fall too low. Report symptoms of hypoglycemia (low blood sugar): nervousness, faintness, weakness, sweating, confusion, cardiac arrhythmias (heart beat irregularities), tachycardia (rapid heart beat), loss of coordination, visual disturbances. Male hormones or anabolic steroids are prescribed for osteoporosis (brittleness or softness of bones often seen in the elderly or in debilitated patients); for some forms of anemia. Male hormone brand names (generic names in parentheses):

Adroyd (oxymetholone)   Anavar (oxandrolone)
Anadrol (oxymetholone)   Danocrine (danazol)

Dianabol (methandrostenolone)   Nandrolin (nandrolone)
Durabolin (nandrolone)   Winstrol (stanozolol)
Maxibolin (ethylestrenol)

*DIABETES DRUGS (ORAL)
....OXYPHENBUTAZONE (Tandearil)

THE EFFECT OF THE DIABETES DRUG MAY BE IN-
CREASED. RESULT: The blood sugar level may fall too low.
Report symptoms of hypoglycemia (low blood sugar): nervousness, faintness, weakness, sweating, confusion, cardiac arrhythmias (heart beat irregularities), tachycardia (rapid heart
beat), loss of coordination, visual disturbances. Oxyphenbutazone
is prescribed for acute inflammatory conditions such as arthritis
or bursitis.

DIABETES DRUG (ORAL)....PEPTO-BISMOL

THE EFFECT OF THE DIABETES DRUG MAY BE IN-
CREASED. RESULT: The blood sugar level may fall too low.
Report symptoms of hypoglycemia (low blood sugar): nervousness, faintness, weakness, sweating, confusion, cardiac arrhythmias (heart beat irregularities), tachycardia (rapid heart
beat), loss of coordination, visual disturbances. Pepto-Bismol, used
for diarrhea, contains a salicylate ingredient which interacts
similarly to aspirin.

*DIABETES DRUGS (ORAL)
....PHENYLBUTAZONE (Azolid, Butazolidin)

THE EFFECT OF THE DIABETES DRUG MAY BE IN-
CREASED. RESULT: The blood sugar level may fall too low.
Report symptoms of hypoglycemia (low blood sugar): nervousness, faintness, weakness, sweating, confusion, cardiac arrhythmias (heart beat irregularities), tachycardia (rapid heart
beat), loss of coordination, visual disturbances. Phenylbutazone is
prescribed for acute inflammatory conditions such as arthritis or
bursitis.

DIABETES DRUGS (ORAL)
....PROBENECID (Benemid, ColBenemid)

THE EFFECT OF THE DIABETES DRUG MAY BE IN-
CREASED. RESULT: The blood sugar level may fall too low.

Report symptoms of hypoglycemia (low blood sugar): nervousness, faintness, weakness, sweating, confusion, cardiac arrhythmias (heart beat irregularities), tachycardia (rapid heart beat), loss of coordination, visual disturbances. Probenecid is prescribed for gout.

DIABETES DRUGS (ORAL)
....SULFONAMIDE ANTIBIOTICS

THE EFFECT OF THE DIABETES DRUG MAY BE INCREASED. RESULT: The blood sugar level may fall too low. Report symptoms of hypoglycemia (low blood sugar): nervousness, faintness, weakness, sweating, confusion, cardiac arrhythmias (heart beat irregularities), tachycardia (rapid heart beat), loss of coordination, visual disturbances. Sulfonamide antibiotics are used to combat infection, especially urinary tract infections. Sulfonamide antibiotic brand names (generic names in parentheses):

Azulfidine (sulfasalazine)—
  prescribed for ulcerative colitis
Bactrim (sulfamethoxazole
  trimethoprim)
Bactrim DS (sulfamethoxazole
  trimethoprim)
Gantanol (sulfamethoxazole)
Gantrisin (sulfisoxazole)
Renoquid (sulfacytine)

SK-Soxazole (sulfisoxazole)
Septra (sulfamethoxazole
  trimethoprim)
Septra DS (sulfamethoxazole
  trimethoprim)
Sulla (sulfameter)
Thiosulfil (sulfamethizole)

II. INTERACTIONS WHICH MAY DECREASE THE EFFECT OF DIABETES DRUGS

DIABETES DRUGS (ORAL AND
INSULIN)....AMPHETAMINES

THE EFFECT OF THE DIABETES DRUG MAY BE ANTAGONIZED. RESULT: The blood sugar level may remain too high. Report symptoms of hyperglycemia (high blood sugar): excessive thirst, large urine output, weight loss, hunger, lethargy, drowsiness, loss of coordination. Amphetamines are used as diet pills (this use is in disfavor), for behavior problems in children, and for narcolepsy (uncontrollable desire to sleep). Amphetamine brand names:

Benzedrine
Biphetamine
Delcobese
Desoxyn
Dexedrine
Didrex
Obetrol

DIABETES DRUGS (ORAL AND INSULIN)....ASTHMA DRUGS (EPINEPHRINE FAMILY)

THE EFFECT OF THE DIABETES DRUG MAY BE ANTAGONIZED. RESULT: The blood sugar level may remain too high. Report symptoms of hyperglycemia (high blood sugar): excessive thirst, large urine output, weight loss, hunger, lethargy, drowsiness, loss of coordination. Asthma drugs are used to make breathing easier in asthma patients. Epinephrine family asthma drug brand names (generic names in parentheses):

Aerolone (isoproterenol)
Alupent (metaproterenol)
AsthmaNefrin (epinephrine)
Brethine (terbutaline)
Bricanyl (terbutaline)
Bronitin (epinephrine)
Bronkaid (epinephrine)
Dispos-a-Med (isoproterenol)
Duo-Medihaler (isoproterenol)
Ephedrine (various companies)

Isuprel (isoproterenol)
Medihaler-Epi (epinephrine)
Medihaler-Iso (isoproterenol)
Metaprel (metaproterenol)
Norisodrine (isoproterenol)
Primatene (epinephrine)
Proventil (albuterol)
Vapo-Iso-Solution (isoproterenol)
Ventolin (albuterol)

*DIABETES DRUGS (ORAL AND INSULIN)....BETA BLOCKER HEART DRUGS

THIS COMBINATION CAN EITHER INCREASE OR DECREASE THE EFFECT OF THE DIABETES DRUG. RESULT: If *increased* diabetes drug effect, the blood sugar level may fall too low. Report symptoms of hypoglycemia (low blood sugar), which will be even more pronounced with physical exertion or exercise: sweating, nervousness, faintness, weakness, confusion, cardiac arrhythmias (heart beat irregularities), tachycardia (rapid heart beat), loss of coordination, visual disturbances—be aware that taking the beta blocker drug can *hide* these warning symptoms. If *decreased* diabetes drug effect, the blood sugar level may remain too high. Report symptoms of hyperglycemia (high blood sugar): excessive thirst, large urine output, weight loss, hunger, lethargy, drowsiness, loss of coordination. Beta blocker heart drugs are prescribed for angina, to restore irregular heart beats to normal rhythm, and to help lower high blood pressure. Beta blocker brand names (generic names in parentheses):

Blocadren (timolol)
Corgard (nadolol)
Inderal (propranolol)
Lopressor (metoprolol)
Tenormin (atenolol)
Visken (pindolol)

DIABETES DRUGS (ORAL AND INSULIN)....COLD/COUGH PRODUCTS CONTAINING DECONGESTANT DRUGS

THE EFFECT OF THE DIABETES DRUG MAY BE ANTAGONIZED. RESULT: The blood sugar level may remain too high. Report symptoms of hyperglycemia (high blood sugar): excessive thirst, large urine output, weight loss, hunger, lethargy, drowsiness, loss of coordination. Be aware that nasal products can be absorbed into the bloodstream and may cause an interaction. Decongestant drugs listed on nonprescription cold/cough product labels (the same drugs are used in prescription-only cold/cough products):

ORAL (tablet, capsule, liquid):
    ephedrine
    methoxyphenamine
    phenylephrine
    phenylpropanolamine
    pseudoephedrine
NASAL (drops, spray, inhaler):
    oxymetazoline
    phenylephrine
    propylhexedrine
    xylometazoline

DIABETES DRUGS (ORAL AND INSULIN)....CORTICOSTEROIDS

THE EFFECT OF THE DIABETES DRUG MAY BE DECREASED. RESULT: The blood sugar level may remain too high.

Report symptoms of hyperglycemia (high blood sugar): excessive thirst, large urine output, weight loss, hunger, lethargy, drowsiness, loss of coordination. Corticosteroids are prescribed for arthritis, severe allergies, asthma, endocrine disorders, leukemia, colitis and enteritis (inflammation of the intestinal tract), and various skin, lung, and eye diseases. Corticosteroid drug brand names (generic names in parentheses):

Aristocort (triamcinolone)   Kenacort (triamcinolone)
Celestone (betamethasone)   Medrol (methylprednisolone)
Cortef (hydrocortisone)   Meticorten (prednisone)
Decadron (dexamethasone)   Orasone (prednisone)
Delta-Cortef (prednisolone)   prednisone (various companies)
Deltasone (prednisone)
hydrocortisone (various
   companies)

DIABETES DRUGS (ORAL AND INSULIN)
....DIET PILLS (NONPRESCRIPTION)
CONTAINING PHENYLPROPANOLAMINE

THE EFFECT OF THE DIABETES DRUG MAY BE ANTAGONIZED. RESULT: The blood sugar level may remain too high. Report symptoms of hyperglycemia (high blood sugar): excessive thirst, large urine output, weight loss, hunger, lethargy, drowsiness, loss of coordination. Phenylpropanolamine is a nasal decongestant drug used as the primary ingredient in the nonprescription diet pills because of its side effect of suppressing the appetite. NOTE: Many of these diet pills also contain caffeine. Nonprescription diet pill brand names:

Anorexin   E-Z Trim
Appedrine   P.P.A.
Appress   P.V.M.
Ayds (capsule, droplets)   Permathene-12
Coffee-Break   Pro Dax 21
Control   Prolamine
Dex-A-Diet II   Resolution
Dexatrim   Super Odrinex
Diadax   Ultra-Lean
Diet Gard   Vita-Slim
Dietac

DIABETES DRUGS (ORAL AND INSULIN)....DIURETICS

THE EFFECT OF THE DIABETES DRUG MAY BE AN-
TAGONIZED. RESULT: The blood sugar level may remain too
high. Report symptoms of hyperglycemia (high blood sugar):
excessive thirst, large urine output, weight loss, hunger, lethargy,
drowsiness, loss of coordination. Diuretics remove excess fluid
from the body and are used to treat high blood pressure and
congestive heart failure. Edecrin (ethacrynic acid) and Lasix
(furosemide) are not as likely to cause this interaction as the other
diuretic drugs listed below. The diuretic drugs taking part in this
interaction are called "potassium-losing" diuretics and the brand
names (generic names in parentheses) are:

Anhydron (cyclothiazide)
Aquatag (benzthiazide)
Aquatensin (methyclothiazide)
Diucardin (hydroflumethiazide)
Diulo (metolazone)
Diuril (chlorothiazide)
Edecrin (ethacrynic acid)
Enduron (methyclothiazide)
Esidrix (hydrochlorothiazide)
Exna (benzthiazide)
Hydrodiuril (hydrochlorothiazide)

Hydromox (quinethazone)
Hygroton (chlorthalidone)
Lasix (furosemide)
Metahydrin (trichlormethiazide)
Naqua (trichlormethiazide)
Naturetin (bendroflumethiazide)
Oretic (hydrochlorothiazide)
Renese (polythiazide)
Saluron (hydroflumethiazide)
Zaroxolyn (metolazone)

NOTE: The combination diuretic products listed below contain a "potassium-sparing" diuretic ingredient to offset the effect
of the "potassium-losing" ingredient, so these products may not
interact as significantly:

Aldactazide (spironolactone, hydrochlorothiazide)
Dyazide (triamterene, hydrochlorothiazide)
Moduretic (amiloride, hydrochlorothiazide)

DIABETES DRUGS (ORAL AND INSULIN)....
METHYLPHENIDATE (Ritalin)

THE EFFECT OF THE DIABETES DRUG MAY BE AN-
TAGONIZED. RESULT: The blood sugar level may remain too
high. Report symptoms of hyperglycemia (high blood sugar):
excessive thirst, large urine output, weight loss, hunger, lethargy,
drowsiness, loss of coordination. Methylphenidate is prescribed

for hyperkinetic behavior and learning disorders in children, narcolepsy (uncontrollable desire to sleep), mild depression, and apathetic or withdrawn senile behavior.

DIABETES DRUGS (ORAL AND INSULIN)....PEMOLINE (Cylert)

THE EFFECT OF THE DIABETES DRUG MAY BE ANTAGONIZED. RESULT: The blood sugar level may remain too high. Report symptoms of hyperglycemia (high blood sugar): excessive thirst, large urine output, weight loss, hunger, lethargy, drowsiness, loss of coordination. Pemoline is prescribed for hyperkinetic behavior and learning disorders.

DIABETES DRUGS (ORAL)....PHENYTOIN (Dilantin)

THE EFFECT OF THE DIABETES DRUG MAY BE ANTAGONIZED. RESULT: The blood sugar level may remain too high. Report symptoms of hyperglycemia (high blood sugar): excessive thirst, large urine output, weight loss, hunger, lethargy, drowsiness, loss of coordination. Phenytoin is prescribed to control seizures in disorders such as epilepsy. Other interacting phenytoin-type drugs are Mesantoin (mephenytoin) and Peganone (ethotoin).

DIABETES DRUGS (ORAL)....RIFAMPIN (Rifadin, Rimactane)

THE EFFECT OF THE DIABETES DRUG MAY BE DECREASED. RESULT: The blood sugar level may remain too high. Report symptoms of hyperglycemia (high blood sugar): excessive thirst, large urine output, weight loss, hunger, lethargy, drowsiness, loss of coordination. Rifampin is used to treat tuberculosis and may be given to suspected meningitis carriers.

DIABETES DRUGS (ORAL AND INSULIN)....THYROID DRUGS

THE EFFECT OF THE DIABETES DRUG MAY BE ANTAGONIZED. RESULT: The blood sugar level may remain too high. Report symptoms of hyperglycemia (high blood sugar): excessive thirst, large urine output, weight loss, hunger, lethargy, drowsiness, loss of coordination. Thyroid hormone is prescribed as thyroid replacement therapy to correct hypothyroidism (insufficient function of the thyroid gland) or goiter (enlargement of the thyroid gland). Thyroid drug brand names (generic names in parentheses):

Armour thyroid (thyroid)
Cytomel (liothyronine)
Euthroid (liotrix)
Levothroid (levothyroxine)

Proloid (thyroglobulin)
Synthroid (levothyroxine)
Thyrar (thyroid)
Thyrolar (liotrix)

12

Drug Interactions in Diarrhea Treatment

Diarrhea is characterized by the frequent passage of unformed or watery stools, often accompanied by cramps or abdominal pain. Acute diarrhea is self-limiting, lasting no longer than one to three days. It may be caused by a bacterial or viral infection, or spoiled food carrying *Salmonella* or other bacteria. Diarrhea sometimes occurs during antibiotic treatment, which will destroy normal "protective" intestinal bacteria along with the infection being treated. In travelers' diarrhea, the normal intestinal bacterial balance is altered by food and drink containing unfamiliar microorganisms.

Nonprescription products for diarrhea contain either *adsorbents* or *adsorbents* and *paregoric* combined. *Adsorbents* "bind" bacteria and toxins so they can be transported through the intestines and excreted in the stool. Adsorbents used in diarrhea products include activated attapulgite, activated charcoal, bismuth salts, kaolin, and pectin. *Paregoric* offsets diarrhea by slowing intestinal motility or movement, providing more time for the formation of a solid stool. You must sign a narcotics registry book when you purchase a paregoric-containing product.

Prescription-only drugs to relieve diarrhea are diphenoxylate and loperamide. These narcotic-like drugs slow intestinal motility or movement, thus providing more time for the formation of a solid stool.

BRAND NAMES

DIARRHEA PRODUCTS CONTAINING ADSORBENTS OR ADSORBENTS/PAREGORIC:

Diar-Aid	Donnagel
Digestalin	Donnagel-PG

| Kaopectate | Pepto-Bismol |
| Parepectolin | Polymagma |

PRESCRIPTION-ONLY PRODUCTS (in most states):

Imodium (loperamide)
Lomotil (diphenoxylate)

DRUG INTERACTIONS

ADSORBENTS....DIGOXIN (Lanoxin)

THE EFFECT OF DIGOXIN MAY BE DECREASED. Adsorbents decrease the body's ability to absorb digoxin. Digoxin is used to treat congestive heart failure or to restore irregular heart beats to normal rhythm. RESULT: The conditions treated may not be controlled properly. To prevent this interaction, do not take an adsorbent within two hours of taking digoxin.

ADSORBENTS....CLINDAMYCIN (Cleocin) and LINCOMYCIN (Lincocin)

THE EFFECT OF CLINDAMYCIN AND LINCOMYCIN MAY BE DECREASED. Adsorbents decrease the body's ability to absorb these two drugs. Clindamycin and Lincomycin are antibiotics reserved for treatment of certain types of serious infections for which the penicillin antibiotics are inappropriate or for patients allergic to penicillin. RESULT: The infection treated may not be cured. To prevent or minimize this interaction, do not take an adsorbent within three or four hours of taking either antibiotic.

DIPHENOXYLATE (Lomotil)....DIGOXIN (Lanoxin)

THE EFFECT OF DIGOXIN MAY BE INCREASED. By slowing intestinal movement, diphenoxylate increases the body's absorption of digoxin. Digoxin is used to treat congestive heart failure or to restore irregular heart beats to normal rhythm. RESULT: Possible adverse side effects caused by too much digoxin. Report symptoms such as nausea, headache, loss of appetite, visual disturbances, confusion, loss of energy, bradycardia (slow heart beat) or tachycardia (rapid heart beat), cardiac arrhythmias (heart beat irregularities). Using a fast-dissolving brand of digoxin such as Lanoxin minimizes this interaction.

LOPERAMIDE (Imodium)....DIGOXIN (Lanoxin)

THE EFFECT OF DIGOXIN MAY BE INCREASED. By slowing intestinal movement, loperamide increases the body's absorption of digoxin. Digoxin is used to treat congestive heart failure or to restore irregular heart beats to normal rhythm. RESULT: Possible adverse side effects caused by too much digoxin. Report symptoms such as nausea, headache, loss of appetite, visual disturbances, confusion, loss of energy, bradycardia (slow heart beat) or tachycardia (rapid heart beat), cardiac arrhythmias (heart beat irregularities). Using a fast-dissolving brand of digoxin such as Lanoxin minimizes this interaction.

PAREGORIC....DIGOXIN (Lanoxin)

THE EFFECT OF DIGOXIN MAY BE INCREASED. By slowing intestinal movement, paregoric increases the body's absorption of digoxin. Digoxin is used to treat congestive heart failure or to restore irregular heart beats to normal rhythm. RESULT: Possible adverse side effects caused by too much digoxin. Report symptoms such as nausea, headache, loss of appetite, visual disturbances, confusion, loss of energy, bradycardia (slow heart beat) or tachycardia (rapid heart beat), cardiac arrhythmias (heart beat irregularities). Using a fast-dissolving brand of digoxin such as *Lanoxin* minimizes this interaction.

13

Drug Interactions in Treatment of Epilepsy and Seizure Disorders

An epileptic seizure results from a "short-circuit" in a part of the brain—a nerve discharge which spills over to other nerves in that area, sometimes causing spasmodic limb and body movements and alterations in consciousness.

Grand mal epilepsy is the seizure disorder most associated with epilepsy. The seizure—sometimes presaged by a distinct smell or odor or some other sensation—begins suddenly and causes jerking of the arms and legs, chewing or gnawing of the teeth, and arching of the neck. The seizure usually runs its course and subsides. The main danger to the victim is from falling, biting the tongue, or choking on saliva or vomit.

Petit mal or "absence" seizure is a sudden loss of awareness of the surroundings—the sufferer may stare blankly ahead for a few seconds, often making random, purposeless movements.

Psychomotor seizures originate in the temporal lobe of the brain and cause a variety of physical and mental effects, usually followed by amnesia about the attack. Psychomotor seizures may presage a grand mal episode.

Flashing lights—such as from a flickering TV screen or computer video game—can precipitate seizures in seizure-prone individuals.

Anticonvulsant drugs are prescribed to prevent seizures. Several types of drugs have anticonvulsant action—including barbiturates and some tranquilizers. This chapter focuses on the drugs used primarily as anticonvulsants.

BRAND NAMES

ANTICONVULSANT DRUGS:

Depakene (valproic acid)
Dilantin (phenytoin)
Mesantoin (mephenytoin)
Mysoline (primidone)

Peganone (ethotoin)
Tegretol (carbamazepine)
Tridione (trimethadione)
Zarontin (ethosuximide)

DRUG INTERACTIONS

I. ANTICONVULSANT DRUG FAMILY INTERACTIONS
(These apply to *all* the anticonvulsant drugs)

ANTICONVULSANTS....OTHER DEPRESSANT DRUGS

The anticonvulsants are central nervous system depressants. They depress or impair functions such as coordination and alertness. Excessive depression or impairment can occur when an anticonvulsant is taken with any other central nervous system depressant. RESULT: Drowsiness, dizziness, loss of muscle coordination and mental alertness; in severe cases, failure of blood circulation and breathing functions causing coma and death. The physician should monitor the patient carefully and adjust the dosages to minimize the excessive depressant effects. Interacting depressant categories and brand names:

ALCOHOL (beer, liquor, wine, etc.)
ANTICHOLINERGICS—Uses and brand names:
> Those used to control tremors resulting from Parkinson's disease or from treatment with antipsychotic drugs—Akineton, Artane, Cogentin, Kemadrin, Pagitane.

> Others—Norflex—a muscle relaxant, Robinul—used for stomach, digestive tract disorders, Transderm-Scop—used for motion sickness.

ANTIHISTAMINES (Used for allergies, colds). Brand names:
> Actidil, Antivert, Atarax, Benadryl, Bendectin, Bonine, Chlor-Trimeton, Clistin, Decapryn, Dimetane, Dramamine, Histadyl, Inhiston, Marezine, Optimine, PBZ, Periactin, Polaramine, Pyronil, Travist, Teldrin, Triten, Vistaril

FENFLURAMINE (Pondimin)—a diet pill
HIGH BLOOD PRESSURE DRUGS—brand names in parentheses:

clonidine (Catapres, Combipres)
guanabenz (Wytensin)
methyldopa (Aldoclor, Aldomet, Aldoril)
reserpine-type drugs:
   deserpidine (Enduronyl, Harmonyl, Oreticyl)
   rauwolfia (Raudixin, Rauzide)
   reserpine (Diupres, Diutensen-R, Hydropres, Rau-Sed, Re-groton, Renese-R, Reserpoid, Salutensin, Sandril, Ser-Ap-Es, Serpasil, Serpasil-Apresoline, Serpasil-Esidrix)

MUSCLE RELAXANTS
Dantrium, Flexeril, Lioresal, Norflex, Norgesic, Norgesic Forte, Paraflex, Parafon Forte, Quinamm, Rela, Robaxin, Robaxisal, Skelaxin, Soma, Soma Compound, Valium

NARCOTICS
Codeine products: Ascriptin w/Codeine, Bancap w/Codeine, Bufferin w/Codeine, Empirin w/Codeine, Empracet w/Codeine, Fiorinal w/Codeine, Phenaphen w/Codeine, Tylenol w/Codeine
Other narcotic or narcotic-like products: Demerol, Dilaudid, Dolophene, morphine, Merpergan Fortis, Norcet, Numorphan, Percocet, Percodan, Synalgos-DC, Talwin, Talwin Compound, Tylox, Vicodan, Zactane, Zactirin

PROPOXYPHENE (pain reliever):
Darvocet-N, Darvon, Dolene, Wygesic

SLEEPING PILLS
Barbiturate sleeping pills: phenobarbital, Alurate, Amytal, Butisol, Buticap, Carbrital, Eskabarb, Lotusate, Luminal, Mebaral, Nembutal, Seconal, Sedadrops, Solfoton, Tuinal
Non-Barbiturate Sleeping pills: Ativan (also used as a tran-quilizer), Dalmane, Doriden, Halcion, Noctec, Noludar, Parest, Placidyl, Quaalude, Restoril, Somnos, Triclos, Valmid

TRANQUILIZERS
Benzodiazepine tranquilizers (the most widely used): Ativan, Centrax, Librium, Limbitrol (also an antidepressant), Paxipam, Serax, SK-Lygen, Tranxene, Valium, Xanax
Non-Benzodiazepine Tranquilizers: Atarax, Equanil, meproba-mate, Meprospan, Meprotab, Miltown, Trancopal, Tybatran, Vistaril

ANTICONVULSANTS....ANTIDEPRESSANTS (CYCLIC TYPE)

THIS COMBINATION MAY BE MUTUALLY ANTAG-ONISTIC. Antidepressants are prescribed to alleviate mental depression and elevate the mood. RESULT: Antidepressants can aggravate seizures and therefore decrease the effect of anticonvulsants; and anticonvulsants can lessen the effect of antidepressants in controlling depression. NOTE: The antidepressant trazadone (Desyrel) may not interact except in the following part of this interaction: Since these drugs are both central nervous system depressants, excessive *physical* depression can occur with symptoms such as drowsiness, dizziness, loss of coordination and mental alertness. Antidepressant brand names (generic names in parentheses):

Adapin (doxepin)
Asendin (amoxapine)
Aventyl (nortriptylene)
Desyrel (trazadone)
Elavil (amitriptyline)
Endep (amitriptyline)
Etrafon (amitriptyline/
   perphenazine)
Limbitrol (amitriptyline/
   chlordiazepoxide)
Ludiomil (maprotiline)

Norpramin (desipramine)
Pamelor (nortriptyline)
Pertofrane (desipramine)
Sinequan (doxepin)
Surmontil (trimipramine)
Tofranil, Tofranil-PM
   (imipramine)
Triavil (amitriptyline/
   perphenazine)
Vivactil (protriptyline)

ANTICONVULSANTS....ANTIPSYCHOTICS

THE EFFECT OF THE ANTICONVULSANT MAY BE DECREASED. RESULT: The seizure disorder may not be controlled properly. Since these drugs are both central nervous system depressants, additive depression can occur with symptoms such as drowsiness, dizziness, loss of coordination and mental alertness. Antipsychotics are major tranquilizers used to treat severe mental disorders such as schizophrenia. Most antipsychotics are of the phenothiazine type. Antipsychotic brand names (generic names in parentheses):

PHENOTHIAZINES
   Compazine (prochlorperazine)
   Mellaril (thioridazine)
   Proketazine (carphenazine)
   Prolixin (fluphenazine)
   Quide (piperacetazine)
   Serentil (mesoridazine)
   Sparine (promazine)
   Stelazine (trifluoperazine)

Thorazine (chlorpromazine)
Tindal (acetophenazine)
Trilafon (perphenazine)
Vesprin (triflupromazine).
OTHERS:
Haldol (haloperidol)
Loxitane (loxapine)
Moban (molindone)
Navane (thiothixene)
Taractan (chlorprothixene).

ANTICONVULSANTS.. ..BIRTH CONTROL PILLS (oral contraceptives)

A. THE EFFECT OF THE BIRTH CONTROL PILL MAY BE DECREASED. RESULT: Approximately twenty-five times increased risk of pregnancy unless an alternate method of contraception is used. Breakthrough bleeding is a symptom of a possible interaction.

B. THE EFFECT OF THE ANTICONVULSANT MAY BE DECREASED. RESULT: The seizure disorder may not be controlled properly. Birth control pill brand names:

Brevicon	Nordette
Demulen	Norinyl
Enovid	Norlestrin
Loestrin	Ortho-Novum
Lo-Ovral	Ovcon
Micronor	Ovral
Modicon	Ovrette
Nor-Q.D.	Ovulen

ANTICONVULSANTS....ESTROGENS (female hormones)

A. THE EFFECT OF THE ESTROGEN MAY BE DECREASED. Estrogens are prescribed for estrogen deficiency during menopause and after hysterectomy (surgical removal of the uterus), to prevent painful swelling of the breasts after pregnancy in women choosing not to nurse, and to treat amenorrhea (failure to menstruate). RESULT: The conditions treated may not be controlled properly.

B. THE EFFECT OF THE ANTICONVULSANT MAY BE DECREASED. RESULT: The seizure disorder may not be controlled properly. Estrogen brand names:

Amen   Menrium
Aygestin   Milprem
DES   Norlutate
Estinyl   Norlutin
Estrace   Ogen
Estratab   PMB
Estrovis   Premarin
Evex   Provera
Feminone   Tace
Menest

II. INDIVIDUAL ANTICONVULSANT DRUG INTERACTIONS
(These apply only to the specific drug listed)

A. CARBAMAZEPINE (Tegretol) INTERACTIONS:

*CARBAMAZEPINE (Tegretol)....ANTICOAGULANTS

THE EFFECT OF THE ANTICOAGULANT MAY BE DECREASED. Anticoagulants are prescribed to thin the blood and prevent it from clotting. RESULT: The blood may clot despite anticoagulant treatment. Anticoagulant brand names (generic names in parentheses):

Athrombin-K (warfarin)   Hedulin (phenindione)
Coufarin (warfarin)   Liquamar (phenprocoumon)
Coumadin (warfarin)   Miradon (anisindione)
dicumarol (various companies)   Panwarfin (warfarin)

CARBAMAZEPINE (Tegretol)....DOXYCYCLINE (Doxychel, Vibramycin, Vibratab)

THE EFFECT OF DOXYCYCLINE MAY BE DECREASED. Doxycycline is an antibiotic used to combat infection. RESULT: The infection may not respond to the doxycycline treatment unless the dosage is raised.

CARBAMAZEPINE (Tegretol) ....ERYTHROMYCIN ANTIBIOTICS

THE EFFECT OF CARBAMAZEPINE MAY BE INCREASED. RESULT: Possible adverse side effects from too much carbamazepine. Report symptoms such as nausea, dizziness, loss of coordination, abdominal pain. Erythromycin is an antibiotic used to combat infection. Erythromycin brand names:

Bristamycin
E.E.S.
E-Mycin
Ery-Tab
Eryc
Erypar
EryPed

Ethril
Ilosone
Ilotycin
Pediamycin
Robimycin
Wyamycin S

CARBAMAZEPINE (Tegretol)....METHADONE (Dolophine)

THE EFFECT OF METHADONE MAY BE DECREASED. Methadone is a narcotic pain reliever used to help free addicts from their dependence on heroin or other narcotics. RESULT: The addiction may not be controlled properly.

CARBAMAZEPINE (Tegretol)....PROPOXYPHENE

THE EFFECT OF CARBAMAZEPINE MAY BE IN-CREASED. RESULT: Possible adverse side effects from too much carbamazepine. Report symptoms such as nausea, dizziness, loss of coordination, abdominal pain. Propoxyphene is a pain reliever. Propoxyphene brand names:

Darvocet-N
Darvon
Dolene
Wygesic

CARBAMAZEPINE (Tegretol)
....TROLEANDOMYCIN (TAO)

THE EFFECT OF CARBAMAZEPINE MAY BE IN-CREASED. RESULT: Possible adverse side effects from too much carbamazepine. Report symptoms such as nausea, dizziness, loss of coordination, abdominal pain. Troleandomycin is an antibiotic used to combat infection.

B. PHENYTOIN (Dilantin) INTERACTIONS
(Apply also phenytoin-type products Mesantoin, Peganone)

PHENYTOIN (Dilantin)....ALCOHOL (beer, liquor, wine, etc.)

THE EFFECT OF PHENYTOIN IS DECREASED. RE-SULT: The seizure disorder may not be controlled properly. Since both drugs are central nervous system depressants, watch for symptoms of excessive depression: drowsiness, dizziness, loss of coordination and mental alertness.

PHENYTOIN.... ANTICOAGULANTS

A. THE EFFECT OF PHENYTOIN MAY BE INCREASED. RESULT: Possible adverse side effects from too much Phenytoin. Report symptoms such as visual disorders, loss of coordination. This interaction occurs primarily with the anticoagulant dicumarol.

B. THE EFFECT OF THE ANTICOAGULANT MAY BE DECREASED. Anticoagulants are used to thin the blood and prevent it from clotting. RESULT: The blood may clot despite anticoagulant treatment. Anticoagulant brand names:

Athrombin-K (warfarin)   Hedulin (phenindione)
Coufarin (warfarin)   Liquamar (phenprocoumon)
Coumadin (warfarin)   Miradon (anisindione)
dicumarol (various companies)   Panwarfin (warfarin)

PHENYTOIN (Dilantin)
....ASTHMA DRUGS (THEOPHYLLINE FAMILY)

THE EFFECT OF PHENYTOIN MAY BE DECREASED. RESULT: The seizure disorder may not be controlled properly. Theophylline family asthma drug brand names (generic names in parentheses):

Accurbron (theophylline)   Sustaire (theophylline)
Bronkodyl (theophylline)   Theobid (theophylline)
Choledyl (oxtriphylline)   Theodur (theophylline)
Dilor (diphylline)   Theolair (theophylline)
Elixicon (theophylline)   Theophyl (theophylline)
Elixophyllin (theophylline)   Theovent (theophylline)
LaBID (theophylline)   Multi-ingredient products
Lufyllin (diphylline)   containing theophylline:
Quibron-T (theophylline)   Amesec, Asbron G,
Respbid (theophylline)   Brondecon, Marax,
Slo-Phyllin (theophylline)   Mudrane, Quibron, Tedral
Somophyllin (aminophylline)   SA
Somophyllin-T (theophylline)

PHENYTOIN (Dilantin)....BARBITURATES

THE EFFECT OF PHENYTOIN MAY BE DECREASED. RESULT: The seizure disorder may not be controlled properly. Barbiturates are sedatives or sleeping pills which also have anticonvulsant action. This interaction varies with the individual patient. In some patients, the effect of phenytoin is increased with larger barbiturate doses; in others, the effect of the barbiturate is increased. Since physicians often prescribe the barbiturate phenobarbital along with phenytoin for seizure control, blood levels should be monitored to determine the proper doses for each individual patient. NOTE: Primidone (Mysoline), also an anticonvulsant, interacts the same as phenobarbital. Barbiturate brand names:

phenobarbital	Luminal
Alurate	Mebaral
Amytal	Nembutal
Butisol	Seconal
Buticap	Sedadrops
Carbrital	Solfoton
Eskabarb	Tuinal
Lotusate	

PHENYTOIN (Dilantin)
....CHLORAMPHENICOL (Chloromycetin, Mychel)

THE EFFECT OF PHENYTOIN MAY BE INCREASED. RESULT: Possible adverse side effects from too much phenytoin. Report symptoms such as visual disorders, loss of coordination. Chloramphenicol is an antibiotic prescribed to combat infection.

PHENYTOIN (Dilantin)....CIMETIDINE (Tagamet)

THE EFFECT OF PHENYTOIN MAY BE INCREASED. RESULT: Possible adverse side effects from too much phenytoin. Report symptoms such as dizziness, drowsiness, visual disorders, loss of coordination. Cimetidine is prescribed for duodenal and gastric ulcers.

PHENYTOIN (Dilantin)....CORTICOSTEROIDS

THE EFFECT OF THE CORTICOSTEROID MAY BE DECREASED. Corticosteroids are used for arthritis, severe allergies, asthma, endocrine disorders, leukemia, colitis and enteritis (inflammation of the intestinal tract), and various skin, lung, and eye diseases. RESULT: The conditions treated may not be controlled properly. Corticosteroid brand names (generic names in parentheses):

Aristocort (triamcinolone)
Celestone (betamethasone)
Cortef (hydrocortisone)
Decadron (dexamethasone)
Delta-Cortef (prednisolone)
Deltasone (prednisone)

hydrocortisone (various companies)
Kenacort (triamcinolone)
Medrol (methylprednisolone)
Meticorten (prednisone)
Orasone (prednisone)
prednisone (various companies)

PHENYTOIN (Dilantin)....DIABETES DRUGS (ORAL)

THE EFFECT OF THE DIABETES DRUG MAY BE ANTAGONIZED. The diabetes drugs are used to lower the blood sugar level in diabetic patients. RESULT: The blood sugar level may remain too high. Report symptoms of hyperglycemia (high blood sugar): excessive thirst or hunger, large urine output, drowsiness, lethargy, loss of coordination. Diabetes drug brand names (generic names in parentheses):

Diabinese (chlorpropamide)
Dymelor (acetohexamide)
Orinase (tolbutamide)
Tolinase (tolazamide)

PHENYTOIN (Dilantin)....DISOPYRAMIDE (Norpace)

THE EFFECT OF DISOPYRAMIDE MAY BE DECREASED. Disopyramide is used to restore irregular heart beats to normal rhythm. RESULT: The heart beat irregularity may not be controlled properly.

*PHENYTOIN (Dilantin)....DISULFIRAM (Antabuse)

THE EFFECT OF PHENYTOIN MAY BE INCREASED. RESULT: Possible adverse side effects from too much phenytoin. Report symptoms such as visual disorders, loss of coordination. Disulfiram, a drug which interacts with alcohol to produce acute adverse side effects, is prescribed to discourage drinking in alcoholics.

PHENYTOIN (Dilantin)....DOXYCYCLINE (Doxychel, Vibramycin, Vibratab)

THE EFFECT OF DOXYCYCLINE MAY BE DECREASED. Doxycycline is an antibiotic used to combat infection. RESULT: The infection may not respond to the doxycycline treatment unless the dosage is raised.

PHENYTOIN (Dilantin)....FOLIC ACID (vitamin B₉)

THE EFFECT OF FOLIC ACID MAY BE DECREASED. Folic acid is one of the B-complex vitamins. RESULT: Possible folic acid deficiency. Be alert for symptoms such as loss of energy, uncommon memory lapses, pale complexion, nervousness and irritability, digestive tract symptoms. To counter the effects of this interaction, take a vitamin supplement containing about 1 mg of folic acid. Taking too much folic acid can, in some cases, decrease the effect of phenytoin—requiring larger doses of phenytoin to control the seizure disorder.

PHENYTOIN (Dilantin)....FUROSEMIDE (Lasix)

THE EFFECT OF FUROSEMIDE MAY BE DECREASED. Furosemide, a strong diuretic which removes excess fluid from the body, is used to treat high blood pressure and congestive heart failure. RESULT: The conditions may not be controlled properly.

*PHENYTOIN (Dilantin)....ISONIAZID (INH, Nydrazid)

THE EFFECT OF PHENYTOIN MAY BE INCREASED. RESULT: Possible adverse side effects from too much phenytoin. Report symptoms such as visual disorders, loss of coordination. Isoniazid is used to treat tuberculosis.

PHENYTOIN (Dilantin)....LEVODOPA (Dopar, Larodopa, Sinemet)

THE EFFECT OF LEVODOPA MAY BE DECREASED. Levodopa is prescribed to control the tremors and other symptoms of Parkinson's disease. RESULT: The condition may not be controlled properly.

PHENYTOIN (Dilantin)....METHADONE (Dolophine)

THE EFFECT OF METHADONE MAY BE DECREASED. Methadone is a narcotic pain reliever used to help free addicts from their dependence on heroin or other narcotics. RESULT: The addiction may not be controlled properly.

PHENYTOIN (Dilantin)....METHYLPHENIDATE (Ritalin)

THE EFFECT OF PHENYTOIN MAY BE INCREASED. RESULT: Possible adverse side effects from too much phenytoin. Report symptoms such as visual disorders, loss of coordination. Methylphenidate is used in hyperkinetic behavior and learning disorders in children; narcolepsy (uncontrollable desire to sleep); mild depression; apathetic or withdrawn senile behavior.

PHENYTOIN (Dilantin)....OXYPHENBUTAZONE (Tandearil)

THE EFFECT OF PHENYTOIN MAY BE INCREASED. RESULT: Possible adverse side effects from too much phenytoin. Report symptoms such as visual disorders, loss of coordination. Oxyphenbutazone is prescribed for acute inflammatory conditions such as arthritis, bursitis, and strains or sprains.

PHENYTOIN (Dilantin)....PHENYLBUTAZONE (Azolid, Butazolidin)

THE EFFECT OF PHENYTOIN MAY BE INCREASED. RESULT: Possible adverse side effects from too much phenytoin. Report symptoms such as visual disorders, loss of coordination. Phenylbutazone is prescribed for acute inflammatory conditions such as arthritis, bursitis, and strains or sprains.

PHENYTOIN (Dilantin)....QUINIDINE

THE EFFECT OF QUINIDINE MAY BE DECREASED. Quinidine is used to restore irregular heart beats to normal rhythm. RESULT: The condition may not be controlled properly. Quinidine brand names:

Cardioquin
Duraquin
Quinaglute Dura-Tabs

Quinidex Extentabs
Quinora

PHENYTOIN (Dilantin)....QUININE (Coco-Quinine, Quinamm, Quine)

THE EFFECT OF QUININE MAY BE DECREASED. Quinine is a nonprescription drug used to treat malaria and nighttime leg cramps. RESULT: The conditions may not be controlled properly.

PHENYTOIN (Dilantin)....SULFONAMIDE ANTIBIOTICS

THE EFFECT OF PHENYTOIN MAY BE INCREASED. RESULT: Possible adverse side effects from too much phenytoin. Report symptoms such as visual disorders, loss of coordination. Sulfonamide antibiotics are prescribed to combat infection, especially urinary tract infections. Sulfonamide antibiotic brand names (generic names in parentheses):

Azulfidine (sulfasalazine)— prescribed for ulcerative colitis
Bactrim (sulfamethoxazole/ trimethoprim)
Bactrim DS (sulfamethoxazole/ trimethoprim)
Gantanol (sulfamethoxazole)
Gantrisin (sulfisoxazole)

Renoquid (sulfacytine)
SK-Soxazole (sulfisoxazole)
Septra (sulfamethoxazole/ trimethoprim)
Septra DS (sulfamethoxazole/ trimethoprim)
Sulla (sulfameter)
Thiosulfil (sulfamethizole)

PHENYTOIN (Dilantin)....TRIMETHADIONE (Tridione)

THE EFFECT OF TRIMETHADIONE MAY BE DECREASED. Trimethadione is also an anticonvulsant used to control seizures. RESULT: Possible loss of seizure control unless dosages are adjusted. Since both drugs are central nervous system depressants, watch for symptoms of excessive depression: drowsiness, dizziness, loss of coordination and mental alertness.

PHENYTOIN (Dilantin)....VALPROIC ACID (Depakene)

THE EFFECT OF PHENYTOIN MAY BE INCREASED. RESULT: Possible adverse side effects from too much phenytoin. Report symptoms such as visual disorders, loss of coordination.

Valproic acid is also an anticonvulsant used to control seizures. Since both drugs are central nervous system depressants, watch for symptoms of excessive depression: drowsiness, dizziness, loss of coordination and mental alertness.

PHENYTOIN (Dilantin).... VITAMIN D

THE EFFECT OF VITAMIN D MAY BE DECREASED. RESULT: Possible vitamin D deficiency, causing rickets in children (bone deformity) or osteomalacia in adults (softening of bones, leading to deformity). To prevent this interaction, eat foods rich in vitamin D: vitamin D-fortified milk, fish, eggs; get sufficient exposure to ultraviolet light via sunlight or sunlamp; or, if okayed by your physician, take a vitamin D supplement (containing calcium).

C. PRIMIDONE (Mysoline) INTERACTIONS

PRIMIDONE (Mysoline).... ALCOHOL (beer, liquor, wine, etc.)

THE EFFECT OF PRIMIDONE MAY BE DECREASED. RESULT: The seizure disorder may not be controlled properly. Since both drugs are central nervous system depressants, watch for symptoms of excessive depression: drowsiness, dizziness, loss of coordination and mental alertness.

*PRIMIDONE (Mysoline).... ANTICOAGULANTS

THE EFFECT OF THE ANTICOAGULANT MAY BE DECREASED. Anticoagulants are prescribed to thin the blood and prevent it from clotting. RESULT: The blood may clot despite anticoagulant treatment. Anticoagulant brand names (generic names in parentheses):

    Athrombin-K (warfarin)
    Coufarin (warfarin)
    Coumadin (warfarin)
    dicumarol (various companies)
    Hedulin (phenindione)
    Miradon (anisindione)
    Panwarfin (warfarin)

PRIMIDONE (Mysoline)
....ASTHMA DRUGS (THEOPHYLLINE FAMILY)

THE EFFECT OF THE ASTHMA DRUG MAY BE DE-CREASED. Asthma drugs open lung air passages to make breathing easier in patients with asthma. RESULT: The asthma may not be controlled properly. Theophylline family asthma drug brand names (generic names in parentheses):

Accurbron (theophylline)
Bronkodyl (theophylline)
Choledyl (oxtriphylline)
Dilor (dyphylline)
Elixicon (theophylline)
Elixophyllin (theophylline)
LaBID (theophylline)
Lufyllin (dyphylline)
Quibron-T (theophylline)
Respbid (theophylline)
Slo-Phyllin (theophylline)
Somophyllin (aminophylline)
Somophyllin-T (theophylline)

Sustaire (theophylline)
Theobid (theophylline)
Theodur (theophylline)
Theolair (theophylline)
Theophyl (theophylline)
Theovent (theophylline)
   Multi-ingredient products
      containing theophylline:
      Amesec, Asbron G,
      Brondecon, Marax,
      Mudrane, Quibron, Tedral
      SA

PRIMIDONE (Mysoline)....BETA BLOCKER HEART DRUGS

THE EFFECT OF THE BETA BLOCKER MAY BE DE-CREASED. Beta blockers are used to treat high blood pressure, angina, and to restore irregular heart beats to normal rhythm. RESULT: The conditions may not be controlled properly. Beta blocker brand names (generic names in parentheses):

Blocadren (timolol)
Corgard (nadolol)
Inderal (propranolol)
Lopressor (metoprolol)
Tenormin (atenolol)
Visken (pindolol)

PRIMIDONE (Mysoline)....CORTICOSTEROIDS

THE EFFECT OF THE CORTICOSTEROID MAY BE DECREASED. Corticosteroids are used for arthritis, severe allergies, asthma, endocrine disorders, leukemia, colitis and enteritis (inflammation of the intestinal tract), and various skin, lung, and eye diseases. RESULT: The conditions treated may not be controlled properly. Corticosteroid brand names (generic names in parentheses):

Aristocort (triamcinolone)
Celestone (betamethasone)
Cortef (hydrocortisone)
Decadron (dexamethasone)
Delta-Cortef (prednisolone)
Deltasone (prednisone)
hydrocortisone (various
   companies)

Kenacort (triamcinolone)
Medrol (methylprednisolone)
Meticorten (prednisone)
Orasone (prednisone)
prednisone (various companies)

PRIMIDONE (Mysoline)....DIGITOXIN (Crystodigin, Purodigin)

THE EFFECT OF DIGITOXIN MAY BE DECREASED. Digitoxin is used to treat congestive heart failure and to restore irregular heart beats to normal rhythm. RESULT: The conditions may not be controlled properly.

PRIMIDONE (Mysoline)....DOXYCYCLINE (Doxychel, Vibramycin, Vibratab)

THE EFFECT OF DOXYCYCLINE MAY BE DECREASED. Doxycycline is an antibiotic used to combat infection. RESULT: The infection may not respond to treatment properly.

PRIMIDONE (Mysoline)....FOLIC ACID (vitamin B₉)

THE EFFECT OF FOLIC ACID MAY BE DECREASED. Folic acid is one of the B-complex vitamins. RESULT: Possible folic acid deficiency. Be alert for symptoms such as loss of energy, uncommon memory lapses, pale complexion, nervousness and irritability, digestive tract symptoms. To counter the effects of this interaction, take a vitamin supplement containing folic acid or eat a fresh fruit and a green leafy vegetable daily.

PRIMIDONE (Mysoline)....GRISEOFULVIN

THE EFFECT OF GRISEOFULVIN MAY BE DECREASED. Griseofulvin is an antifungal drug prescribed orally for fungal infections of the skin, hair, and fingernails and toenails.

RESULT: The infections may not respond to treatment properly. Griseofulvin brand names:

Fulvicin P/G
Fulvicin-U/F
Grifulvin V
Grisactin
Gris-PEG

PRIMIDONE (Mysoline)....METHADONE (Dolophine)

THE EFFECT OF METADONE MAY BE DECREASED. Methadone is a narcotic pain reliever used to help free addicts from their dependence on heroin or other narcotics. RESULT: The addictions may not be controlled properly.

PRIMIDONE (Mysoline)....PHENYTOIN (Dilantin)

THE EFFECT OF PHENYTOIN MAY BE DECREASED. Phenytoin is also an anticonvulsant used to control seizures. RESULT: The seizure disorder may not be controlled as expected. This interaction varies with the individual patient. In some patients, the effect of phenytoin is increased with larger primidone doses; in others, the effect of primidone may be increased.

PRIMIDONE (Mysoline)....QUINIDINE

THE EFFECT OF QUINIDINE MAY BE DECREASED. Quinidine is used to restore irregular heart beats to normal rhythm. RESULT: The condition may not be controlled properly. Quinidine brand names:

Cardioquin
Duraquin
Quinaglute Dura-Tabs
Quinidex Extentabs
Quinora

PRIMIDONE (Mysoline)....QUININE (Coco-Quinine, Quinamm, Quine)

THE EFFECT OF QUININE MAY BE DECREASED. Quinine is a nonprescription drug used to treat malaria and nighttime leg cramps. RESULT: The condition may not be controlled properly.

PRIMIDONE (Mysoline)....RIFAMPIN (Rifadin, Rimactane)

THE EFFECT OF PRIMIDONE MAY BE DECREASED.
RESULT: The seizure disorder may not be controlled properly.
Rifampin is used to treat tuberculosis and is given to suspected
carriers of meningitis.

PRIMIDONE (Mysoline)....VALPROIC ACID (Depakene)

THE EFFECT OF PRIMIDONE MAY BE INCREASED.
Valproic acid is also an anticonvulsant used to control seizures.
RESULT: Adverse side effects caused by too much primidone.
Report symptoms such as confusion, loss of coordination, excessive sedation, drowsiness, dizziness, loss of mental alertness.

D. TRIMETHADIONE (Tridione) INTERACTION

TRIMETHADIONE (Tridione)....PHENYTOIN (Dilantin)

THE EFFECT OF TRIMETHADIONE MAY BE DE-
CREASED. Phenytoin is also an anticonvulsant used to control
seizures. RESULT: Possible loss of seizure control unless dosages
are adjusted. Since both drugs are central nervous system depressants, watch for symptoms of excessive depression: drowsiness,
dizziness, loss of coordination and mental alertness.

E. VALPROIC ACID (Depakene) INTERACTIONS

VALPROIC ACID (Depakene)....PHENOBARBITAL

THE EFFECT OF PHENOBARBITAL MAY BE IN-
CREASED. Phenobarbital is a sedative or sleeping pill which also
has anticonvulsant action. RESULT: Since both drugs are central
nervous system depressants, watch for symptoms of excessive
depression: excessive sedation, drowsiness, dizziness, loss of coordination and mental alertness.

VALPROIC ACID (Depakene)....PHENYTOIN (Dilantin)

THE EFFECT OF PHENYTOIN MAY BE INCREASED.
RESULT: Possible adverse side effects from too much phenytoin.
Report symptoms such as visual disorders, loss of coordination.
Valproic acid is also an anticonvulsant used to control seizures.
Since both drugs are central nervous system depressants, watch

for symptoms of excessive depression: drowsiness, dizziness, loss of coordination and mental alertness.

VALPROIC ACID (Depakene)....PRIMIDONE (Mysoline)

THE EFFECT OF PRIMIDONE MAY BE INCREASED. Primidone is also an anticonvulsant used to control seizures. RESULT: Adverse side effects caused by too much primidone. Report symptoms such as confusion, loss of coordination, excessive sedation, drowsiness, dizziness, loss of mental alertness.

14

Drug Interactions in Treatment of Heart Disorders

The most common disorders of the heart are angina, heart beat irregularities (cardiac arrhythmias), and congestive heart failure.

Angina pain results when the heart itself does not receive enough oxygen-carrying blood. This happens when blood flow through coronary arteries becomes impeded, usually because of obstructive plaques lining the inside of these arteries. The discomfort is usually brought on in situations demanding more work by the heart, such as physical exertion and emotional stress.

Heart beat irregularities are disturbances in the heart's normal rhythm. The various types are fibrillation, flutter, palpitation (skipped beats), "premature beat," and paroxysmal tachycardia (episodes of very rapid heart beat).

Congestive heart failure occurs when the heart fails to pump blood out as fast as it comes in. This causes blood to back up and overfill the lungs, resulting in shortness of breath and accumulation of fluid in body tissues.

HEART DRUG CATEGORIES:

Angina drugs
Anti-arrhythmics
Beta blocker heart drugs
Calcium blocker heart drugs
Digitalis heart drugs
Diuretics

BRAND NAMES

ANGINA DRUGS

Angina drugs relieve angina pain by improving the supply of blood and oxygen to the heart. Angina drug brand names (generic names in parentheses):

Cardilate (erythrityl tetranitrate)
Duotrate (pentaerythritol tetranitrate)
Isordil (isosorbide dinitrate)
Nitro-BID (nitroglycerin)
Nitro-Dur (nitroglycerin, transmucosal)
Nitrodisc (nitroglycerin, transmucosal)
nitroglycerin (various companies)
Nitroglyn (nitroglycerin)
Nitrol ointment (nitroglycerin)
Nitrospan (nitroglycerin)
Nitrostat (nitroglycerin)
Pentritol (pentaerythritol tetranitrate)
Peritrate (pentaerythritol tetranitrate)
Persantine (dipyridamole)
Sorbitrate (isosorbide dinitrate)
Susadrin (nitroglycerin, transmucosal)
Transderm-Nitro (nitroglycerin, transmucosal)

ANTI-ARRHYTHMICS

These drugs restore irregular heart beats to normal rhythm.

Cardioquin (quinidine)
Duraquin (quinidine)
Norpace (disopyramide)
Procan (procainamide)
Pronestyl (procainamide)
Quinaglute Dura-Tabs (quinidine)
Quinidex Extentabs (quinidine)
quinidine (various companies)
Quinora (quinidine)

BETA BLOCKER HEART DRUGS

Beta blockers are the most versatile heart drugs. In addition to relieving angina pain and restoring irregular heart beats to normal rhythm, they are effective in lowering blood pressure. Beta blockers are finding other uses also, such as in the prevention of migraine headaches. Beta blocker brand names (generic names in parentheses):

Blocadren (timolol)
Corgard (nadolol)
Inderal (propranolol)
Lopressor (metroprolol)

Tenormin (atenolol)
Visken (pindolol)

CALCIUM BLOCKER HEART DRUGS

The calcium blockers are the newest development in heart drugs. They may relieve angina pain unresponsive to other treatment. Verapamil is effective against certain types of heart beat irregularities.

Calan (verapamil)
Cardizem (diltiazem)
Isoptin (verapamil)
Procardia (nifedipine)

DIGITALIS HEART DRUGS

Digitalis-type drugs improve the strength and efficiency of the heart and are used to treat congestive heart failure and to restore irregular heart beats to normal rhythm.

Crystodigin (digitoxin)
Digifortis (digitalis)
Lanoxin (digoxin)
Purodigin (digitoxin)

DIURETICS

Diuretics remove excess body fluid and are often used to treat congestive heart failure. NOTE: For diuretic brand names and interactions, see *High Blood Pressure* chapter.

DRUG INTERACTIONS

I. ANGINA DRUG/ANTI-ARRHYTHMIC DRUG INTERACTIONS

ANGINA DRUG/ANTI-ARRHYTHMIC DRUG....BETA BLOCKER HEART DRUGS

THIS COMBINATION MAY CAUSE THE BLOOD PRESSURE TO DROP TOO LOW. RESULT: Postural hypotension (sudden drop in blood pressure when changing positions, especially when rising after sitting or lying down) with associated symptoms: dizziness, weakness, faintness; a severe drop in blood pressure may cause seizures or shock. Beta blocker drugs are prescribed for angina, to restore irregular heart beats to normal, and to lower high blood pressure. Beta blocker brand names (generic names in parentheses):

Blocadren (timolol)
Corgard (nadolol)
Inderal (propranolol)
Lopressor (metoprolol)
Tenormin (atenolol)
Visken (pindolol)

ANGINA DRUG/ANTI-ARRHYTHMIC DRUG....DIURETIC DRUGS

THIS COMBINATION MAY CAUSE THE BLOOD PRESSURE TO DROP TOO LOW. RESULT: Postural hypotension (sudden drop in blood pressure when changing positions, especially when rising after sitting or lying down) with associated symptoms: dizziness, weakness, faintness; a severe drop in blood pressure may cause seizures or shock. Diuretics remove excess fluid from the body and are used to treat high blood pressure and congestive heart failure. Diuretic drug brand names (generic names in parentheses):

Aldactazide (spironolactone, hydrochlorothiazide)
Aldactone (spironolactone)
Anhydron (cyclothiazide)
Aquatag (benzthiazide)
Aquatensin (methyclothiazide)
Diucardin (hydroflumethiazide)
Diulo (metolazone)
Diuril (chlorothiazide)
Dyazide (triamterene, hydrochlorothiazide)
Dyrenium (triamterene)
Edecrin (ethacrynic acid)
Enduron (methyclothiazide)
Esidrix (hydrochlorothiazide)

Exna (benzthiazide)
Hydrodiuril (hydrochlorothiazide)
Hydromox (quinethazone)
Hygroton (chlorthalidone)
Lasix (furosemide)
Metahydrin (trichlormethiazide)
Midamor (amiloride)
Moduretic (amiloride, hydrochlorothiazide)
Naqua (trichlormethiazide)
Naturetin (bendroflumethiazide)
Oretic (hydrochlorothiazide)
Renese (polythiazide)
Saluron (hydroflumethiazide)
Zaroxolyn (metolazone)

ANGINA DRUG/ANTI-ARRHYTHMIC DRUG....HIGH BLOOD PRESSURE DRUGS

THIS COMBINATION MAY CAUSE THE BLOOD PRESSURE TO DROP TOO LOW. RESULT: Postural hypotension (sudden drop in blood pressure when changing positions, especially when rising after sitting or lying down) with associated symptoms: dizziness, weakness, faintness; a severe drop in blood pressure may cause seizures or shock. High blood pressure drugs are used to lower high blood pressure. High blood pressure drugs (brand names in parentheses):

> clonidine (Catapres, Combipres)
> guanabenz (Wytensin)
> guanethidine (Esimil, Ismelin)
> hydralazine (Apresoline, Ser-Ap-Es, Serpasil-Apresoline)
> methyldopa (Aldoclor, Aldomet, Aldoril)
> minoxidil (Loniten)
> prazosin (Minipress)
> reserpine-type drugs:
>> deserpidine (Enduronyl, Harmonyl, Oreticyl)
>> rauwolfia (Raudixin, Rauzide)
>> reserpine (Diupres, Diutensen-R, Hydropres, Rau-Sed, Regroton, Renese-R, Reserpoid, Salutensin, Sandril, Ser-Ap-Es, Serpasil, Serpasil-Apresoline, Serpasil-Esidrix)

ANGINA DRUG....ALCOHOL (beer, liquor, wine, etc.)

THIS COMBINATION MAY CAUSE THE BLOOD PRESSURE TO DROP TOO LOW. RESULT: Postural hypotension (sudden drop in blood pressure when changing positions, especially when rising after sitting or lying down) with associated symptoms: dizziness, weakness, faintness; a severe drop in blood pressure may cause seizures or shock. Limiting alcohol ingestion to small amounts minimizes this interaction.

ANGINA DRUG....VASODILATOR DRUGS

THIS COMBINATION MAY CAUSE THE BLOOD PRESSURE TO DROP TOO LOW. RESULT: Postural hypotension (sudden drop in blood pressure when changing positions, especially when rising after sitting or lying down) with associated symptoms: dizziness, weakness, faintness; a severe drop in blood pressure may cause seizures or shock. Vasodilators dilate the blood vessels and are used to treat problems associated with poor blood circulation, such as arteriosclerosis (hardening of the arteries). Vasodilator drugs (brand names in parentheses):

cyclandelate (Cyclospasmol)
ethaverine (Cebral, Ethaquin, Ethatab, Pavaspan)
isoxsuprine (Vasodilan)
nicotinyl alcohol (Roniacol)
nylidrin (Arlidin)
papaverine (Cerespan, Pavabid, Pavacap, Paverine, P-200, Therapav)
tolazoline (Priscoline)

ANTI-ARRHYTHMIC DRUG ....ANTIDEPRESSANTS (CYCLIC TYPE)

THIS COMBINATION MAY CAUSE ADVERSE EFFECTS ON THE HEART. RESULT: Possible cardiac arrhythmias (heart beat irregularities). Antidepressants are prescribed to alleviate mental depression and elevate the mood. NOTE: The antidepressant trazadone (Desyrel) may not interact. Antidepressant brand names (generic names in parentheses):

Adapin (doxepin)
Asendin (amoxapine)
Aventyl (nortriptyline)
Desyrel (trazadone)
Elavil (amitriptyline)
Endep (amitriptyline)
Etrafon (amitriptyline/
  perphenazine)
Limbitrol (amitriptyline/
  chlordiazepoxide)
Ludiomil (maprotiline)

Norpramin (desipramine)
Pamelor (nortriptyline)
Pertofrane (desipramine)
Sinequan (doxepin)
Surmontil (trimipramine)
Tofranil, Tofranil-PM
  (imipramine)
Triavil (amitriptyline/
  perphenazine)
Vivactil (protriptyline)

DISOPYRAMIDE (Norpace)....BENZTROPINE (Cogentin)

THIS COMBINATION MAY CAUSE EXCESSIVE "ANTI-CHOLINERGIC" EFFECTS. RESULT: dry mouth, blurry vision, dizziness, loss of coordination, stomach discomfort, constipation, difficult urination, possible toxic psychosis (disorientation, agitation, delirium). Benztropine is used to control tremors resulting from Parkinson's disease or from treatment with antipsychotic drugs.

DISOPYRAMIDE (Norpace)....BIPERIDEN (Akineton)

THIS COMBINATION MAY CAUSE EXCESSIVE "ANTI-CHOLINERGIC" EFFECTS. RESULT: dry mouth, blurry vision, dizziness, loss of coordination, stomach discomfort, constipation, difficult urination, possible toxic psychosis (disorientation, agitation, delirium). Biperiden is used to control tremors resulting from Parkinson's disease or from treatment with antipsychotic drugs.

DISOPYRAMIDE (Norpace)....CYCRIMINE (Pagitane)

THIS COMBINATION MAY CAUSE EXCESSIVE "ANTICHOLINERGIC" EFFECTS. RESULT: dry mouth, blurry vision, dizziness, loss of coordination, stomach discomfort, constipation, difficult urination, possible toxic psychosis (disorientation, agitation, delirium). Cycrimine is used to control tremors resulting from Parkinson's disease or from treatment with antipsychotic drugs.

DISOPYRAMIDE (Norpace)....DICYCLOMINE (Bentyl)

THIS COMBINATION MAY CAUSE EXCESSIVE "ANTICHOLINERGIC" EFFECTS. RESULT: dry mouth, blurry vision, dizziness, loss of coordination, stomach discomfort, constipation, difficult urination, possible toxic psychosis (disorientation, agitation, delirium). Dicyclomine is used in stomach and digestive tract disorders.

DISOPYRAMIDE (Norpace) ....DIPHENHYDRAMINE (Benadryl, Benylin)

THIS COMBINATION MAY CAUSE EXCESSIVE "ANTICHOLINERGIC" EFFECTS. RESULT: dry mouth, blurry vision, dizziness, loss of coordination, stomach discomfort, constipation, difficult urination, possible toxic psychosis (disorientation, agitation, delirium)). Diphenhydramine is an antihistamine used in products for allergy, cold, cough, and in nonprescription sleeping pills.

DISOPYRAMIDE (Norpace) ....GLYCOPYRROLATE (Robinul)

THIS COMBINATION MAY CAUSE EXCESSIVE "ANTICHOLINERGIC" EFFECTS. RESULT: dry mouth, blurry vision, dizziness, loss of coordination, stomach discomfort, constipation, difficult urination, possible toxic psychosis (disorientation, agitation, delirium). Glycopyrrolate is used in stomach and digestive tract disorders.

DISOPYRAMIDE (Norpace)....ISOPROPAMIDE (Combid)

THIS COMBINATION MAY CAUSE EXCESSIVE "ANTI-CHOLINERGIC" EFFECTS. RESULT: dry mouth, blurry vision, dizziness, loss of coordination, stomach discomfort, constipation, difficult urination, possible toxic psychosis (disorientation, agitation, delirium). Isopropamide is used in stomach and digestive tract disorders.

DISOPYRAMIDE (Norpace)....ORPHENADRINE (Norflex, Norgesic)

THIS COMBINATION MAY CAUSE EXCESSIVE "ANTI-CHOLINERGIC" EFFECTS. RESULT: dry mouth, blurry vision, dizziness, loss of coordination, stomach discomfort, constipation, difficult urination, possible toxic psychosis (disorientation, agitation, delirium). Orphenadrine is a muscle relaxant.

DISOPYRAMIDE (Norpace)....PHENYTOIN (Dilantin)

THE EFFECT OF DISOPYRAMIDE MAY BE DE-CREASED. RESULT: The heart beat irregularity may not be controlled properly. Phenytoin is used to control seizures in disorders such as epilepsy. Other interacting phenytoin-like drugs are Mesantoin (mephenytoin) and Peganone (ethotoin).

DISOPYRAMIDE (Norpace)....PROCYCLIDINE (Kemadrin)

THIS COMBINATION MAY CAUSE EXCESSIVE "ANTI-CHOLINERGIC" EFFECTS. RESULT: dry mouth, blurry vision, dizziness, loss of coordination, stomach discomfort, constipation, difficult urination, possible toxic psychosis (disorientation, agitation, delirium). Procyclidine is used to control tremors resulting from Parkinson's disease or from treatment with antipsychotic drugs.

DISOPYRAMIDE (Norpace)....PROPANTHELINE (Pro-Banthine)

THIS COMBINATION MAY CAUSE EXCESSIVE "ANTI-CHOLINERGIC" EFFECTS. RESULT: dry mouth, blurry vision, dizziness, loss of coordination, stomach discomfort, constipation, difficult urination, possible toxic psychosis (disorientation, agitation, delirium). Propantheline is used in stomach and digestive tract disorders.

DISOPYRAMIDE (Norpace)....RIFAMPIN (Rifadin, Rimactane)

THE EFFECT OF DISOPYRAMIDE MAY BE DE-CREASED. RESULT: The heart beat irregularity may not be controlled properly. Rifampin is used to treat tuberculosis and is given to suspected carriers of meningitis.

DISOPYRAMIDE (Norpace)....SCOPOLAMINE (Transderm-Scop)

THIS COMBINATION MAY CAUSE EXCESSIVE "ANTI-CHOLINERGIC" EFFECTS. RESULT: dry mouth, blurry vision, dizziness, loss of coordination, stomach discomfort, constipation, difficult urination, possible toxic psychosis (disorientation, agitation, delirium). Scopolamine is used for motion sickness.

DISOPYRAMIDE (Norpace) ....TRIHEXYPHENIDYL (Artane)

THIS COMBINATION MAY CAUSE EXCESSIVE "ANTI-CHOLINERGIC" EFFECTS. RESULT: dry mouth, blurry vision, dizziness, loss of coordination, stomach discomfort, constipation, difficult urination, possible toxic psychosis (disorientation, agitation, delirium). Trihexyphenidyl is used to control tremors resulting from Parkinson's disease or from treatment with antipsychotic drugs.

PROCAINAMIDE (Procan, Pronestyl) ....ACETAZOLAMIDE (Diamox)

THE EFFECT OF PROCAINAMIDE MAY BE IN-CREASED. RESULT: Too much procainamide can cause a fall in blood pressure; heart block (disruption in the nerve transmission required for proper heart beat); or a very serious heart beat irregularity called ventricular fibrillation. Acetazolamide is used to treat glaucoma and some seizure disorders.

PROCAINAMIDE (Procan, Pronestyl)....ANTACIDS

THE EFFECT OF PROCAINAMIDE MAY BE IN-
CREASED. RESULT: Too much procainamide can cause a fall in
blood pressure; heart block (disruption in the nerve transmission
required for proper heart beat); or a very serious heart beat
irregularity called ventricular fibrillation. Antacid brand names:

AlternaGel	Maalox
Delcid	Mylanta
Di-Gel	Riopan
Gelusil	WinGel
Kudrox	

PROCAINAMIDE (Procan, Pronestyl)....MILK OF MAGNESIA

THE EFFECT OF PROCAINAMIDE MAY BE IN-
CREASED. RESULT: Too much procainamide can cause a fall in
blood pressure; heart block (disruption in the nerve transmission
required for proper heart beat); or a very serious heart beat
irregularity called ventricular fibrillation. Milk of magnesia is a
laxative.

QUINIDINE....ACETAZOLAMIDE (Diamox)

THE EFFECT OF QUINIDINE MAY BE INCREASED.
RESULT: Too much quinidine can cause a fall in blood pressure;
heart block (disruption in the nerve transmission required for
proper heart beat); or a very serious heart beat irregularity called
ventricular fibrillation. Acetazolamide is used to treat glaucoma
and some seizure disorders.

QUINIDINE.... ANTACIDS

THE EFFECT OF QUINIDINE MAY BE INCREASED.
RESULT: Too much quinidine can cause a fall in blood pressure;
heart block (disruption in the nerve transmission required for
proper heart beat); or a very serious heart beat irregularity called
ventricular fibrillation. Antacid brand names:

AlternaGel	Maalox
Delcid	Mylanta
Di-Gel	Riopan
Gelusil	WinGel
Kudrox	

QUINIDINE....ANTICOAGULANTS

THE EFFECT OF THE ANTICOAGULANT MAY BE INCREASED. Anticoagulants are used to thin the blood and prevent it from clotting. RESULT: Increased risk of hemorrhage. Report symptoms such as bruising or bleeding anywhere on the body, black or tarry stools. Anticoagulant brand names (generic names in parentheses):

Athrombin-K (warfarin)   Hedulin (phenindione)
Coufarin (warfarin)   Liquamar (phenprocoumon
Coumadin (warfarin)   Miradon (anisindione)
dicumarol (various companies)   Panwarfin (warfarin)

QUINIDINE.... BARBITURATES

THE EFFECT OF QUINIDINE MAY BE INCREASED. RESULT: The heart beat irregularity may not be controlled properly. Barbiturate are used as sedatives or sleeping pills. Barbiturate brand names:

phenobarbital   Luminal
Alurate   Mebaral
Amytal   Nembutal
Butisol   Seconal
Buticap   Sedadrops
Carbrital   Solfoton
Eskabarb   Tuinal
Lotusate

QUINIDINE....BENZTROPINE (Cogentin)

THIS COMBINATION MAY CAUSE EXCESSIVE "ANTI-CHOLINERGIC" EFFECTS. RESULT: dry mouth, blurry vision, dizziness, loss of coordination, stomach discomfort, constipation, difficult urination, possible toxic psychosis (disorientation, agitation, delirium). Benztropine is used to control tremors resulting from Parkinson's disease or from treatment with antipsychotic drugs.

QUINIDINE....BIPERIDEN (Akineton)

THIS COMBINATION MAY CAUSE EXCESSIVE "ANTI-CHOLINERGIC" EFFECTS. RESULT: dry mouth, blurry vision, dizziness, loss of coordination, stomach discomfort, constipation, difficult urination, possible toxic psychosis (disorientation, agitation, delirium). Biperiden is used to control tremors resulting from Parkinson's disease or from treatment with antipsychotic drugs.

QUINIDINE....CYCRIMINE (Pagitane)

THIS COMBINATION MAY CAUSE EXCESSIVE "ANTICHOLINERGIC" EFFECTS. RESULT: dry mouth, blurry vision, dizziness, loss of coordination, stomach discomfort, constipation, difficult urination, possible toxic psychosis (disorientation, agitation, delirium). Cycrimine is used to control tremors resulting from Parkinson's disease or from treatment with antipsychotic drugs.

QUINIDINE....DICYCLOMINE (Bentyl)

THIS COMBINATION MAY CAUSE EXCESSIVE "ANTICHOLINERGIC" EFFECTS. RESULT: dry mouth, blurry vision, dizziness, loss of coordination, stomach discomfort, constipation, difficult urination, possible toxic psychosis (disorientation, agitation, delirium). Dicyclomine is used in stomach and digestive tract disorders.

QUINIDINE.... DIGOXIN (Lanoxin)

THE EFFECT OF DIGOXIN MAY BE INCREASED. Digoxin is used to treat congestive heart failure and to restore irregular heart beats to normal rhythm. RESULT: Possible adverse side effects from too much digoxin. Report symptoms such as nausea, visual disturbances, headache, loss of energy, loss of appetite, confusion, bradycardia (slow heart beat) or tachycardia (rapid heart beat), cardiac arrhythmias (heart beat irregularities). NOTE: Physicians who decide to prescribe these two heart drugs together should reduce the digoxin dosage by half and then adjust it thereafter as needed.

QUINIDINE....DIPHENHYDRAMINE (Benadryl, Benylin)

THIS COMBINATION MAY CAUSE EXCESSIVE "ANTICHOLINERGIC" EFFECTS. RESULT: dry mouth, blurry vision, dizziness, loss of coordination, stomach discomfort, constipation, difficult urination, possible toxic psychosis (disorientation, agitation, delirium). Diphenhydramine is an antihistamine used in products for allergy, cold, cough, and in nonprescription "sleeping pills."

QUINIDINE....GLYCOPYRROLATE (Robinul)

THIS COMBINATION MAY CAUSE EXCESSIVE "ANTICHOLINERGIC" EFFECTS. RESULT: dry mouth, blurry vision, dizziness, loss of coordination, stomach discomfort, constipation, difficult urination, possible toxic psychosis (disorientation, agitation, delirium). Glycopyrrolate is used in stomach and digestive tract disorders.

QUINIDINE....ISOPROPAMIDE (Combid)

THIS COMBINATION MAY CAUSE EXCESSIVE "ANTICHOLINERGIC" EFFECTS. RESULT: dry mouth, blurry vision, dizziness, loss of coordination, stomach discomfort, constipation, difficult urination, possible toxic psychosis (disorientation, agitation, delirium). Isopropamide is used in stomach and digestive tract disorders.

QUINIDINE....MILK OF MAGNESIA

THE EFFECT OF QUINIDINE MAY BE INCREASED. RESULT: Too much quinidine can cause a fall in blood pressure; heart block (disruption in the nerve transmission required for proper heart beat); or a very serious heart beat irregularity called ventricular fibrillation. Milk of magnesia is a laxative.

QUINIDINE....ORPHENADRINE (Norflex, Norgesic)

THIS COMBINATION MAY CAUSE EXCESSIVE "ANTICHOLINERGIC" EFFECTS. RESULT: dry mouth, blurry vision, dizziness, loss of coordination, stomach discomfort, constipation, difficult urination, possible toxic psychosis (disorientation, agitation, delirium). Orphenadrine is a muscle relaxant.

QUINIDINE....PHENYTOIN (Dilantin)

THE EFFECT OF QUINIDINE MAY BE DECREASED. RESULT: The heart beat irregularity may not be controlled properly. Phenytoin is used to control seizures in disorders such as epilepsy. Other interacting phenytoin-like drugs are Mesantoin (mephenytoin) and Peganone (ethotoin).

QUINIDINE....PRIMIDONE (Mysoline)

THE EFFECT OF QUINIDINE MAY BE DECREASED. RESULT: The heart beat irregularity may not be controlled properly. Primidone is used to control seizures in disorders such as epilepsy.

QUINIDINE....PROCYCLIDINE (Kemadrin)

THIS COMBINATION MAY CAUSE EXCESSIVE "ANTI-CHOLINERGIC" EFFECTS. RESULT: dry mouth, blurry vision, dizziness, loss of coordination, stomach discomfort, constipation, difficult urination, possible toxic psychosis (disorientation, agitation, delirium). Procyclidine is used to control tremors resulting from Parkinson's disease or from treatment with antipsychotic drugs.

QUINIDINE....PROPANTHELINE (Pro-Banthine)

THIS COMBINATION MAY CAUSE EXCESSIVE "ANTI-CHOLINERGIC" EFFECTS. RESULT: dry mouth, blurry vision, dizziness, loss of coordination, stomach discomfort, constipation, difficult urination, possible toxic psychosis (disorientation, agitation, delirium). Propantheline is used in stomach and digestive tract disorders.

QUINIDINE....RIFAMPIN (Rifadin, Rimactane)

THE EFFECT OF QUINIDINE MAY BE DECREASED. RESULT: The heart beat irregularity may not be controlled properly. Rifampin is used to treat tuberculosis and is given to suspected carrier of meningitis.

QUINIDINE....SCOPOLAMINE (Transderm-Scop)

THIS COMBINATION MAY CAUSE EXCESSIVE "ANTI-CHOLINERGIC" EFFECTS. RESULT: dry mouth, blurry vision, dizziness, loss of coordination, stomach discomfort, constipation, difficult urination, possible toxic psychosis (disorientation, agitation, delirium). Scopolamine is used for motion sickness.

QUINIDINE....TRIHEXYPHENIDYL (Artane)

THIS COMBINATION MAY CAUSE EXCESSIVE "ANTI-CHOLINERGIC" EFFECTS. RESULT: dry mouth, blurry vision, dizziness, loss of coordination, stomach discomfort, constipation, difficult urination, possible toxic psychosis (disorientation, agitation, delirium). Trihexyphenidyl is used to control tremors resulting from Parkinson's disease or from treatment with antipsychotic drugs.

II. BETA BLOCKER HEART DRUG INTERACTIONS

BETA BLOCKER....ALCOHOL (beer, liquor, wine, etc.)

THIS COMBINATION MAY CAUSE THE BLOOD PRESSURE TO DROP TOO LOW. RESULT: Postural hypotension (sudden drop in blood pressure when changing positions, especially when rising after sitting or lying down) with associated symptoms: dizziness, weakness, faintness; a severe drop in blood pressure may cause seizures or shock. Limiting alcohol ingestion to small amounts minimizes this interaction.

BETA BLOCKER....AMPHETAMINES

THE EFFECT OF THE BETA BLOCKER MAY BE ANTAGONIZED. RESULT: The disorders treated by the beta blocker may not be controlled properly. This combination can also cause a paradoxical dangerous increase in blood pressure with symptoms such as fever, headache, visual disturbances. Amphetamines are used as diet pills (this use is in disfavor); for behavior problems in children; and for narcolepsy (uncontrollable desire to sleep). Amphetamine brand names:

Benzedrine
Biphetamine
Delcobese
Desoxyn
Dexedrine
Didrex
Obetrol

BETA BLOCKER....ANGINA DRUGS/ANTI-ARRHYTHMIC DRUGS

THIS COMBINATION MAY CAUSE THE BLOOD PRES-SURE TO DROP TOO LOW. RESULT: Postural hypotension (sudden drop in blood pressure when changing positions, especially when rising after sitting or lying down) with associated symptoms: dizziness, weakness, faintness; a severe drop in blood pressure may cause seizures or shock.

ANGINA DRUG BRAND NAMES:
    Cardilate (erythrityl tetranitrate)
    Duotrate (pentaerythritol tetranitrate)
    Isordil (isosorbide dinitrate)
    Nitro-BID (nitroglycerin)
    Nitro-Dur (nitroglycerin, transmucosal)
    Nitrodisc (nitroglycerin, transmucosal)
    nitroglycerin (various companies)
    Nitroglyn (nitroglycerin)
    Nitrol ointment (nitroglycerin)
    Nitrospan (nitroglycerin)
    Nitrostat (nitroglycerin)
    Pentritol (pentaerythritol tetranitrate)
    Peritrate (pentaerythritol tetranitrate)
    Persantine (dipyridamole)
    Sorbitrate (isosorbide dinitrate)
    Susadrin (nitroglycerin, transmucosal)
    Transderm-Nitro (nitroglycerin, transmucosal)
ANTI-ARRHYTHMIC DRUG BRAND NAMES:
    Cardioquin (quinidine)
    Duraquin (quinidine)
    Norpace (disopyramide)
    Procan (procainamide)
    Pronestyl (procainamide)
    Quinaglute Dura-Tabs (quinidine)
    Quinidex Extentabs (quinidine)
    quinidine (various companies)
    Quinora (quinidine)

BETA BLOCKER....ANTACIDS

THE EFFECT OF THE BETA BLOCKER MAY BE DE-CREASED. RESULT: The heart condition treated may not be controlled properly. NOTE: The beta blocker metoprolol (Lopressor) does not interact. Antacid brand names:

AlternaGel   Maalox
Delcid   Mylanta
Di-Gel   Riopan
Gelusil   WinGel
Kudrox

BETA BLOCKER....ANTIDEPRESSANTS (MAOI TYPE)

THIS COMBINATION MAY CAUSE A SIGNIFICANT RISE IN BLOOD PRESSURE. Report symptoms such as heart beat irregularities, fever, headache, visual disturbances. MAOI depressants, used to alleviate mental depression and elevate the mood, are not used much since the development of the cyclic antidepressants such as Elavil and Sinequan. MAOI antidepressant brand names (generic names in parentheses):

Marplan (isocarboxazid)
Nardil (phenelzine)
Eutonyl (pargyline)
Parnate (tranylcypromine)

BETA BLOCKER....ANTIDEPRESSANTS (CYCLIC TYPE)

THE EFFECT OF THE BETA BLOCKER MAY BE DE-CREASED. RESULT: The heart condition may not be controlled properly. Antidepressants are used to alleviate mental depression and elevate the mood. NOTE: The antidepressant trazadone (Desyrel) may not interact. Antidepressant brand names (generic names in parentheses):

Adapin (doxepin)   Norpramin (desipramine)
Asendin (amoxapine)   Pamelor (nortriptyline)
Aventyl (nortriptyline)   Pertofrane (desipramine)
Desyrel (trazadone)   Sinequan (doxepin)
Elavil (amitriptyline)   Surmontil (trimipramine)
Endep (amitriptyline)   Tofranil, Tofranil-PM
Etrafon (amitriptyline/   (imipramine)
   perphenazine)   Triavil (amitriptyline/
Limbitrol (amitriptyline/   perphenazine)
   chlordiazepoxide)   Vivactil (protriptyline)
Ludiomil (maprotiline)

BETA BLOCKER....ANTIPSYCHOTIC DRUGS

THIS COMBINATION MAY CAUSE THE BLOOD PRESSURE TO DROP TOO LOW AND AN INCREASE IN THE EFFECT OF THE BETA BLOCKER. Report low blood pressure symptoms: dizziness, weakness, faintness. Report symptoms of too much beta blocker drug: bradycardia (slow heart beat), fatigue, cardiac arrhythmias (heart beat irregularities), asthma-like wheezing or difficulty breathing. Antipsychotics are "major" tranquilizers used to treat severe mental disorders such as schizophrenia. Most antipsychotics are of the phenothiazine type. Antipsychotic brand names (generic names in parentheses):

PHENOTHIAZINES:
    Compazine (prochlorperazine)
    Mellaril (thioridazine)
    Proketazine (carphenazine)
    Prolixin (fluphenazine)
    Quide (piperacetazine)
    Serentil (mesoridazine)
    Sparine (promazine)
    Stelazine (trifluoperazine)
    Thorazine (chlorpromazine)
    Tindal (acetophenazine)
    Trilafon (perphenazine)
    Vesprin (triflupromazine)
OTHERS:
    Haldol (haloperidol)
    Loxitane (loxapine)
    Moban (molindone)
    Navane (thiothixene)
    Taractan (chlorprothixene)

BETA BLOCKER....ASTHMA DRUGS (EPINEPHRINE FAMILY)

EACH DRUG ANTAGONIZES THE EFFECTS OF THE OTHER.

A. The asthma drugs are used to open lung air passages and make breathing easier in bronchial asthma. RESULT: Lung bronchial tubes may not be opened enough to relieve the asthmatic episode. NOTE: Beta blocker drugs which minimally antagonize epinephrine's effect on the lungs are Lopressor (metoprolol) and Tenormin (atenolol).

B. The beta blocker may not control the disorder treated. This combination may also cause a paradoxical dangerous increase in blood pressure with associated symptoms: fever, headache, visual disturbances.

Epinephrine family asthma drug brand names (generic names in parentheses):

Aerolone (isoproterenol)
Alupent (metaproterenol)
AsthmaNefrin (epinephrine)
Brethine (terbutaline)
Bricanyl (terbutaline)
Bronitin (epinephrine)
Bronkaid (epinephrine)
Dispos-a-Med (isoproterenol)
Duo-Medihaler (isoproterenol)
Ephedrine (various companies)

Isuprel (isoproterenol)
Medihaler-Epi (epinephrine)
Medihaler-Iso (isoproterenol)
Metaprel (metaproterenol)
Norisodrine (isoproterenol)
Primatene (epinephrine)
Proventil (albuterol)
Vapo-Iso-Solution (isoproterenol)
Ventolin (albuterol)

BETA BLOCKER....ASTHMA DRUGS (THEOPHYLLINE FAMILY)

THE EFFECT OF THEOPHYLLINE ON ASTHMA MAY BE ANTAGONIZED. Asthma drugs are used to open lung air passages and make breathing easier in asthmatic conditions. RESULT: Lung bronchial tubes may not be opened enough to relieve the asthmatic episode. NOTE: Beta blocker drugs which minimally antagonize epinephrine's effect on the lungs are Lopressor (metoprolol) and Tenormin (atenolol). Theophylline family asthma drug brand names (generic names in parentheses):

Accurbron (theophylline)
Bronkodyl (theophylline)
Choledyl (oxtriphylline)
Dilor (dyphylline)
Elixicon (theophylline)
LaBID (theophylline)
Lufyllin (dyphylline)
Quibron-T (theophylline)
Respbid (theophylline)
Slo-Phyllin (theophylline)
Somophyllin (aminophylline)
Somophyllin-T (theophylline)

Sustaire (theophylline)
Theobid (theophylline)
Theodur (theophylline)
Theophyl (theophylline)
Theovent (theophylline)
Theolair (theophylline)
Multi-ingredient products
   containing theophylline:
   Amesec, Asbron G,
   Brondecon, Marax,
   Mudrane, Quibron, Tedral
SA

BETA BLOCKER....BARBITURATES

THE EFFECT OF THE BETA BLOCKER MAY BE DE-CREASED. RESULT: The condition treated by the beta blocker may not be controlled properly. NOTE: The beta blockers Tenormin (atenolol) and Corgard (nadolol) do not interact. Barbiturates are used as sedatives or sleeping pills. Barbiturate brand names:

phenobarbital	Luminal
Alurate	Mebaral
Amytal	Nembutal
Butisol	Seconal
Buticap	Sedadrops
Carbrital	Solfoton
Eskabarb	Tuinal
Lotusate	

BETA BLOCKER....CALCIUM BLOCKER HEART DRUGS

THIS COMBINATION MAY HAVE ADVERSE EFFECTS ON THE HEART. When these two drugs are given together, the physician should carefully monitor the effects on the patient. The calcium blockers are given for certain types of angina. Calcium blocker brand names (generic names in parentheses):

Calan (verapamil)
Cardizem (diltiazem)
Isoptin (verapamil)
Procardia (nifedipine)

BETA BLOCKER....CIMETIDINE (Tagamet)

THE EFFECT OF THE BETA BLOCKER MAY BE IN-CREASED. RESULT: Possible adverse side effects from too much beta blocker. Report symptoms such as bradycardia (slow heart beat), fatigue, cardiac arrhythmias (heart beat irregularities), asthma-like wheezing or difficulty breathing. Cimetidine is prescribed for duodenal and peptic ulcers.

BETA BLOCKER....CLONIDINE (Catapres, Combipres)

THIS COMBINATION MAY CAUSE A "REBOUND" RISE IN BLOOD PRESSURE. This can occur when clonidine treatment is stopped suddenly—causing symptoms of high blood pressure crisis: restlessness and irritabiity, tremors, tachycardia (rapid heart beat), headache, nausea, fever, visual disturbances. Clonidine is used to treat high blood pressure.

BETA BLOCKER....COLD/COUGH PRODUCTS CONTAINING DECONGESTANT DRUGS

THE EFFECT OF THE BETA BLOCKER MAY BE AN-TAGONIZED. RESULT: The condition treated by the beta blocker may not be controlled properly. Be aware that decongestant nasal products can be absorbed into the bloodstream and may cause an interaction. Decongestant drugs listed on nonprescription cold/cough product labels (the same drugs are used in prescription-only cold/cough products):

ORAL (tablet, capsule, liquid):
  ephedrine
  methoxyphenamine
  phenylephrine
  phenylpropanolamine
  pseudoephedrine
NASAL (drops, spray, inhaler):
  oxymetazoline
  phenylephrine
  propylhexedrine
  xylometazoline

*BETA BLOCKER....DIABETES DRUGS

THIS COMBINATION CAN EITHER INCREASE OR DECREASE THE EFFECT OF THE DIABETES DRUG. RESULT: If INCREASED diabetes drug effect, the blood sugar level may fall too low. Report symptoms of hypoglycemia (low blood sugar), which will be even more pronounced with physical exertion or exercise: sweating, nervousness, faintness, weakness, confusion, cardiac arrhythmias (heart beat irregularities), tachycardia (rapid heart beat), loss of coordination, visual disturbances—be aware that taking the beta blocker drug can *hide* these warning symptoms. If DECREASED diabetes drug effect, the blood sugar level may remain too high. Report symptoms of hyperglycemia (high blood sugar): excessive thirst, large urine output, weight loss, hunger, lethargy, drowsiness, loss of coordination. Beta blocker heart drugs are prescribed for angina, to restore irregular heart beats to normal rhythm, and to help lower high blood pressure. Diabetes drug brand names (generic names in parentheses):

Diabinese (chlorpropamide)
Dymelor (acetohexamide)
Orinase (tolbutamide)
Tolinase (tolazamide)
Insulin (several brands)

BETA BLOCKER....DIET PILLS (NONPRESCRIPTION) CONTAINING PHENYLPROPANOLAMINE

THE EFFECT OF THE BETA BLOCKER MAY BE ANTAGONIZED. RESULT: The condition treated by the beta blocker may not be controlled properly. Phenylpropanolamine is a nasal decongestant drug used as the primary ingredient in the nonprescription diet pills because of its side effect of supressing the appetite. NOTE: Many of these diet pills also contain caffeine. Nonprescription diet pill brand names:

Anorexin	Dietac
Appredrine	E-Z Trim
Appress	P.P.A.
Ayds (capsule, droplets)	P.V.M.
Coffee-Break	Permathene-12
Control	Pro Dax 21
Dex-A-Diet II	Prolamine Resolution
Dexatrim	Super Odrinex
Diadax	Ultra-Lean
Diet Gard	Vita-Slim

BETA BLOCKER....METHYLPHENIDATE (Ritalin)

THE EFFECT OF THE BETA BLOCKER MAY BE ANTAGONIZED. RESULT: The heart condition treated by the beta blocker may not be controlled properly. Methylphenidate is used in hyperkinetic behavior and learning disorders in children, narcolepsy (uncontrollable desire to sleep), mild depression, and apathetic or withdrawn senile behavior.

BETA BLOCKER....PRAZOSIN (Minipress)

THE BETA BLOCKER MAY INTENSIFY THE "FIRST DOSE" ADVERSE EFFECTS OF PRAZOSIN. Prazosin is used to lower the blood pressure. RESULT: Severe postural hypotension (sudden drop in blood pressure when changing positions, especially when rising after sitting or lying down) with associated symptoms: dizziness, weakness, faintness.

BETA BLOCKER....PRIMIDONE (Mysoline)

THE EFFECT OF THE BETA BLOCKER MAY BE DECREASED. RESULT: The condition treated by the beta blocker may not be controlled properly. NOTE: The beta blockers Tenormin (atenolol) and Corgard (nadolol) do not interact. Primidone is used to control seizures in disorders such as epilepsy.

BETA BLOCKER....RESERPINE-TYPE DRUGS

THE EFFECT OF EACH DRUG MAY BE INCREASED. Reserpine is used to treat high blood pressure. RESULT: Bradycardia (slow heart beat) and a fall in blood pressure. Report symptoms such as dizziness, weakness, faintness, postural hypotension (sudden drop in blood pressure when changing positions, especially when rising after sitting or lying down—with above symptoms). Reserpine-type drugs (brand names in parentheses):

deserpidine (Enduronyl, Harmonyl, Oreticyl)
rauwolfia (Raudixin, Rauzide)
reserpine (Diupres, Diutensen-R, Hydropres, Rau-Sed, Regroton, Renese-R, Reserpoid, Salutensin, Sandril, Ser-Ap-Es, Serpasil, Serpasil-Apresoline, Serpasil-Esidrix)

BETA BLOCKER....VASODILATOR DRUGS

THIS COMBINATION MAY CAUSE THE BLOOD PRESSURE TO DROP TOO LOW. RESULT: Postural hypotension (sudden drop in blood pressure when changing positions, especially when rising after sitting or lying down) with associated symptoms: dizziness, weakness, faintness; a severe drop in blood pressure may cause seizures or shock. Vasodilators dilate the blood vessels and are used to treat disorders associated with poor blood circulation, such as arteriosclerosis (hardening of the arteries). Vasodilator drugs (brand names in parentheses):

cyclandelate (Cyclospasmol)
ethaverine (Cebral, Ethaquin, Ethatab, Pavaspan)
isoxsuprine (Vasodilan)
nicotinyl alcohol (Roniacol)
nylidrin (Arlidin)
papaverine (Cerespan, Pavabid, Pavacap, Paverine, P-200, Therapav)
tolazoline (Priscoline)

III. DIGITALIS DRUG INTERACTIONS

A. DIGITALIS FAMILY INTERACTIONS
(Apply to digitalis, digitoxin, digoxin)

DIGITALIS FAMILY....ACETAZOLAMIDE (Diamox)

THIS COMBINATION CAN CAUSE ADVERSE EFFECTS ON THE HEART. Acetazolamide, used in glaucoma and certain seizure disorders, depletes the body of potassium. Lack of potassium makes the heart extra sensitive to digitalis and increases the risk of digitalis toxicity with associated symptoms: nausea, confusion, visual disturbances, headache, lack of energy, loss of appetite, bradycardia (slow heart beat), tachycardia (rapid heart beat), cardiac arrhythmias (heart beat irregularities). Be aware of symptoms of potassium loss: muscular weakness or cramps, large urine output, dizziness, faintness.

DIGITALIS FAMILY....AMPHETAMINES

THIS COMBINATION MAY CAUSE CARDIAC AR-RHYTHMIAS (HEART BEAT IRREGULARITIES). Amphetamines are used as diet pills (this use is in disfavor); for behavior problems in children; and for narcolepsy (uncontrollable desire to sleep). Amphetamine brand names:

Benzedrine
Biphetamine
Delcobese
Desoxyn
Dexedrine
Didrex
Obetrol

DIGITALIS FAMILY....ASTHMA DRUGS (EPINEPHRINE FAMILY)

THIS COMBINATION MAY CAUSE CARDIAC AR-RHYTHMIAS (HEART BEAT IRREGULARITIES). Asthma drugs are used to open lung air passages and make breathing easier in bronchial asthma. Epinephrine family asthma drug brand names (generic names in parentheses):

Aerolone (isoproterenol)
Alupent (metaproterenol)
AsthmaNefrin (epinephrine)
Brethine (terbutaline)
Bricanyl (terbutaline)
Bronitin (epinephrine)
Bronkaid (epinephrine)
Dispos-a-Med (isoproterenol)
Duo-Medihaler (isoproterenol)
Ephedrine (various companies)

Isuprel (isoproterenol)
Medihaler-Epi (epinephrine)
Medihaler-Iso (isoproterenol)
Metaprel (metaproterenol)
Norisodrine (isoproterenol)
Primatene (epinephrine)
Proventil (albuterol)
Vapo-Iso-Solution (isoproterenol)
Ventolin (albuterol)

DIGITALIS FAMILY....CHOLESTYRAMINE (Cuemid, Questran)

THE EFFECT OF DIGITALIS MAY BE DECREASED. RESULT: The heart disorder may not respond to treatment properly. Cholestyramine is used to lower blood levels of cholesterol. This interaction is prevented by not giving one drug within three hours of the other.

DIGITALIS FAMILY....COLD/COUGH PRODUCTS CONTAINING DECONGESTANT DRUGS

THIS COMBINATION MAY CAUSE CARDIAC AR-RHYTHMIAS (HEART BEAT IRREGULARITIES). Be aware that decongestant nasal products can be absorbed into the blood-stream and cause an interaction. Decongestant drugs listed on nonprescription cold/cough product labels (the same drugs are used in prescription-only cold/cough products):

ORAL (tablet, capsule, liquid):
  ephedrine
  methoxyphenamine
  phenylephrine
  phenylpropanolamine
  pseudoephedrine

NASAL (drops, spray, inhaler):
  oxymetazoline
  phenylephrine
  propylhexedrine
  xylometazoline

DIGITALIS FAMILY....CORTICOSTEROIDS

THIS COMBINATION CAN CAUSE ADVERSE EFFECTS ON THE HEART. Corticosteroids are used for arthritis, severe allergies, asthma, endocrine disorders, leukemia, colitis and enteritis (inflammation of the intestinal tract), and various skin, lung, and eye diseases. Corticosteroids deplete the body of potassium. Lack of potassium makes the heart extra sensitive to digitalis and increases the risk of digitalis toxicity with associated symptoms: nausea, confusion, visual disturbances, headache, lack of energy, loss of appetite, bradycardia (slow heart beat), tachycardia (rapid heart beat), cardiac arrhythmias (heart beat irrregularities). Be aware of symptoms of potassium loss: muscular weakness or cramps, large urine output, dizziness, faintness. Corticosteroid brand names (generic names in parentheses):

Aristocort (triamcinolone)
Celestone (betamethasone)
Cortef (hydrocortisone)
Decadron (dexamethasone)
Delta-Cortef (prednisolone)
Deltasone (prednisone)

hydrocortisone (various
  companies)
Kenacort (triamcinolone)
Medrol (methylprednisolone)
Meticorten (prednisone)
Orasone (prednisone)
prednisone (various companies)

DIGITALIS FAMILY....DIET PILLS (NONPRESCRIPTION) CONTAINING PHENYLPROPANOLAMINE

THIS COMBINATION MAY CAUSE CARDIAC ARRHYTHMIAS (HEART BEAT IRREGULARITIES). Phenylpropanolamine is a nasal decongestant drug used as the primary ingredient in the nonprescription diet pills because of its side effect of suppressing the appetite. NOTE: Many of these diet pills also contain caffeine. Nonprescription diet pill brand names:

Anorexin
Appedrine
Appress

Ayds (capsule, droplets)
Coffee-Break
Control

Dex-A-Diet II
Dexatrim
Diadax
Diet Gard
Dietac
E-Z Trim
P.P.A.
P.V.M.

Permathene-12
Pro Dax 21
Prolamine
Resolution
Super Odrinex
Ultra-Lean
Vita-Slim

DIGITALIS FAMILY....DIURETICS

THIS COMBINATION CAN CAUSE ADVERSE EFFECTS ON THE HEART. Diuretics remove excess body fluid and are prescribed for congestive heart failure and high blood pressure. Most diuretics depelete the body of potassium. Lack of potassium makes the heart extra sensitive to digitalis and increases the risk of digitalis toxicity with associated symptoms: nausea, confusion, visual disturbances, headache, loss of energy, loss of appetite, bradycardia (slow heart beat), tachycardia (rapid heart beat), cardiac arrhythmias (heart beat irregularities). Be aware of symtpoms of potassium loss: muscular weakness or cramps, large urine output, dizziness, faintness. The diuretics involved in this interaction are "potassium-losing" and brand names (generic names in parentheses) are:

Anhydron (cyclothiazide)
Aquatag (benzthiazide)
Aquatensin (methyclothiazide)
Diucardin (hydroflumethiazide)
Diulo (metolazone)
Diuril (chlorothiazide)
Edecrin (ethacrynic acid)
Enduron (methyclothiazide)
Esidrix (hydrochlorothiazide)
Exna (benzthiazide)
Hydrodiuril (hydrochlorothiazide)

Hydromox (quinethazone)
Hygroton (chlorthalidone)
Lasix (furosemide)
Metahydrin (trichlormethiazide)
Naqua (trichlormethiazide)
Naturetin (bendroflumethiazide)
Oretic (hydrochlorothiazide)
Renese (polythiazide)
Saluron (hydroflumethiazide)
Zaroxolyn (metolazone)

NOTE: The combination diuretic products listed below contain a "potassium-sparing" diuretic ingredient to offset the effect of the "potassium-losing" ingredient, so these products may not interact as significantly:

Aldactazide (spironolactone, hydrochlorothiazide)
Dyazide (triamterene, hydrochlorothiazide)
Moduretic (amiloride, hydrochlorothiazide)

DIGITALIS FAMILY....LAXATIVES

THIS COMBINATION CAN CAUSE ADVERSE EFFECTS ON THE HEART. Laxatives deplete the body of potassium. Lack of potassium makes the heart extra sensitive to digitalis and increases the risk of digitalis toxicity with associated symptoms: nausea, confusion, visual disturbances, headache, lack of energy, loss of appetite, bradycardia (slow heart beat), tachycardia (rapid heart beat), cardiac arrhythmias (heart beat irregularities). Be aware of symptoms of potassium loss: muscular weakness or cramps, large urine output, dizziness, faintness.

DIGITALIS FAMILY....LEVODOPA (Dopar, Larodopa, Sinemet)

THIS COMBINATION MAY CAUSE ADVERSE EFFECTS ON THE HEART. Levodopa, used to control the tremors and other symptoms of Parkinson's Disease, depletes the body of potassium. Lack of potassium makes the heart extra sensitive to digitalis and increases the risk of digitalis toxicity with associated symptoms: nausea, confusion, visual disturbances, headache, lack of energy, loss of appetite, bradycardia (slow heart beat), tachycardia (rapid heart beat), cardiac arrhythmias (heart beat irregularities). Be aware of symptoms of potassium loss: muscular weakness or cramps, large urine output, dizziness, faintness.

DIGITALIS FAMILY....METHYLPHENIDATE (Ritalin)

THIS COMBINATION MAY CAUSE CARDIAC ARRHYTHMIAS (HEART BEAT IRREGULARITIES). Methylphenidate is used in hyperkinetic behavior and learning disorders in children, narcolepsy (uncontrollable desire to sleep), mild depression, and apathetic or withdrawn senile behavior.

B. INDIVIDUAL DIGITALIS DRUG INTERACTIONS
(Apply only to the digitalis drug listed)

DIGITOXIN (Crystodigin, Purodigin)....BARBITURATES

THE EFFECT OF DIGITOXIN MAY BE DECREASED. RESULT: The heart condition treated by digitoxin may not be controlled properly. Barbiturates are used as sedatives or sleeping pills. Barbiturate brand names:

phenobarbital
Alurate
Amytal
Butisol
Buticap
Carbrital
Eskabarb
Lotusate

Luminal
Mebaral
Nembutal
Seconal
Sedadrops
Solfoton
Tuinal

DIGITOXIN (Crystodigin,Purodigin)....PRIMIDONE (Mysoline)

THE EFFECT OF DIGITOXIN MAY BE DECREASED. RESULT: The heart condition treated by digitoxin may not be controlled properly. Primidone is used to control seizures in conditions such as epilepsy.

DIGITOXIN (Crystodigin, Purodigin)....RIFAMPIN (Rifadin, Rimactane)

THE EFFECT OF DIGITOXIN MAY BE DECREASED. RESULT: The heart condition treated by digitoxin may not be controlled properly. Rifampin is used to treat tuberculosis and is given to suspected meningitis carriers.

DIGOXIN (Lanoxin)....ANTACIDS

THE EFFECT OF DIGOXIN MAY BE DECREASED. RESULT: The heart condition treated by digoxin may not be controlled properly. NOTE: Sodium bicarbonate antacids such as Alka-Seltzer do not interact. Antacid brand names:

AlternaGel
Delcid
Di-Gel
Gelusil
Kudrox

Maalox
Mylanta
Riopan
WinGel

DIGOXIN (Lanoxin)....CALCIUM BLOCKER HEART DRUGS

THE EFFECT OF DIGOXIN MAY BE INCREASED. RESULT: Possible adverse side effects from too much digoxin. Report symptoms such as nausea, confusion, visual disturbances, headache, lack of energy, loss of appetite, bradycardia (slow heart beat) or tachycardia (rapid heart beat), cardiac arrhythmias (heart beat irregularities). Calcium blockers are used for certain types of angina and heart beat irregularities. Calcium blocker brand names (generic names in parentheses):

Calan (verpamil)
Cardizem (diltiazem)
Isoptin (verapamil)
Procardia (nifedipine)

DIGOXIN (Lanoxin)
....DIARRHEA PRODUCTS CONTAINING ADSORBENTS

THE EFFECT OF DIGOXIN MAY BE DECREASED. RESULT: The heart condition treated by digoxin may not be controlled properly. Interacting Diarrhea products:

Diar-Aid	Kaopectate
Digestalin	Parepectolin
Donnagel	Pepto-Bismol
Donnagel-PG	Polymagma

DIGOXIN (Lanoxin)....ERYTHROMYCIN ANTIBIOTICS

THE EFFECT OF DIGOXIN MAY BE INCREASED. RESULT: Possible adverse side effects from too much digoxin. Report symptoms such as nausea, confusion, visual disturbances, headache, lack of energy, loss of appetite, bradycardia (slow heart beat), tachycardia (rapid heart beat), cardiac arrhythmias (heart beat irregularities). Erythromycin antibiotics are used to combat infection. Erythromycin brand names:

Bristamycin	Ethril
E.E.S.	Ilosone
E-Mycin	Ilotycin
Ery-Tab	Pediamycin
Eryc	Robimycin
Erypar	Wyamycin S
EryPed	

DIGOXIN (Lanoxin)....METHYLDOPA (Aldomet, Aldoril)

THIS COMBINATION MAY CAUSE ADVERSE EFFECTS ON THE HEART. Methyldopa is used to treat high blood pressure. Report symptoms such as bradycardia (slow heart beat), dizziness, faintness, confusion, forgetfulness.

DIGOXIN (Lanoxin)....METOCLOPRAMIDE (Reglan)

THE EFFECT OF DIGOXIN MAY BE DECREASED. RE-SULT: The heart condition treated by digoxin may not be controlled properly. Metoclopramide is used to combat vomiting.

DIGOXIN (Lanoxin)....NEOMYCIN (Oral—various companies)

THE EFFECT OF DIGOXIN MAY BE DECREASED. RE-SULT: The heart condition treated by digoxin may not be controlled properly. Neomycin is an antibiotic prescribed for certain types of diarrhea and other highly specific infections.

DIGOXIN (Lanoxin)....QUINIDINE

THE EFFECT OF DIGOXIN MAY BE INCREASED. RE-SULT: Possible adverse side effects from too much digoxin. Report symptoms such as nausea, visual disturbances, headache, loss of energy, loss of appetite, confusion, bradycardia (slow heart beat) or tachycardia (rapid heart beat), cardiac arrhythmias (heart beat irregularities). Quinidine is used to restore irregular heart beats to normal rhythm. NOTE: Physicians who decide to prescribe these two heart drugs together should reduce the digoxin dosage by half and then adjust it thereafter as needed. Quinidine brand names:

> Cardioquin
> Duraquin
> Quinaglute Dura-Tabs
> Quinidex Extentabs
> Quinora

DIGOXIN (Lanoxin)....QUININE (Coco-Quinine, Quinamm, Quine)

THE EFFECT OF DIGOXIN MAY BE INCREASED. RE-SULT: Possible adverse side effects from too much digoxin. Report symptoms such as nausea, visual disturbances, headache, loss of energy, loss of appetite, confusion, bradycardia (slow heart beat) or tachycardia (rapid heart beat), cardiac arrhythmias (heart beat irregularities). Quinine is a nonprescription drug used for malaria and nighttime leg cramps.

DIGOXIN (Lanoxin)....SPIRONOLACTONE (Aldactazide, Aldactone)

THE EFFECT OF DIGOXIN MAY BE INCREASED. RESULT: Possible adverse side effects from too much digoxin. Report symptoms such as nausea, visual disturbances, headache, loss of energy, loss of appetite, confusion, bradycardia (slow heart beat) or tachycardia (rapid heart beat), cardiac arrhythmias (heart beat irregularities). Spironolactone, a diuretic, removes excess fluid from the body and is used to treat congestive heart failure and high blood pressure.

DIGOXIN (Lanoxin)....SULFASALAZINE (Azulfidine)

THE EFFECT OF DIGOXIN MAY BE DECREASED. RESULT: The heart condition treated by digoxin may not be controlled properly. Sulfasalazine is prescribed for ulcerative colitis (inflammation of the large bowel or colon).

DIGOXIN (Lanoxin)....TETRACYCLINE ANTIBIOTICS

THE EFFECT OF DIGOXIN MAY BE INCREASED. RESULT: Possible adverse side effects from too much digoxin. Report symptoms such as nausea, confusion, visual disturbances, headache, lack of energy, loss of appetite, bradycardia (slow heart beat) or tachycardia (rapid heart beat), cardiac arrhythmias (heart beat irregularities). Tetracycline antibiotics are used to combat infection. Tetracycline brand names (generic names in parentheses):

Achromycin (tetracycline)
Aureomycin (chlortetracyline)
Bristacycline (tetracycline)
Cyclopar (tetracycline)
Declomycin (demeclocycline)
Doxychel (doxycycline)
Minocin (minocycline)
Panmycin (tetracycline)
Retet-S (tetracycline)
Robitet (tetracycline)

Rondomycin (methacycline)
Sumycin (tetracycline)
Terramycin (oxytetracycline)
Tetra-Bid (tetracycline)
Tetrachel (tetracycline)
tetracycline (various companies)
Tetracyn (tetracycline)
Tetrex (tetracycline)
Vibramycin (doxycycline)
Vibratab (doxycycline)

IV. CALCIUM BLOCKER INTERACTIONS

CALCIUM BLOCKER....BETA BLOCKER HEART DRUGS

THIS COMBINATION MAY CAUSE ADVERSE EFFECTS ON THE HEART. When these two drugs are given together, the physician should carefully monitor the effects on the patient. Beta blockers are used to treat heart disorders and for high blood pressure. Beta blocker brand names (generic names in parentheses):

Blocadren (timolol)
Corgard (nadolol)
Inderal (propranolol)
   Lopressor (metoprolol)
   Tenormin (atenolol)
   Visken (pindolol)

CALCIUM BLOCKER....DIGOXIN (Lanoxin)

THE EFFECT OF DIGOXIN MAY BE INCREASED. Digoxin is used to treat heart disorders. RESULT: Possible adverse side effects from too much digoxin. Report symptoms such as nausea, confusion, visual disturbances, headache, lack of energy, loss of appetite, bradycardia (slow heart beat) or tachycardia (rapid heart beat), cardiac arrhythmias (heart beat irregularities).

15

Drug Interactions in Treatment of High Blood Pressure

Hypertension, or high blood pressure, is referred to as *essential* hypertension, and its cause remains unknown. What we do know is that untreated high blood pressure increases the risk of heart attack and stroke. Since the condition may cause no obvious symptoms, it is usually discovered by a routine physical examination.

A reading of $120/80$ is a typical "normal" blood pressure reading for a young adult. 120 is the *systolic* pressure and 80 is the *diastolic* pressure. The systolic number indicates the pumping pressure in the arteries; the diastolic number, the resting pressure.

Treatment for high blood pressure is usually begun when the diastolic pressure consistently exceeds ninety in readings taken over several days.

Generally, the physician first recommends nondrug measures to lower blood pressure: dietary salt restriction (salt causes the body to retain fluid, thereby adding to blood volume and increasing pressure within the vessels), weight reduction, and giving up smoking. If satisfactory results aren't achieved, drug treatment is begun.

Drug treatment traditionally follows the "stepped-care" regimen consisting of four graduated steps. In step one, a simple diuretic is prescribed to reduce the volume of body fluid. Often, this is sufficient to control mild high blood pressure. If not, the physician moves to step two and adds a beta blocker or other type of nerve blocker to block the nerve impulses which raise blood pressure. In step three, a vasodilator is added to relax and dilate the blood vessels. Step four, reserved for severe high blood pressure, consists of adding the potent nerve blocker guanethidine. This stepped-care approach aims at controlling high blood pressure while keeping adverse side effects to a minimum.

HIGH BLOOD PRESSURE DRUG CATEGORIES

> beta blocker heart drugs
> captopril
> diuretics
> nerve blockers
> vasodilators

BRAND NAMES

BETA BLOCKER HEART DRUGS

Beta blockers lower blood pressure in a variety of ways—including slowing the heart rate and decreasing the amount of blood pumped per beat. Beta blocker brand names (generic names in parentheses):

> Blocadren (timolol)
> Corgard (nadolol)
> Inderal (propranolol)
> Lopressor (metporolol)
> Tenormin (atenolol)
> Visken (pindolol)

CAPTOPRIL (Capoten)

Captopril works by preventing the conversion of a chemical released by the kidney into a form that raises blood pressure. This drug has also been approved to treat congestive heart failure.

DIURETICS

Diuretics lower blood pressure by removing excess body fluid. Diuretic brand names (generic names in parentheses):

Aldactazide (spironolactone,   Aldactone (spironolactone)
   hydrochlorothiazide)   Anhydron (cyclothiazide)

Aquatag (benzthiazide)
Aquatensin (methyclothiazide)
Diucardin (hydroflumethiazide)
Diulo (metolazone)
Diuril (chlorothiazide)
Dyazide (triamterene, hydrochlorothiazide)
Dyrenium (triamterene)
Edecrin (ethacrynic acid)
Enduron (methyclothiazide)
Esidrix (hydrochlorothiazide)
Exna (benzthiazide)
Hydrodiuril (hydrochlorothiazide)
Hydromox (quinethazone)
Hygroton (chlorthalidone)
Lasix (furosemide)
Metahydrin (trichlormethiazide)
Midamor (amiloride)
Moduretic (amiloride, hydrochlorothiazide)
Naqua (trichlormethiazide)
Naturetin (bendroflumethiazide)
Oretic (hydrochlorothiazide)
Renese (polythiazide)
Saluron (hydroflumethiazide)
Zaroxolyn (metolazone)

NERVE BLOCKERS

The nerve blockers block the nerve impulses that raise blood pressure. Nerve blocker drugs (brand names in parentheses):

clonidine (Catapres, Combipres)
guanabenz (Wytensin)
guanethidine (Esimil, Ismelin)
methyldopa (Aldoclor, Aldomet, Aldoril)
prazosin (Minipress)
reserpine-type drugs:
    deserpidine (Enduronyl, Harmonyl, Oreticyl)
    rauwolfia (Raudixin, Rauzide)
    reserpine (Diupres, Diutensen-R, Hydropres, Rau-Sed, Regroton, Renese-R, Reserpoid, Salutensin, Sandril, Ser-Ap-Es, Serpasil, Serpasil-Apresoline, Serpasil-Esidrix)

VASODILATORS

Vasodilators lower blood pressure by relaxing and dilating blood vessels. Vasodilator brand names (generic names in parentheses):

Apresoline (hydralazine)
    (Other products containing hydralazine: Apresazide, Apresoline-Esidrix, Dralserp, Dralzine, Ser-Ap-Es, Serpasil-Apresoline, Unipres)
Loniten (minoxidil)

DRUG INTERACTIONS

I. HIGH BLOOD PRESSURE DRUG FAMILY INTERACTIONS
(Apply to ALL the high blood pressure drugs)

HIGH BLOOD PRESSURE DRUGS (ALL)
....AMPHETAMINES

THE EFFECT OF THE BLOOD PRESSURE DRUG MAY BE ANTAGONIZED. RESULT: The blood pressure may not be controlled properly. Amphetamines are used as diet pills (this use is in disfavor); for behavior problems in children; and for narcolepsy (uncontrollable desire to sleep). Amphetamine brand names:

> Benzedrine
> Biphetamine
> Delcobese
> Desoxyn
> Dexedrine
> Didrex
> Obetrol

HIGH BLOOD PRESSURE DRUGS (ALL)
....ANGINA HEART DRUGS

THIS COMBINATION MAY CAUSE THE BLOOD PRESSURE TO DROP TOO LOW. RESULT: Postural hypotension (sudden drop in blood pressure when changing positions, especially when rising after sitting or lying down) with associated symptoms: dizziness, weakness, faintness; a severe drop in blood pressure may cause seizures or shock. Angina drugs are used to relieve angina pain. Angina drug brand names (generic names in parentheses):

Cardilate (erythrityl tetranitrate)
Duotrate (pentaerythritol tetranitrate)
Isordil (isosorbide dinitrate)
Nitro-BID (nitroglycerin)
Nitro-Dur (nitroglycerin, transmucosal)
Nitrodisc (nitroglycerin, transmucosal)
nitroglycerin (various companies)
Nitroglyn (nitroglycerin)
Nitrol ointment (nitroglycerin)
Nitrospan (nitroglycerin)
Nitrostat (nitroglycerin)

Pentritol (pentaerythritol tetranitrate)
Peritrate (pentaerythritol tetranitrate)
Persantine (dipyridamole)

Sorbitrate (isosorbide dinitrate)
Susadrin (nitroglycerin, transmucosal)
Transderm-Nitro (nitroglycerin, transmucosal)

HIGH BLOOD PRESSURE DRUGS (ALL)
....ANTI-ARRHYTHMIC HEART DRUGS

THIS COMBINATION MAY CAUSE THE BLOOD PRESSURE TO DROP TOO LOW. RESULT: Postural hypotension (sudden drop in blood pressure when changing positions, especially when rising after sitting or lying down) with associated symptoms: dizziness, weakness, faintness; a severe drop in blood pressure may cause seizures or shock. Anti-arrhythmic drugs are used to restore irregular heart beats to normal rhythm. Anti-arrhythmic drug brand names (generic names in parentheses):

Cardioquin (quinidine)
Duraquin (quinidine)
Norpace (disopyramide)
Procan (procainamide)
Pronestyl (procainamide)

Quinaglute Dura-Tabs (quinidine)
Quinidex Extentabs (quinidine)
quinidine (various companies)
Quinora (quinidine).

HIGH BLOOD PRESSURE DRUGS (ALL)
....ANTIPSYCHOTIC DRUGS

THIS COMBINATION MAY CAUSE THE BLOOD PRESSURE TO DROP TOO LOW. RESULT: dizziness, weakness, faintness; a severe drop in blood pressure may cause seizure or shock. Antipsychotics are "major" tranquilizers used to treat severe mental disorders such as schizophrenia. Most antipsychotics are of the phenothiazine family. Antipsychotic brand names (generic names in parentheses):

PHENOTHIAZINES
Compazine (prochlorperazine)
Mellaril (thioridazine)
Proketazine (carphenazine)
Prolixin (fluphenazine)
Quide (piperacetazine)
Serentil (mesoridazine)

Sparine (promazine)
Stelazine (trifluoperazine)
Thorazine (chlorpromazine)
Tindal (acetophenazine)
Trilafon (perphenazine)
Vesprin (triflupromazine)
OTHERS
Haldol (haloperidol)
Loxitane (loxapine)
Moban (molindone)
Navane (thiothixene)
Taractan (chlorprothixene)

HIGH BLOOD PRESSURE DRUGS (ALL)....ASTHMA DRUGS (EPINEPHRINE FAMILY)

THE EFFECT OF THE BLOOD PRESSURE DRUG MAY BE ANTAGONIZED. RESULT: The blood pressure may not be controlled properly. Asthma drugs are used to open lung air passages and make breathing easier in asthmatics. Epinephrine family asthma drug brand names (generic names in parentheses):

Aerolone (isoproterenol)
Alupent (metaproterenol)
AsthmaNefrin (epinephrine)
Brethine (terbutaline)
Bricanyl (terbutaline)
Bronitin (epinephrine)
Bronkaid (epinephrine)
Dispos-a-Med (isoproterenol)
Duo-Medihaler (isoproterenol)
Ephedrine (various companies)
Isuprel (isoproterenol)
Medihaler-Epi (epinephrine)
Medihaler-Iso (isoproterenol)
Metaprel (metaproterenol)
Norisodrine (isoproterenol)
Primatene (epinephrine)
Proventil (albuterol)
Vapo-Iso-Solution (isoproterenol)
Ventolin (albuterol)

HIGH BLOOD PRESSURE DRUGS (ALL)....COLD/COUGH PRODUCTS CONTAINING DECONGESTANT DRUGS

THE EFFECT OF THE BLOOD PRESSURE DRUG MAY BE ANTAGONIZED. RESULT: The blood pressure may not be controlled properly. Be aware that decongestant nasal products are absorbed into the bloodstream and may cause an interaction. Decongestant drugs listed on nonprescription cold/cough product labels (the same drugs are used in prescription-only cold/cough products):

ORAL (tablet, capsule, liquid):
  ephedrine
  methoxyphenamine
  phenylephrine
  phenylpropanolamine
  pseudoephedrine
NASAL (drops, spray, inhaler):
  oxymetazoline
  phenylephrine
  propylhexedrine
  xylometazoline

HIGH BLOOD PRESSURE DRUGS (ALL)
....DIET PILLS (NONPRESCRIPTION)
CONTAINING PHENYLPROPANOLAMINE

THE EFFECT OF THE BLOOD PRESSURE DRUG MAY BE ANTAGONIZED. RESULT: The blood pressure may not be controlled properly. Phenylpropanolamine is a nasal decongestant drug used as the primary ingredient in the nonprescription diet pills because of its side effect of suppressing the appetite. NOTE: Many of these diet pills also contain caffeine. Nonprescription diet pill brand names:

Anorexin	E-Z Trim
Appedrine	P.P.A.
Appress	P.V.M.
Ayds (capsule, droplets)	Permathene-12
Coffee-Break	Pro Dax 21
Control	Prolamine
Dex-A-Diet II	Resolution
Dexatrim	Super Odrinex
Diadax	Ultra-Lean
Diet Gard	Vita-Slim
Dietac	

HIGH BLOOD PRESSURE DRUGS (ALL)
....METHYLPHENIDATE (Ritalin)

THE EFFECT OF THE BLOOD PRESSURE DRUG MAY BE ANTAGONIZED. RESULT: The blood pressure may not be controlled properly. Methylphenidate is used in hyperkinetic behavior and learning disorders in children, narcolepsy (uncontrollable desire to sleep), mild depression, and apathetic or withdrawn senile behavior.

II. BETA BLOCKER HEART DRUG INTERACTIONS

BETA BLOCKER....ALCOHOL (beer, liquor, wine, etc.)

THIS COMBINATION MAY CAUSE THE BLOOD PRESSURE TO DROP TOO LOW. RESULT: Postural hypotension (sudden drop in blood pressure when changing positions, especially when rising after sitting or lying down) with associated symptoms: dizziness, weakness, faintness; a severe drop in blood pressure may cause seizures or shock. Patients on angina drugs should limit alcohol consumption to less than four ounces in any twenty-four hour period.

BETA BLOCKER....AMPHETAMINES

THE EFFECT OF THE BETA BLOCKER MAY BE ANTAGONIZED. RESULT: The blood pressure treated by the beta blocker may not be controlled properly. This combination can also cause a paradoxical dangerous increase in blood pressure with symptoms such as fever, headache, visual disturbances. Amphetamines are used as diet pills (this use is in disfavor); for behavior problems in children; and for narcolepsy (uncontrollable desire to sleep). Amphetamine brand names:

Benzedrine
Biphetamine
Delcobese
Desoxyn
Dexedrine
Didrex
Obetrol

BETA BLOCKER....ANGINA DRUGS/ANTI-ARRHYTHMIC DRUGS

THIS COMBINATION MAY CAUSE THE BLOOD PRESSURE TO DROP TOO LOW. RESULT: Postural hypotension (sudden drop in blood pressure when changing positions, especially when rising after sitting or lying down) with associated symptoms: dizziness, weakness, faintness; a severe drop in blood pressure may cause seizures or shock.

A. Angina drug brand names (generic names in parentheses):
    Cardilate (erythrityl tetranitrate)
    Duotrate (pentaerythritol tetranitrate)
    Isordil (isosorbide dinitrate)
    Nitro-BID (nitroglycerin)
    Nitro-Dur (nitroglycerin, transmucosal)
    Nitrodisc (nitroglycerin, transmucosal)
    nitroglycerin (various companies)
    Nitroglyn (nitroglycerin)
    Nitrol ointment (nitroglycerin)
    Nitrospan (nitroglycerin)
    Nitrostat (nitroglycerin)
    Pentritol (pentaerythritol tetranitrate)
    Peritrate (pentaerythritol tetranitrate)
    Persantine (dipyridamole)
    Sorbitrate (isosorbide dinitrate)
    Susadrin (nitroglycerin, transmucosal)
    Transderm-Nitro (nitroglyerin, transmucosal)
B. Anti-arrhythmic drug brand names (generic names in parentheses):
    Cardioquin (quinidine)
    Duraquin (quinidine)
    Norpace (disopyramide)
    Procan (procainamide)
    Pronestyl (procainamide)
    Quinaglute Dura-Tabs (quinidine)
    Quinidex Extentabs (quinidine)
    quinidine (various companies)
    Quinora (quinidine)

BETA BLOCKER....ANTACIDS

THE EFFECT OF THE BETA BLOCKER MAY BE DE-CREASED. RESULT: The blood pressure treated by the beta blocker may not be controlled properly. NOTE: The beta blocker metoprolol (Lopressor) does not interact. Antacid brand names:

Alka-Seltzer	Kudrox
AlternaGel	Maalox
Delcid	Mylanta
Di-Gel	Riopan
Gelusil	WinGel

BETA BLOCKER....ANTIDEPRESSANTS (MAOI TYPE)

THIS COMBINATION MAY CAUSE A SIGNIFICANT RISE IN BLOOD PRESSURE. Report symptoms such as heart beat irregularities, fever, headache, visual disturbances. MAOI antidepressants, used to alleviate mental depression and elevate the mood, are not used much now that the safer cyclic antidepressants like Elavil and Sinequan are available. MAOI antidepressant brand names (generic names in parentheses):

Eutonyl (pargyline)
Marplan (isocarboxazid)
Nardil (phenelzine)
Parnate (tranylcypromine)

BETA BLOCKER....ANTIDEPRESSANTS (CYCLIC TYPE)

THE EFFECT OF THE BETA BLOCKER MAY BE DECREASED. RESULT: The blood pressure treated by the beta blocker may not be controlled properly. Antidepressants are used to alleviate mental depression and elevate the mood. NOTE: The antidepressant trazadone (Desyrel) may not interact. Antidepressant brand names (generic names in parentheses):

Adapin (doxepin)
Asendin (amoxapine)
Aventyl (nortriptyline)
Desyrel (trazadone)
Elavil (amitriptyline)
Endep (amitriptyline)
Etrafon (amitriptyline/perphenazine)
Limbitrol (amitriptyline/chlordiazepoxide)
Ludiomil (maprotiline)
Norpramin (desipramine)
Pamelor (nortriptyline)
Pertofrane (desipramine)
Sinequan (doxepin)
Surmontil (trimipramine)
Tofranil, Tofranil-PM (imipramine)
Triavil (amitriptyline/perphenazine)
Vivactil (protriptyline)

BETA BLOCKER....ANTIPSYCHOTIC DRUGS

THIS COMBINATION MAY CAUSE THE BLOOD PRESSURE TO DROP TOO LOW AND ALSO MAY INCREASE THE

EFFECT OF THE BETA BLOCKER. Report low blood pressure symptoms: dizziness, weakness, faintness. Report symptoms of too much beta blocker drug: bradycardia (slow heart beat), fatigue, cardiac arrhythmias (heart beat irregularities), asthma-like wheezing or difficulty breathing. Antipsychotics are major tranquilizers used to treat severe mental disorders such as schizophrenia. Most antipsychotics are of the phenothiazine type. Antipsychotic brand names (generic names in parentheses):

PHENOTHIAZINES
   Compazine (prochlorperazine)
   Mellaril (thioridazine)
   Proketazine (carphenazine)
   Prolixin (fluphenazine)
   Quide (piperacetazine)
   Serentil (mesoridazine)
   Sparine (promazine)
   Stelazine (trifluoperazine)
   Thorazine (chlorpromazine)
   Tindal (acetophenazine)
   Trilafon (perphenazine)
   Vesprin (triflupromazine)
OTHERS
   Haldol (haloperidol)
   Loxitane (loxapine)
   Moban (molindone)
   Navane (thiothixene)
   Taractan (chlorprothixene)

BETA BLOCKER....ASTHMA DRUGS (EPINEPHRINE FAMILY)

EACH DRUG MAY ANTAGONIZE THE EFFECTS OF THE OTHER.

A. The asthma drugs are used to open lung air passages and make breathing easier in bronchial asthma. RESULT: The asthmatic episode may not be relieved properly. NOTE: Beta blocker drugs that minimally antagonize epinephrine's effect on the lungs are Lopressor (metoprolol) and Tenormin (atenolol).

B. The beta blocker may not control the blood pressure properly. This combination may also cause a paradoxical dangerous increase in blood pressure with associated symptoms: fever, headache, visual disturbances.

Epinephrine family asthma drug brand names (generic names in parentheses):

Aerolone (isoproterenol)
Alupent (metaproterenol)
AsthmaNefrin (epinephrine)
Brethine (terbutaline)
Bricanyl (terbutaline)
Bronitin (epinephrine)
Bronkaid (epinephrine)
Dispos-a-Med (isoproterenol)
Duo-Medihaler (isoproterenol)
Ephedrine (various companies)

Isuprel (isoproterenol)
Medihaler-Epi (epinephrine)
Medihaler-Iso (isoproterenol)
Metaprel (metaproterenol)
Norisodrine (isoproterenol)
Primatene (epinephrine)
Proventil (albuterol)
Vapo-Iso-Solution (isoproterenol)
Ventolin (albuterol)

BETA BLOCKER....ASTHMA DRUGS (THEOPHYLLINE FAMILY)

THE EFFECT OF THEOPHYLLINE ON ASTHMA MAY BE ANTAGONIZED. Asthma drugs are used to open lung air passages and make breathing easier in asthmatic conditions. RESULT: The asthmatic episode may not be relieved properly. NOTE: Beta blocker drugs which minimally antagonize epinephrine's effect on the lungs are Lopressor (metoprolol) and Tenormin (atenolol). Theophylline family asthma drug brand names (generic names in parentheses):

Accurbron (theophylline)
Bronkodyl (theophylline)
Choledyl (oxtriphylline)
Dilor (dyphylline)
Elixicon (theophylline)
Elixophyllin (theophylline)
LaBID (theophylline)
Lufyllin (dyphylline)
Quibron-T (theophylline)
Respbid (theophylline)
Slo-Phyllin (theophylline)

Somophyllin (aminophylline)
Somophyllin-T (theophylline)
Sustaire (theophylline)
Theobid (theophylline)
Theodur (theophylline)
Theolair (theophylline)
Theophyl (theophylline)
Theovent (theophylline)
   Multi-ingredient products
   containing theophylline:
   Amesec, Asbron G,
   Brondecon, Marax,
   Mudrane, Quibron, Tedral
   SA

BETA BLOCKER....BARBITURATES

THE EFFECT OF THE BETA BLOCKER MAY BE DE-CREASED. RESULT: The blood pressure treated by the beta blocker may not be controlled properly. NOTE: The beta blockers Tenormin (atenolol) and Corgard (nadolol) do not interact. Barbiturates are used as sedatives or sleeping pills. Barbiturate brand names:

Phenobarbital	Luminal
Alurate	Mebaral
Amytal	Nembutal
Butisol	Seconal
Buticap	Sedadrops
Carbrital	Solfoton
Eskabarb	Tuinal
Lotusate	

BETA BLOCKER....CALCIUM BLOCKER HEART DRUGS

THIS COMBINATION MAY HAVE ADVERSE EFFECTS ON THE HEART. When these two drugs are given together, the physician should carefully monitor the effects on the patient. The calcium blockers are given for certain types of angina. Calcium blocker brand names (generic names in parentheses):

Calan (verapamil)
Cardizem (diltiazem)
Isoptin (verapamil)
Procardia (nifedipine)

BETA BLOCKER....CIMETIDINE (Tagamet)

THE EFFECT OF THE BETA BLOCKER MAY BE IN-CREASED. RESULT: Possible adverse side effects from too much beta blocker. Report symptoms such as bradycardia (slow heart beat), fatigue, cardiac arrhythmias (heart beat irregularities), asthma-like wheezing or difficulty breathing. Cimetidine is prescribed for duodenal and peptic ulcers.

BETA BLOCKER....CLONIDINE (Catapres, Combipres)

THIS COMBINATION MAY CAUSE A "REBOUND" RISE IN BLOOD PRESSURE. This can occur when clonidine treatment is stopped suddenly—causing symptoms of high blood pressure crisis: restlessness and irritability, tremors, tachycardia (rapid heart beat), headache, nausea, fever, visual disturbances. Clonidine is used to treat high blood pressure.

BETA BLOCKER....COLD/COUGH PRODUCTS CONTAINING DECONGESTANT DRUGS

THE EFFECT OF THE BETA BLOCKER MAY BE ANTAGONIZED. RESULT: The blood pressure treated by the beta blocker may not be controlled properly. Be aware that decongestant nasal products can be absorbed into the bloodstream and cause an interaction. Decongestant drugs listed on nonprescription cold/cough product labels (the same drugs are used in prescription-only cold/cough products):

> ORAL (tablet, capsule, liquid):
>   ephedrine
>   methoxyphenamine
>   phenylephrine
>   phenylpropanolamine
>   pseudoephedrine
> NASAL (drops, spray, inhaler):
>   oxymetazoline
>   phenylephrine
>   propylhexedrine
>   xylometazoline

BETA BLOCKER....DIABETES DRUGS

THIS COMBINATION CAN EITHER INCREASE OR DECREASE THE EFFECT OF THE DIABETES DRUG. RESULT: If INCREASED diabetes drug effect, the blood sugar level may fall too low. Report symptoms of hypoglycemia (low blood sugar), which will be even more pronounced with physical exertion or exercise: sweating, nervousness, faintness, weakness, confusion, cardiac arrhythmias (heart beat irregularities), tachycardia (rapid heart beat), loss of coordination, visual disturbances—be aware that taking the beta blocker drug can *hide* these warning symptoms. If DECREASED diabetes drug effect, the blood sugar level may remain too high. Report symptoms of hyperglycemia (high blood sugar): excessive thirst, large urine output, weight loss, hunger, lethargy, drowsiness, loss of coordination. Beta blocker heart drugs are prescribed for angina, to restore irregular heart beats to normal rhythm, and to help lower high blood pressure. Diabetes drug brand names (generic names in parentheses):

Diabinese (chlorpropamide)
Dymelor (acetohexamide)
Orinase (tolbutamide)
Tolinase (tolazamide)
Insulin (several brands)

BETA BLOCKER....DIET PILLS (NONPRESCRIPTION) CONTAINING PHENYLPROPANOLAMINE

THE EFFECT OF THE BETA BLOCKER MAY BE ANTAGONIZED. RESULT: The condition treated by the beta blocker may not be controlled properly. Phenylpropanolamine is a nasal decongestant drug used as the primary ingredient in the nonprescription diet pills because of its side effect of suppressing the appetite. NOTE: Many of these diet pills also contain caffeine. Nonprescription diet pill brand names:

Anorexin	E-Z Trim
Appedrine	P.P.A.
Appress	P.V.M.
Ayds (capsule, droplets)	Permathene-12
Coffee-Break	Pro Dax 21
Control	Prolamine
Dex-A-Diet II	Resolution
Dexatrim	Super Odrinex
Diadax	Ultra-Lean
Diet Gard	Vita-Slim
Dietac	

BETA BLOCKER....METHYLPHENIDATE (Ritalin)

THE EFFECT OF THE BETA BLOCKER MAY BE ANTAGONIZED. RESULT: The condition treated by the beta blocker may not be controlled properly. Methylphenidate is used in hyperkinetic behavior and learning disorders in children, narcolepsy (uncontrollabe desire to sleep), mild depression, and apathetic or withdrawn senile behavior.

BETA BLOCKER....PRAZOSIN (Minipress)

THE BETA BLOCKER MAY INTENSIFY THE "FIRST DOSE" ADVERSE EFFECTS OF PRAZOSIN. Prazosin is used to treat high blood pressure. RESULT: Severe postural hypotension (sudden drop in blood pressure when changing positions, especially when rising after sitting or lying down) with associated symptoms: dizziness, weakness, faintness.

BETA BLOCKER....PRIMIDONE (Mysoline)

THE EFFECT OF THE BETA BLOCKER MAY BE DECREASED. RESULT: The blood pressure treated by the beta blocker may not be controlled properly. NOTE: The beta blockers Tenormin (atenolol) and Corgard (nadolol) do not interact. Primidone is used to control seizures in disorders such as epilepsy.

BETA BLOCKER....RESERPINE-TYPE DRUGS

THE EFFECT OF EACH DRUG MAY BE INCREASED. Reserpine is used to treat high blood pressure. RESULT: Bradycardia (slow heart beat) and a fall in blood pressure. Report symptoms such as dizziness, weakness, faintness, postural hypotension (sudden drop in blood pressure when changing positions, especially when rising after sitting or lying down—with above symptoms). Reserpine-type drugs (brand names in parentheses):

deserpidine (Enduronyl, Harmonyl, Oreticyl)
rauwolfia (Raudixin, Rauzide)
reserpine (Diupres, Diutensen-R, Hydropres, Rau-Sed, Regroton, Renese-R, Reserpoid, Salutensin, Sandril, Ser-Ap-Es, Serpasil, Serpasil-Apresoline, Serpasil-Esidrix

BETA BLOCKER....VASODILATOR DRUGS

THIS COMBINATION MAY CAUSE THE BLOOD PRESSURE TO DROP TOO LOW. RESULT: Postural hypotension (sudden drop in blood pressure when changing positions, especially when rising after sitting or lying down) with associated symptoms: dizziness, weakness, faintness; a severe drop in blood pressure may cause seizures or shock. This type of vasodilator dilates the blood vessels and is used to treat problems associated with poor blood circulation, such as arteriosclerosis (hardening of the arteries). Vasodilator drugs (brand names in parentheses):

cyclandelate (Cyclospasmol)
ethaverine (Cebral, Ethaquin, Ethatab, Pavaspan)
isoxsuprine (Vasodilan)
nicotinyl alcohol (Roniacol)

nylidrin (Arlidin)
papaverine (Cerespan, Pavabid, Pavacap, Paverine, Therapav)
tolazoline (Priscoline)

III. CAPTOPRIL DRUG INTERACTIONS

CAPTOPRIL (CAPOTEN)....ANTIDEPRESSANTS (MAOI TYPE)

THIS COMBINATION MAY CAUSE THE BLOOD PRESSURE TO DROP TOO LOW. RESULT: Postural hypotension (sudden drop in blood pressure when changing positions, especially when rising after sitting or lying down) with associated symptoms: dizziness, weakness, faintness. MAOI antidepressants, used to alleviate mental depression and elevate the mood, are not used much since the development of the safer cyclic antidepressants such as Elavil and Sinequan. MAOI antidepressant brand names (generic names in parentheses):

Eutonyl (pargyline)
Marplan (isocarboxazid)
Nardil (phenelzine)
Parnate (tranylcypromine)

CAPTOPRIL (CAPOTEN)....DIURETICS

THIS COMBINATION MAY CAUSE A SEVERE DROP IN BLOOD PRESSURE. RESULT: dizziness, weakness, faintness; possible seizures or shock. Diuretics remove excess body fluid and are used to treat high blood pressure and congestive heart failure. The diuretics amiloride (Midamor), spironolactone (Aldactone), and triamterene (Dyrenium) interact with captopril to make the body hold too much potassium, causing adverse side effects such as muscular weakness, numbness or paralysis, bradycardia (slow heart beat), cardiac arrhythmias (heart beat irregularities). Diuretic drug brand names (generic names in parentheses):

Aldactazide (spironolactone, hydrochlorothiazide)
Aldactone (spironolactone)
Anydron (cyclothiazide)
Aquatag (benzthiazide)
Aquatensin (methylclothiazide)
Diucardin (hydroflumethiazide)

Diulo (metolazone)
Diuril (chlorothiazide)
Dyazide (triamterne, hydrochlorothiazide)
Dyrenium (triamterene)
Edecrin (ethacrynic acid)
Enduron (methyclothiazide)

Esidrix (hydrochlorothiazide)
Exna (benzthiazide)
Hydrodiuril (hydrochlorothiazide)
Hydromox (quinethazone)
Hygroton (chlorthalidone)
Lasix (furosemide)
Metahydrin (trichlormethiazide)
Midamor (amiloride)

Moduretic (amiloride,
  hydrochlorothiazide)
Naqua (trichlormethiazide)
Naturetin (bendroflumethiazide)
Oretic (hydrochlorothiazide)
Renese (polythiazide)
Saluron (hydroflumethiazide)
Zaroxolyn (metolazone)

CAPTOPRIL (CAPOTEN)....PENICILLIN (POTASSIUM TYPE)

THIS COMBINATION MAY CAUSE A MARKED IN-CREASE IN BODY POTASSIUM. RESULT: Adverse side effects from too much potassium. Report symptoms such as muscular weakness, numbness or paralysis, bradycardia (slow heart beat), cardiac arrhythmias (heart beat irregularities). Penicillin is an antibiotic used to combat infection. Interacting penicillin brand names:

Betapen VK
Ledercillin VK
Pentids
Pen Vee K

Pfizerpen G
Pfizerpen VK
Robicillin VK
V-Cillin K

CAPTOPRIL (CAPOTEN)....POTASSIUM SUPPLEMENTS

THIS COMBINATION MAY CAUSE A MARKED IN-CREASE IN BODY POTASSIUM. RESULT: Adverse side effects from too much potassium. Report symptoms such as muscular weakness, numbness or paralysis, bradycardia (slow heart beat), cardiac arrhythmias (heart beat irregularities). Potassium supplements are often prescribed for patients taking diuretic drugs. Potassium supplement brand names:

K-Lyte
Kaochlor
Kaon
Kato
Kay-Ciel

Klorvess
Klotrix
Kolyum
Slow-K
Twin-K

CAPTOPRIL (CAPOTEN)
....SALT SUBSTITUTES (CONTAIN POTASSIUM)

THIS COMBINATION MAY CAUSE A MARKED IN-CREASE IN BODY POTASSIUM. RESULT: Adverse side effects from too much potassium. Report symptoms such as muscular weakness, numbness or paralysis, bradycardia (slow heart beat), cardiac arrhythmias (heart beat irregularities). Salt substitutes are often used by those on low sodium (salt) diets. Salt substitute brand names:

Adolph's Salt Substitute
Morton Salt Substitute
NoSalt
Neocurtasal
Nu-Salt

IV. DIURETIC DRUG INTERACTIONS

DIURETIC....ANTIDEPRESSANTS (MAOI TYPE)

THIS COMBINATION MAY CAUSE THE BLOOD PRES-SURE TO DROP TOO LOW. RESULT: Postural hypotension (sudden drop in blood pressure when changing positions, especially when rising after sitting or lying down) with associated symptoms: dizziness, weakness, faintness. MAOI antidepressants, used to alleviate mental depression and elevate the mood, are not used much since the development of the safer tricyclic antidepressants such as Elavil and Sinequan. MAOI antidepressant brand names (generic names in parentheses):

Eutonyl (pargyline)
Marplan (isocarboxazid)
Nardil (phenelzine)
Parnate (tranylcypromine)

DIURETIC....CAPTOPRIL (Capoten)

THIS COMBINATION MAY CAUSE A SEVERE DROP IN BLOOD PRESSURE. RESULT: dizziness, weakness, faintness; possible seizures or shock. Captopril is used to lower blood pressure and may be used for congestive heart failure. The diuretics amiloride (Midamor), spironolactone (Aldactone), and triamterene (Dyrenium) interact with captopril to make the body hold too much potassium, causing adverse side effects such as muscular weakness, numbness or paralysis, bradycardia (slow heart beat), cardiac arrhythmias (heart beat irregularities).

DIURETIC....CORTICOSTEROIDS

THIS COMBINATION MAY CAUSE THE BODY TO LOSE TOO MUCH POTASSIUM AND HOLD TOO MUCH SODIUM. Report symptoms of potassium depletion: muscular weakness or cramps, large urine output, bradycardia (slow heart beat) or tachycardia (rapid heart beat), cardiac arrhythmias (heart beat irregularities), low blood pressure with dizziness, faintness. Report symptoms of too much sodium: edema (excess body fluid), thirst, scant urine output, confusion, high blood pressure, hyperexcitability. Corticosteroids are used for arthritis, severe allergies, asthma, endocrine disorders, leukemia, colitis and enteritis (inflammation of the intestinal tract), and various skin, lung, and eye diseases. Interacting diuretics include all except those containing the "potassium-sparing" diuretic drugs amiloride, spironolactone, and triamterene. Corticosteroid brand names (generic names in parentheses):

Aristocort (triamcinolone)   Kenacort (triamcinolone)
Celestone (betamethasone)   Medrol (methylprednisolone)
Cortef (hydrocortisone)   Meticorten (prednisone)
Decadron (dexamethasone)   Orasone (prednisone)
Delta-Cortef (prednisolone)   prednisone (various companies)
hydrocortisone (various
   companies)

DIURETIC....DIABETES DRUGS

THE EFFECT OF THE DIABETES DRUG MAY BE ANTAGONIZED. The diabetes drugs are used to lower the blood sugar level in diabetics. RESULT: The blood sugar level may remain too high. Report symptoms of hyperglycemia (high blood sugar): large urine output, excessive thirst and hunger, weight loss, loss of coordination, lethargy, drowsiness. The interacting diuretic drugs are those causing the body to lose its potassium, and this interaction is minimized by adding extra potassium to the diet. Interacting diuretics include all except those containing the "potassium-sparing" diuretic drugs amiloride, spironolactone, and triamterene. Diabetes drug brand names (generic names in parentheses):

Diabinese (chlorpropamide)
Dymelor (acetohexamide)
Orinase (tolbutamide)
Tolinase (tolazamide)
Insulin injection

DIURETIC....DIGITALIS HEART DRUGS

THIS COMBINATION CAN CAUSE ADVERSE EFFECTS ON THE HEART. Digitalis is used to treat congestive heart failure and to restore irregular heart beats to normal rhythm. Most diuretics deplete the body of potassium. Lack of potassium makes the heart extra sensitive to digitalis and increases the risk of digitalis toxicity with associated symptoms: nausea, confusion, visual disturbances, headache, loss of energy, loss of appetite, bradycardia (slow heart beat) or tachycardia (rapid heart beat), cardiac arrhythmias (heart beat irregularities). Be aware of symptoms of potassium loss: muscular weakness or cramps, large urine output, dizziness, faintness. Interacting diuretics include all except those containing the "potassium-sparing" diuretic drugs amiloride, spironolactone, and triamterene. This interaction is prevented by taking a potassium supplement. Digitalis heart drug brand names (generic names in parentheses):

Crystodigin (digitoxin)
Digifortis (digitalis)
Lanoxin (digoxin)
Purodigin (digitoxin)

DIURETIC....LITHIUM

THE EFFECT OF LITHIUM MAY BE INCREASED. Lithium is an antipsychotic used to treat manic-depressive disorders. RESULT: Possible adverse side effects from too much lithium. Report symptoms such as dizziness, nausea, confusion, weakness, lethargy, dry mouth, appetite loss, stomach or abdominal pain, loss of coordination. Interacting diuretics include all except those containing the "potassium-sparing" diuretic drugs amiloride, spironolactone, and triamterene. This interaction is minimized by taking a potassium supplement to offset the potassium loss caused by the diuretics. Lithium brand names:

Eskalith
Lithane
Lithonate
Lithobid
Lithonate-S
Lithotabs

DIURETIC....NON-CORTICOSTEROID PAIN AND INFLAMMATION DRUGS

THE EFFECT OF THE DIURETIC DRUG MAY BE DECREASED. RESULT: The blood pressure treated by the diuretic may not be controlled properly. The non-corticosteroids are used to alleviate pain and inflammation in arthritic conditions and to relieve pain in general. Non-corticosteroid drug brand names (generic names in parentheses):

Anaprox (naproxen)   Nalfon (fenoprofen)
aspirin (various brands)   Naprosyn (naproxen)
Butazolidin (phenylbutazone)   Ponstel (mefenamic acid)
Clinoril (sulindac)   Rufen (ibuprofen)
Feldene (piroxicam)   Tandearil (oxyphenbutazone)
Indocin (indomethacin)   Tolectin (tolmetin)
Meclomen (meclofenamate)   Zomax (zomepirac)
Motrin (ibuprofen)

DIURETIC....PRAZOSIN (Minipress)

THE DIURETIC MAY INTENSIFY THE "FIRST DOSE" ADVERSE EFFECTS OF PRAZOSIN. Prazosin is used to lower the blood pressure. RESULT: Severe postural hypotension (sudden drop in blood pressure when changing positions, especially when rising after sitting or lying down) with associated symptoms: dizziness, weakness, faintness.

V. NERVE BLOCKER INTERACTIONS

NOTE: Four of the nerve blocker high blood pressure drugs (clonidine, guanabenz, methyldopa, reserpine) are central nervous system depressants. They depress or impair functions such as coordination and alertness. Excessive depression or impairment can occur when one of these nerve blockers is taken with any other central nervous system depressant. Therefore, in addition to the other specific interactions, be aware of this general interaction.

CLONIDINE/GUANABENZ/METHYLDOPA/RESERPINE.... OTHER DEPRESSANT DRUGS

RESULT: Drowsiness, dizziness, loss of muscle coordination and mental alertness; in severe cases, failure of blood circulation and breathing functions causing coma and death. The physician should monitor the patient carefully and adjust the dosages to minimize the excessive depressant effects. Interacting *depressant* drugs:

ALCOHOL (beer, liquor, wine, etc.)
ANTICHOLINERGICS—uses and brand names:
   Those used to control tremors resulting from Parkinson's disease
   or from treatment with antipsychotic drugs:
      Akineton, Artane, Cogentin, Kemadrin, Pagitane
   Others:
      Norflex (a muscle relaxant)
      Robinul (used for stomach, digestive tract disorders)
      Transderm-Scop (used for motion sickness)
ANTICONVULSANTS (Used to control seizures in disorders such
   as epilepsy). Brand names: Depakene, Dilantin, Mesantoin, My-
   soline, Peganone, Tegretol, Tridione, Zarontin
ANTIDEPRESSANTS (CYCLIC TYPE) Used to alleviate mental
   depression. Brand names: Adapin, Asendin, Aventyl, Desyrel,
   Elavil, Endep, Etrafon, Limbitrol, Ludiomil, Norpramin, Pam-
   elor, Pertofrane, Sinequan, Surmontil Tofranil, Tofranil-PM,
   Triavil, Vivactil
ANTIHISTAMINES (Used for allergies, colds). Brand names:
   Actidil, Antivert, Atarax, Benadryl, Bendectin, Bonine, Chlor-
   Trimeton, Clistin, Decapryn, Dimetane, Dramamine, Histadyl,
   Inhiston, Marezine, Optimine, PBZ, Periactin, Polaramine,
   Pyronil, Tavist, Teldrin, Triten, Vistaril
ANTIPSYCHOTICS (Used for severe mental disorders). Antipsy-
   chotic brand names: Compazine, Haldol, Loxitane, Mellaril,
   Moban, Navane, Proketazine, Prolixin, Quide, Serentil, Sparine,
   Stelazine, Taractan, Thorazine, Tindal, Trilafon, Vesprin
FENFLURAMINE (Pondimin) (a diet pill)

MUSCLE RELAXANTS
  Dantrium, Flexeril, Lioresal, Norflex, Norgesic, Norgesic Forte, Paraflex, Parafon Forte, Quinamm, Rela, Robaxin, Robaxisal, Skelaxin, Soma, Soma Compound, Valium
NARCOTICS
  Codeine products: Ascriptin w/Codeine, Bancap w/Codeine, Bufferin w/Codeine, Empirin w/Codeine, Empracet w/Codeine, Fiorinal w/Codeine, Phenaphen w/Codeine, Tylenol w/ Codeine

  Other narcotic or narcotic-like products: Demerol, Dilaudid, Dolophene, morphine, Merpergan Fortis, Norcet, Numorphan, Percocet, Percodan, Synalgos-DC, Talwin, Talwin Compound, Tylox, Vicodan, Zactane, Zactirin
PROPOXYPHENE (pain reliever):
  Darvocet-N, Darvon, Dolene, Wygesic
SLEEPING PILLS
  Barbiturate sleeping pills: phenobarbital, Alurate, Amytal, Butisol, Buticap, Carbrital, Eskabarb, Lotusate, Luminal, Mebaral, Nembutal, Seconal, Sedadrops, Solfoton, Tuinal
  Non-Barbiturate sleeping pills: Ativan (also used as a tranquilizer), Dalmane, Doriden, Halcion, Noctec, Noludar, Parest, Placidyl, Quaalude, Restoril, Somnos, Triclos, Valmid
TRANQUILIZERS
  Benzodiazepine tranquilizers: Ativan, Centrax, Librium, Limbitrol (also an antidepressant), Paxipam, Serax, SK-Lygen, Tranxene, Valium, Xanax
  Non-Benzodiazepine tranquilizers: Atarax, Equanil, meprobamate, Meprospan, Meprotab, Miltown, Trancopal, Tybatran, Vistaril

CLONIDINE (Catapres, Combipres)
....ANTIDEPRESSANTS (CYCLIC TYPE)

THE EFFECT OF CLONIDINE MAY BE DECREASED. RESULT: The high blood pressure may not be controlled properly. Also, since both drugs are central nervous system depressants, additive "physical" depression can occur with associated symptoms: drowsiness, dizziness, loss of muscle coordination and mental alertness. The antidepressant trazadone (Desyrel) may not decrease the effect of clonidine, but may cause excessive physical depression. Antidepressants are prescribed to alleviate mental depression and elevate the mood. Antidepressant brand names (generic names in parentheses):

Adapin (doxepin)
Asendin (amoxapine)
Aventyl (nortriptyline)
Desyrel (trazadone)
Elavil (amitriptyline)
Endep (amitriptyline)
Etrafon (amitriptyline/
　perphenazine)
Limbitrol (amitriptyline/
　chlordiazepoxide)
Ludiomil (maprotiline)

Norpramin (desipramine)
Pamelor (nortriptyline)
Pertofrane (desipramine)
Sinequan (doxepin)
Surmontil (trimipramine)
Tofranil, Tofranil-PM
　(imipramine)
Triavil (amitriptyline/
　perhpenazine)
Vivactil (protriptyline)

CLONIDINE (Catapres, Combipres)
....BETA BLOCKER HEART DRUGS

THIS COMBINATION MAY CAUSE A "REBOUND" RISE IN BLOOD PRESSURE. This occurs when clonidine treatment is stopped suddenly—causing symptoms of hypertensive crisis: restlessness and irritability, tremors, tachycardia (rapid heart beat), headache, nausea, fever, visual disturbances. Beta blocker heart drugs are used to treat high blood pressure, angina, and to restore irregular heart beats to normal rhythm. Beta blocker brand names (generic names in parentheses):

Blocadren (timolol)
Corgard (nadolol)
Inderal (propranolol)
Lopessor (metoprolol)
Tenormin (atenolol)
Visken (pindolol)

CLONIDINE (Catapres, Combipres)....LEVODOPA (Dopar, Larodopa, Sinemet)

THE EFFECT OF LEVODOPA MAY BE DECREASED. Levodopa is used to treat Parkinson's disease. RESULT: The disorder may not be controlled properly.

CLONIDINE (Catapres, Combipres)
....TOLAZOLINE (Priscoline)

THE EFFECT OF CLONIDINE MAY BE DECREASED. RESULT: The blood pressure may not be controlled properly. Tolazoline is used to treat disorders associated with poor blood circulation, such as arteriosclerosis (hardening of the arteries).

GUANABENZ (Wytensin)

See *Clonidine* interactions.

GUANETHIDINE (Esimil, Ismelin)....ALCOHOL (beer, liquor, wine, etc.)

THIS COMBINATION MAY CAUSE THE BLOOD PRESSURE TO DROP TOO LOW. RESULT: Postural hypotension (sudden drop in blood pressure when changing positions, especially when rising after sitting or lying down) with associated symptoms: dizziness, weakness, faintness; a severe drop in blood pressure may cause seizures or shock. Limiting alcohol ingestion to small amounts minimizes this interaction.

GUANETHIDINE (Esimil, Ismelin) ....ANTIDEPRESSANTS (MAOI TYPE)

THE EFFECT OF GUANETHIDINE MAY BE DECREASED. RESULT: The blood pressure may not be controlled properly. In some cases, a severe increase in blood pressure can occur with confusion and headache. MAOI antidepressants, used to alleviate mental depression and elevate the mood, are not used much since the development of the safer tricyclic antidepressants such as Elavil and Sinequan. MAOI antidepressant brand names (generic names in parentheses):

Eutonyl (pargyline)
Marplan (isocarboxazid)
Nardil (phenelzine)
Parnate (tranylcypromine)

*GUANETHIDINE (Esimil, Ismelin) ....ANTIDEPRESSANTS (CYCLIC TYPE)

THE EFFECT OF GUANETHIDINE MAY BE DECREASED. RESULT: The blood pressure may not be controlled properly. NOTE: The antidepressant doxepin (Adapin, Sinequan), in lower doses, may not interact, and the antidepressant trazadone (Desyrel) may not interact at all. Antidepressants are prescribed to alleviate mental depression and elevate the mood. Antidepressant brand names (generic names in parentheses):

Adapin (doxepin)
Asendin (amoxapine)
Aventyl (nortriptyline)
Desyrel (trazadone)
Elavil (amitriptyline)
Endep (amitriptyline)
Etrafon (amitriptyline/
  perphenazine)
Limbitrol (amitriptyline/
  chlordiazepoxide)
Ludiomil (maprotiline)

Norpramin (desipramine)
Pamelor (nortriptyline)
Pertofrane (desipramine)
Sinequan (doxepin)
Surmontil (trimipramine)
Tofranil, Tofranil-PM
  (imipramine)
Triavil (amitriptyline/
  perphenazine)
Vivactil (protriptyline)

GUANETHIDINE (Esimil, Ismelin) ....ANTIPSYCHOTICS (PHENOTHIAZINE FAMILY)

THE EFFECT OF GUANETHIDINE MAY BE DE-CREASED. RESULT: The blood pressure may not be controlled properly. The phenothiazines are antipsychotics or "major" tranquilizers used to treat severe mental disorders such as schizophrenia. Phenothiazine brand names (generic names in parentheses):

Compazine (prochlorperazine)
Mellaril (thioridazine)
Proketazine (carphenazine)
Prolixin (fluphenazine)
Quide (piperacetazine)
Serentil (mesoridazine)

Sparine (promazine)
Stelazine (trifluoperazine)
Thorazine (chlorpromazine)
Tindal (acetophenazine)
Trilafon (perphenazine)
Vesprin (triflupromazine)

GUANETHIDINE (Esimil, Ismelin) ....CHLORPROTHIXENE(Taractan)

THE EFFECT OF GUANETHIDINE MAY BE DE-CREASED. RESULT: The blood pressure may not be controlled properly. Chlorprothixene is an antipsychotic or major tranquilizer used to treat severe mental disorders such as schizophrenia.

GUANETHIDINE (Esimil, Ismelin)....DIABETES DRUGS

THE EFFECT OF THE DIABETES DRUG MAY BE IN-CREASED. Diabetes drugs are used to lower the blood sugar level in diabetics. RESULT: The blood sugar level may fall too low. Report symptoms of hypoglycemia (low blood sugar): nervousness, faintness, weakness, sweating, confusion, tachycardia (rapid heart beat), cardiac arrhythmias (heart beat irregularities), loss of coordination, visual disturbances. Diabetes drug brand names (generic names in parentheses):

Diabinese (chlorpropamide)
Dymelor (acetohexamide)
Orinase (tolbutamide)
Tolinase (tolazamide)
Insulin injection

GUANETHIDINE (Esimil, Ismelin) ....HALOPERIDOL (Haldol)

THE EFFECT OF GUANETHIDINE MAY BE DE-CREASED. RESULT: The blood pressure may not be controlled properly. Haloperidol is an antipsychotic or "major" tranquilizer used to treat severe mental disorders such as schizophrenia.

GUANETHIDINE (Esimil, Ismelin)....LEVODOPA (Dopar, Larodopa, Sinemet)

THIS COMBINATION MAY CAUSE THE BLOOD PRES-SURE TO DROP TOO LOW. RESULT: Postural hypotension (sudden drop in blood pressure when changing positions, especially when rising after sitting or lying down) with associated symptoms: dizziness, weakness, faintness; a severe drop in blood pressure may cause seizures or shock. Levodopa is used to treat Parkinson's disease.

GUANETHIDINE (Esimil, Ismelin)....LOXAPINE (Loxitane)

THIS COMBINATION MAY CAUSE THE BLOOD PRES-SURE TO DROP TOO LOW. RESULT: Postural hypotension (sudden drop in blood pressure when changing positions, especially when rising after sitting or lying down) with associated symptoms: dizziness, weakness, faintness; a severe drop in blood pressure may cause seizures or shock. Loxapine is an antipsychotic or "major" tranquilizer used to treat severe mental disorders such as schizophrenia.

GUANETHIDINE (Esimil, Ismelin)....MINOXIDIL (Loniten)

THIS COMBINATION MAY CAUSE A SEVERE DROP IN BLOOD PRESSURE. RESULT: Postural hypotension (sudden drop in blood pressure when changing positions, especially when rising after sitting or lying down) with associated symptoms: dizziness, weakness, faintness; possible seizures or shock. Minoxidil is used to lower the blood pressure.

GUANETHIDINE (Esimil, Ismelin)....MOLINDONE (Moban)

THIS COMBINATION MAY CAUSE THE BLOOD PRESSURE TO DROP TOO LOW. RESULT: Postural hypotension (sudden drop in blood pressure when changing positions, especially when rising after sitting or lying down) with associated symptoms: dizziness, weakness, faintness; a severe drop in blood pressure may cause seizures or shock. Molindone is an antipsychotic or "major" tranquilizer used to treat severe mental disorders such as schizophrenia.

GUANETHIDINE (Esimil, Ismelin)....THIOTHIXENE (Navane)

THE EFFECT OF GUANETHIDINE MAY BE DECREASED. RESULT: The blood pressure may not be controlled properly. Thiothixene is an antipsychotic or "major" tranquilizer used to treat severe mental disorders such as schizophrenia.

METHYLDOPA (Aldoclor, Aldomet, Aldoril).... ANTIDEPRESSANTS (MAOI TYPE)

THE EFFECT OF METHYLDOPA MAY BE DECREASED. RESULT: The blood pressure may not be controlled properly. MAOI depressants, used to alleviate mental depression and elevate the mood, are not used much since the development of the safer cyclic antidepressants such as Elavil and Sinequan. MAOI antidepressant brand names (generic names in parentheses):

Eutonyl (pargyline)
Marplan (isocarboxazid)
Nardil (phenelzine)
Parnate (tranylcypromine)

METHYLDOPA (Aldoclor, Aldomet, Aldoril) ....DIGOXIN (Lanoxin)

THIS COMBINATION MAY CAUSE ADVERSE EFFECTS ON THE HEART. Digoxin is used to treat congestive heart failure and to restore irregular heart beats to normal rhythm.

Report symptoms such as bradycardia (slow heart beat), dizziness, faintness, confusion, forgetfulness.

METHYLDOPA (Aldoclor, Aldomet, Aldoril)....
HALOPERIDOL (Haldol)

A. THE EFFECT OF HALOPERIDOL MAY BE IN-CREASED. Haloperidol is an antipsychotic or major tranquilizer used to treat severe mental disorders such as schizophrenia. RESULT: Increased risk of adverse side effects from too much haloperidol. Report symptoms such as tremors, insomnia, toxic psychosis (agitation, disorientation, delirium).

B. THIS COMBINATION MAY CAUSE THE BLOOD PRESSURE TO DROP TOO LOW. RESULT: Postural hypotension (sudden drop in blood pressure when changing positions, especially when rising after sitting or lying down) with associated symptoms: dizziness, weakness, faintness; a severe drop in blood pressure may cause seizures or shock.

METHYLDOPA (Aldoclor, Aldomet, Aldoril)....LEVODOPA

THIS COMBINATION MAY CAUSE THE BLOOD PRESSURE TO DROP TOO LOW. RESULT: Postural hypotension (sudden drop in blood pressure when changing positions, especially when rising after sitting or lying down) with associated symptoms: dizziness, weakness, faintness.

B. THE EFFECT OF LEVODOPA MAY BE DECREASED. Levodopa is used to treat Parkinson's disease. RESULT: The disorder may not be controlled properly. Levodopa brand names:

Dopar
Larodopa
Sinemet

METHYLDOPA (Aldoclor, Aldomet, Aldoril)....LITHIUM

THE EFFECT OF LITHIUM MAY BE INCREASED. Lithium is an antipsychotic used to treat manic-depressive disorders. RESULT: Possible adverse side effects from too much lithium. Report symptoms such as dizziness, nausea, confusion, weakness, lethargy, dry mouth, appetite loss, stomach or abdominal pain, loss of coordination. Lithium brand names:

Eskalith
Lithane
Lithonate
Lithobid
Lithonate-S
Lithotabs

PRAZOSIN (Minipress)....ANTIDEPRESSANTS (MAOI TYPE)

THIS COMBINATION MAY CAUSE THE BLOOD PRESSURE TO DROP TOO LOW. RESULT: Postural hypotension (sudden drop in blood pressure when changing positions, especially when rising after sitting or lying down) with associated symptoms: dizziness, weakness, faintness. MAOI depressants, used to alleviate mental depression and elevate the mood, are not used much since the development of the safer cyclic antidepressants such as Elavil and Sinequan. MAOI antidepressant brand names (generic names in parentheses):

Eutonyl (pargyline)
Marplan (isocarboxazid)
Nardil (phenelzine)
Parnate (tranylcypromine)

PRAZOSIN (Minipress)....BETA BLOCKER HEART DRUGS

THE BETA BLOCKER MAY INTENSIFY THE "FIRST DOSE" ADVERSE EFFECTS OF PRAZOSIN. RESULT: Severe postural hypotension (sudden drop in blood pressure when changing positions, especially when rising after sitting or lying down) with associated symptoms: dizziness, weakness, faintness. Beta blockers are used to treat high blood pressure, angina, and to restore irregular heart beats to normal rhythm. Beta blocker brand names (generic names in parentheses):

Blocadren (timolol)
Corgard (nadolol)
Inderal (propranolol)

Lopressor (metoprolol)
Tenormin (atenolol)
Visken (pindolol)

PRAZOSIN (Minipress)....DIURETICS

THE DIURETIC MAY INTENSIFY THE "FIRST DOSE" ADVERSE EFFECTS OF PRAZOSIN. Diuretics remove excess body fluid and are used to treat high blood pressure and congestive heart failure. RESULT: Severe postural hypotension (sudden drop in blood pressure when changing positions, especially when rising after sitting or lying down) with associated symptoms: dizziness, weakness, faintness. Diuretic drug brand names (generic names in parentheses):

Aldactazide (spironolactone,
 hydrochlorothiazide)
Aldactone (spironolactone)
Anhydron (cyclothiazide)
Aquatag (benzthiazide)
Aquatensin (methyclothiazide)
Diucardin (hydroflumethiazide)
Diulo (metolazone)
Diuril (chlorothiazide)
Dyazide (triamterene,
 hydrochlorothiazide)
Dyrenium (triamterene)
Edecrin (ethacrynic acid)
Enduron (methyclothiazide)
Esidrix (hydrochlorothiazide)

Exna (benzthiazide)
Hydrodiuril (hydrochlorothiazide)
Hydromox (quinethazone)
Hygroton (chlorthalidone)
Lasix (furosemide)
Metahydrin (trichlormethiazide)
Midamor (amiloride)
Moduretic (amiloride,
 hydrochlorothiazide)
Naqua (trichlormethiazide)
Naturetin (bendroflumethiazide)
Oretic (hydrochlorothiazide)
Renese (polythiazide)
Saluron (hydroflumethiazide)
Zaroxolyn (metolazone)

RESERPINE....ANTIDEPRESSANTS (MAOI TYPE)

THIS COMBINATION MAY CAUSE EXCESSIVE STIMULATION. RESULT: Possible dangerous increase in blood pressure with confusion, headache, fever, hyperexcitability. MAOI depressants, used to alleviate mental depression and elevate the mood, are not used much since the development of the safer cyclic antidepressants such as Elavil and Sinequan. MAOI antidepressant brand names (generic names in parentheses):

Eutonyl (pargyline)
Marplan (isocarboxazid)
Nardil (phenelzine)
Parnate (tranylcypromine)

RESERPINE... .ANTIDEPRESSANTS (CYCLIC TYPE)

THIS COMBINATION MAY CAUSE EXCESSIVE STIM-ULATION. RESULT: Hyperexcitability, aberrant or psychotic behavior. Antidepressants are prescribed to alleviate mental depression and elevate the mood. The antidepressant trazadone (Desyrel) may not interact. Antidepressant brand names (generic names in parentheses):

Adapin (doxepin)
Asendin (amoxapine)
Aventyl (nortriptyline)
Desyrel (trazadone)
Elavil (amitriptyline)
Endep (amitriptyline)
Etrafon (amitriptyline/
　perphenazine)
Limbitrol (amitriptyline/
　chlordiazepoxide)
Ludiomil (maprotiline)

Norpramin (desipramine)
Pamelor (nortriptyline)
Pertofrane (desipramine)
Sinequan (doxepin)
Surmontil (trimipramine)
Tofranil, Tofranil-PM
　(imipramine)
Triavil (amitriptyline/
　perphenazine)
Vivactil (protriptyline)

RESERPINE....BETA BLOCKER HEART DRUGS

THE EFFECT OF EACH DRUG MAY BE INCREASED. Beta blockers are prescribed for angina, to restore irregular heart beats to normal rhythm, and to help lower high blood pressure. RESULT: Bradycardia (slow heart beat) and a fall in blood pressure. Report symptoms such as dizziness, weakness, faintness, postural hypotension (sudden drop in blood pressure when changing positions, especially when rising after sitting or lying down—with above symptoms). Beta blocker brand names (generic names in parentheses):

Blocadren (timolol)
Corgard (nadolol)
Inderal (propranolol)
Lopressor (metoprolol)
Tenormin (atenolol)
Visken (pindolol)

RESERPINE....LEVODOPA (Dopar, Larodopa, Sinemet)

THE EFFECT OF LEVODOPA MAY BE DECREASED. Levodopa is used to treat Parkinson's disease. RESULT: The disorder may not be controlled properly.

VI. VASODILATOR INTERACTIONS

HYDRALAZINE or MINOXIDIL ....ANTIDEPRESSANTS (MAOI TYPE)

THIS COMBINATION MAY CAUSE THE BLOOD PRESSURE TO DROP TOO LOW. RESULT: Postural hypotension (sudden drop in blood pressure when changing positions, especially when rising after sitting or lying down) with associated symptoms: dizziness, weakness, faintness. MAOI antidepressants, used to alleviate mental depression and elevate the mood, are not used much since the development of the safer tricyclic antidepressants such as Elavil and Sinequan. MAOI antidepressant brand names (generic names in parentheses):

Eutonyl (pargyline)
Marplan (isocarboxazid)
Nardil (phenelzine)
Parnate (tranylcypromine)

HYDRALAZINE or MINOXIDIL....PYRIDOXINE (vitamin B₆)

THE EFFECT OF PYRIDOXINE MAY BE DECREASED. Pyridoxine is one of the B-complex vitamins. RESULT: Possible pyridoxine deficiency. Watch for symptoms such as numbness or tingling of the feet or lower legs, tenderness, weakness, skin lesions, anemia. To counter the effects of this interaction, take a vitamin supplement containing pyridoxine. Foods containing pyridoxine include whole grain cereals and legumes (peas, beans, etc.).

MINOXIDIL (Loniten)....GUANETHIDINE (Esimil, Ismelin)

THIS COMBINATION MAY CAUSE A SEVERE DROP IN BLOOD PRESSURE. RESULT: Postural hypotension (sudden drop in blood pressure when changing positions, especially when rising after sitting or lying down) with associated symptoms: dizziness, weakness, faintness; possible seizures or shock. Guanethidine is used to lower the blood pressure.

16

Drug Interactions in Treatment of Indigestion (Antacid Therapy)

Everyone suffers from the discomforts of indigestion—also called dyspepsia—now and then. It can be caused by overindulgence in food or drink, poor chewing habits (chewing is the first step in digestion), swallowing air while eating, or the use of stomach-irritating drugs.

Symptoms include heartburn, sour or acid stomach, cramps, nausea, and excessive gas. The drugs used to treat indigestion are called *antacids*. Most cases of indigestion are uncomplicated and respond readily to treatment with these nonprescription agents.

Antacids work by helping to neutralize excess hydrochloric acid in stomach fluids.

ANTACID PRODUCT INGREDIENTS:

sodium bicarbonate
calcium carbonate
aluminum hydroxide
magnesium hydroxide
magnesium oxide
magnesium trisilicate
magnesium carbonate
dihydroxyaluminum sodium carbonate

DRUG INTERACTIONS

(Primarily two types of interactions occur. In one, antacids interefere with the body's absorption of some drugs, causing a *decrease* in their effects. In the other, the antacid changes the acidity of the urine, causing certain drugs to be reabsorbed by the body instead of eliminated, which *increases* their effects.) Most interactions can be prevented by not taking an interacting drug within one to two hours of taking the antacid.

ANTACIDS....AMPHETAMINES

THE EFFECT OF THE AMPHETAMINE MAY BE IN-CREASED. RESULT: Possible adverse side effects from too much amphetamine: nervousness, irritability, dizziness, exaggerated movements, heart palpitations, blurred vision, mouth dryness. The amphetamines are used as diet pills (this use is in disfavor); for narcolepsy (uncontrollable desire to sleep); and for hyperkinetic behavior problems in children. Amphetamine brand names:

Benzedrine
Biphetamine
Delcobese
Desoxyn
Dexedrine
Didrex
Obetrol

ANTACIDS....ANTIPSYCHOTICS (PHENOTHIAZINE FAMILY)

THE EFFECT OF THE ANTIPSYCHOTIC MAY BE DE-CREASED. Antipsychotics are major tranquilizers used to treat severe mental disorders such as schizophrenia. RESULT: The condition treated may not be controlled properly. All antacids interact except sodium bicarbonate antacids such as Alka-Seltzer. Phenothiazine antipsychotic brand names (generic names in parentheses):

Compazine (prochlorperazine)
Mellaril (thioridazine)
Proketazine (carphenazine)
Prolixin (fluphenazine)
Quide (piperacetazine)
Serentil (mesoridazine)
Sparine (promazine)
Stelazine (trifluoperazine)
Thorazine (chlorpromazine)
Tindal (acetophenazine)
Trilafon (perphenazine)
Vesprin (triflupromazine)

ANTACIDS....ANTICHOLINERGIC DRUGS

THE EFFECT OF THE ANTICHOLINGERIC MAY BE DECREASED. RESULT: The condition treated by the anticholinergic may not be controlled properly. Anticholinergic uses and brand names:

Benadryl (an antihistamine)
Norflex (a muscle relaxant)
Transderm-Scop (a small disk attached behind the ear for motion sickness)

Those used to control tremors resulting from Parkinson's disease or from treatment with antipsychotic drugs:

Akineton
Artane
Cogentin
Kemadrin
Pagitane

Those used in stomach and digestive tract disorders:

Bentyl
Combid
Probanthine
Robinul

NOTE: There are dozens of brands of stomach anticholinergics—others are: Anaspaz, Barbidonna, Belladenal, Bellergal, Butibel, Cantil, Chardonna, Cystospaz, Daricon, Donnatal, Enarax, Kinesed, Levsin, Levsinex, Librax, Milpath, Pamine, Pathibamate, Pathilon, Sidonna, Valpin, Vistrax.

ANTACIDS....ASPIRIN

(Anacin, Ascriptin, Aspergum, Bayer, Bufferin, CAMA, Ecotrin, Empirin, Measurin, Momentum, Pabirin, Persistin, St. Joseph Aspirin)

THE EFFECT OF ASPIRIN MAY BE DECREASED. Aspirin is a nonprescription pain reliever. RESULT: The pain may not be relieved properly. NOTE: Other salicylate-like pain relievers which intract similarly to aspirin: Arthralgen, Arthropan, Calurin, Disalcid, Dolobid, Magan, Mobidin, Pabalate, Salrin, Uracel, Uromide.

ANTACIDS....BETA BLOCKER HEART DRUGS

THE EFFECT OF THE BETA BLOCKER MAY BE DE-CREASED. Beta blockers are used to treat angina, to restore irregular heartbeats to normal rhythm, and to lower blood pressure. RESULT: The condition treated may not be controlled properly. NOTE: The beta blocker metoprolol (Lopressor) does not interact. Beta blocker brand names (generic names in parentheses):

Blocadren (timolol)
Corgard (nadolol)
Inderal (propranolol)
Lopressor (metoprolol)
Tenormin (atenolol)
Visken (pindolol)

ANTACIDS.... CIMETIDINE (Tagamet)

THE EFFECT OF CIMETIDINE MAY BE DECREASED. Cimetidine is used to treat stomach and duodenal ulcers. RE-SULT: The ulcer may not be controlled properly.

ANTACIDS (containing MAGNESIUM) ....CORTICOSTEROIDS

THIS COMBINATION CAN CAUSE THE BODY TO LOSE TOO MUCH POTASSIUM AND HOLD TOO MUCH SODIUM. Report symptoms of potassium depletion: muscular weakness or cramps, large urine output, bradycardia (slow heart beat) or tachycardia (rapid heart beat), cardiac arrhythmias (heart beat irregularities), low blood pressure with dizziness, faintness. Report symptoms of too much sodium: edema (excess body fluid), thirst, scant urine output, confusion, high blood pressure, hyper-excitability. Corticosteroids are prescribed for arthritis, severe allergies, asthma, endocrine disorders, leukemia, colitis and en-teritis (inflammation of the intestinal tract), and various skin, lung, and eye diseases. Most antacid products contain magne-sium: Alkets, Aludrox, BiSoDol, Camalox, Creamalin, Delcid, Di-Gel, Gelusil, Kolantyl, Kudrox, Maalox, Magnatril, Milk of Mag-nesia, Mylanta, Riopan, Silain-Gel, Simeco, WinGel. Cortico-steroid brand names (generic names in parentheses):

Aristocort (triamcinolone)
Celestone (betamethasone)
Cortef (hydrocortisone)
Decadron (dexamethasone)
Delta-Cortef (prednisolone)
Deltasone (prednisone)

hydrocortisone (various companies)
Kenacort (triamcinolone)
Medrol (methylprednisolone)
Meticorten (prednisone)
Orasone (prednisone)
prednisone (various companies)

ANTACIDS....DIGOXIN (Lanoxin)

THE EFFECT OF DIGOXIN MAY BE DECREASED. Digoxin is used for congestive heart failure and to restore irregular heart beats to normal rhythm. RESULT: The heart conditions treated may not be controlled properly. All antacids interact except sodium bicarbonate antacids such as Alka-Seltzer.

ANTACIDS....IRON

THE EFFECT OF IRON MAY BE DECREASED. Iron is sometimes taken as a mineral supplement. RESULT: The body may not get the amount of iron intended. All antacids interact, but especially those containing magnesium trisilicate:A-M-T, Gaviscon, Gelumina, Magnatril, Pama.

ANTACIDS (containing ALUMINUM)....ISONIAZID

THE EFFECT OF ISONIAZID MAY BE DECREASED. Isoniazid is used to treat tuberculosis. RESULT: The tuberculosis may not be controlled properly. Most antacids contain aluminum: Aludrox, AlternaGel, Amphojel, Camalox, Creamalin, Delcid, Di-Gel, Gaviscon, Gelusil, Kolantyl, Kudrox, Maalox, Magnatril, Mylanta, Riopan, Rolaids, Silain-Gel, Simeco, WinGel. Isoniazid brand names:

INH
Nydrazid
Rifamate
Triniad
Uniad

ANTACIDS.... METHENAMINE (Hiprex, Mandelamine)

THE EFFECT OF METHENAMINE MAY BE DECREASED. Methenamine is used to treat urinary tract (bladder and kidney) infections. RESULT: The infection may not be controlled properly.

ANTACIDS (containing MAGNESIUM TRISILICATE) ....NITROFURANTOIN

THE EFFECT OF NITROFURANTOIN MAY BE DE-CREASED. Nitrofurantoin is used to treat urinary tract (bladder and kidney) infections. RESULT: The infection may not be controlled properly. Magnesium trisilicate-containing antacids:A-M-T, Gaviscon, Gelumina, Magnatril, Pama. Nitrofurantoin brand names:

> Furadantin
> Macrodantin

ANTACIDS....PROCAINAMIDE (Procan, Pronestyl)

THE EFFECT OF PROCAINAMIDE MAY BE IN-CREASED. Procainamide is an antiarrhythmic used to restore irregular heart beats to normal rhythm. RESULT: Possible adverse side effects from too much procainamide with associated symptoms: faintness (from lowered blood pressure), ventricular arrhythmias (a serious heart beat irregularity).

ANTACIDS....PSEUDOEPHEDRINE

THE EFFECT OF PSEUDOEPHEDRINE MAY BE IN-CREASED. Pseudoephedrine is a decongestant drug used in Novafed, Sudafed, and many other cold/cough products (read product label list of ingredients). RESULT: Possible adverse side effects from too much pseudoephedrine. Report symptoms such as heart palpitations, nervousness and irritability, dizziness, hallucinations, aberrant behavior.

ANTACIDS....QUINIDINE

THE EFFECT OF QUINIDINE MAY BE INCREASED. Quinidine is an antiarrhythmic used to restore irregular heart beats to normal rhythm. RESULT: Possible adverse side effects from too much quinidine with associated symptoms: ventricular arrhythmias (a serious heart beat irregularity), heart palpitations, headache, dizziness, visual disturbances, ringing in the ears. Quinidine brand names:

Cardioquin
Duraquin
Quinaglute Dura-Tabs
Quinidex
Extentabs
Quinora

ANTACIDS....QUININE (Coco-quinine, Quinamm, Quine)

THE EFFECT OF QUININE MAY BE INCREASED. Quinine is a nonprescription drug used for malaria and nighttime leg cramps. RESULT: Possible adverse side effects from too much quinine. Report symptoms such as headache, dizziness, visual disturbances, ringing in the ears.

ANTACIDS....TETRACYCLINE ANTIBIOTICS

THE EFFECT OF THE TETRACYCLINE MAY BE DE-CREASED. Tetracycline is an antibiotic used to combat infection. RESULT: The infection treated may not be controlled properly. Tetracycline brand names (generic names in parentheses):

Achromycin (tetracycline)
Aureomycin (chlortetracycline)
Bristacycline (tetracycline)
Cyclopar (tetracycline)
Declomycin (demeclocycline)
Doxychel (doxycycline)
Minocin (minocycline)
Panmycin (tetracycline)
Retet-S (tetracycline)
Robitet (tetracycline)
Rondomycin (methacycline)
Sumycin (tetracycline)
Terramycin (oxytetracycline)
Tetra-Bid (tetracycline)
Tetrachel (tetracycline)
tetracycline (various companies)
Tetracyn (tetracycline)
Tetrex (tetracycline)
Vibramycin (doxycycline)
Vibratab (doxycycline)

17

Drug Interactions in Treatment of Bacterial Infections (Antibiotic Interactions)

This chapter focuses on the antibiotics used to treat bacterial infections—including bronchitis, pneumonia, strep throat, tonsillitis, cystitis or urinary tract (bladder and kidney) infections, ear infections, sinusitis, syphilis, gonorrhea, vaginitis, cholera, Rocky Mountain Spotted Fever, chancre sores, conjunctivitis of the eye, and intestinal amebiasis.

Many people think that antibiotics are prescribed for colds or the flu. They may indeed be prescribed at the same time—but only for the purpose of warding off a secondary *bacterial* infection such as strep throat—not for the cold or flu, which are caused by viruses, not bacteria.

ANTIBIOTIC CATEGORIES AND USES

Aminoglycosides are used for certain types of diarrhea and other highly specific conditions.

Cephalosporins are related to the penicillins and are used for upper respiratory tract infections (nose and throat) such as strep throat; pneumonia; infections of the ear, skin and soft tissue, bone, and urinary tract (bladder and kidney).

Chloramphenicol is prescribed for serious infections for which less potentially dangerous antibiotics are ineffective.

Clindamycin and *Lincomycin* are reserved for serious infections in patients who are allergic to penicillin or in cases for which penicillin is inappropriate.

Erythromycin is used for upper respiratory tract infections such as strep throat and ear infections; for lower respiratory tract infections such as pneumonia; for skin and soft tissue infections; for syphilis; it is effective in treating Legionnaire's Disease. Erythromycin is often used in patients allergic to penicillin.

Griseofulvin is given orally to combat fungal infections of the skin, hair, fingernails, and toenails.

Ketoconazole is given orally to combat fungal infections of the skin, hair, fingernails, and toenails.

Metronidazole is given orally to treat trichomoniasis, a type of vaginitis. Both sexual partners are treated.

Penicillin is prescribed for upper respiratory tract (nose and throat) infections such as strep throat; ear infections; chronic bronchitis; pneumonia; urinary tract (bladder and kidney) infections; and syphilis and gonorrhea.

Sulfonamides are prescribed primarily for cystitis or urinary tract (bladder and kidney) infections.

Tetracyclines are prescribed for some of the same type of infections as penicillin and also for other infections such as cholera, Rocky Mountain Spotted Fever, chancre sores, conjunctivitis of the eye, and intestinal amebiasis. Dermatologists prescribe it for severe acne.

Troleandomycin is used for certain infections of the upper respiratory tract (nose and throat) and for pneumonia.

BRAND NAMES

AMINOGLYCOSIDES

Kantrex (kanamycin)
Klebcil (kanamycin)
Mycifradin (neomycin)
Neobiotic (neomycin)
neomycin (various companies)

CEPHALOSPORINS

Anspor (cephradine)
Ceclor (cefaclor)
Duricef (cefadroxil)
Kafocin (cephaloglycin)
Keflex (cephalexin)
Ultracef (cefadroxil)
Velosef (cephradine)

CHLORAMPHENICOL

Chloromycetin
Mychel

CLINDAMYCIN and LINCOMYCIN

Cleocin
Lincocin

ERYTHROMYCIN

Bristamycin
E.E.S.
E-Mycin
Ery-Tab
Eryc
Erypar
EryPed
Ethril
Ilosone
Ilotycin
Pedamycin
Robimycin
Wyamycin S

GRISEOFULVIN

Fulvicin P/G
Fulvicin U/F
Grifulvin V
Grisactin
Gris-PEG

KETOCONAZOLE

Nizoral

METRONIDAZOLE

Flagyl
Metryl
Satric

PENICILLINS

Amcill (ampicillin)
amoxicillin (various companies)
Amoxil (amoxicillin)
ampicillin (various companies)
Betapen-VK (penicillin VK)
Cyclapen-W (cyclacillin)
Dynapen (dicloxacillin)
Geocillin (carbenicillin)
Larotid (amoxicillin)
Ledercillin VK (penicillin VK)

Nafcil (nafcillin)
Omnipen (ampicillin)
Pathocil (dicloxacillin)
Pen-Vee K (penicillin VK)
Penapar VK (penicillin VK)
Penbritin (ampicillin)
penicillin VK (various companies)
Pensyn (ampicillin)
Pfizerpen A (ampicillin)
Pfizerpen VK (penicillin VK)
Polycillin (ampicillin)
Polymox (amoxicillin)
Principen (ampicillin)
Prostaphlin (oxacillin)

Robamox (amoxicillin)
Robicillin VK (penicillin VK)
Spectrobid (bacampicillin)
Supen (ampicillin)
Tegopen (cloxacillin)
Totacillin (ampicillin)
Trimox (amoxicillin)
Utimox (amoxicillin)
Unipen (nafcillin)
V-Cillin K (penicillin VK)
Veracillin (dicloxacillin)
Versapen (hetacillin)
Wymox (amoxicillin)

SULFONAMIDES

Azulfidine (sulfasalazine)—
  prescribed for ulcerative colitis
Bactrim (sulfamethoxazole/
  trimethoprim)
Bactrim DS (sulfamethoxazole/
  trimethoprim)
Gantanol (sulfamethoxazole)
Gantrisin (sulfisoxazole)
Renoquid (sulfacytine)

SK-Soxazole (sulfisoxazole)
Septra (sulfamethoxazole/
  trimethoprim)
Septra DS (sulfamethoxazole/
  trimethoprim)
Sulla (sulfameter)
Thiosulfil (sulfamethizole)

TETRACYCLINES

Achromycin (tetracycline)
Aureomycin (chlortetracycline)
Bristacycline (tetracycline)
Cyclopar (tetracycline)
Declomycin (demeclocycline)
Doxychel (doxycycline)
Minocin (minocycline)
Panmycin (tetracycline)
Retet-S (tetracycline)
Robitet (tetracycline)

Rondomycin (methacycline)
Sumycin (tetracycline)
Terramycin (oxytetracycline)
Tetra-Bid (tetracycline)
Tetrachel (tetracycline)
tetracycline (various companies)
Tetracyn (tetracycline)
Tetrex (tetracycline)
Vibramycin (doxycycline)
Vibratab (doxycycline)

TROLEANDOMYCIN

TAO

DRUG INTERACTIONS

AMINOGLYCOSIDE.....AMINOGLYCOSIDES (OTHER)

THE ADVERSE EFFECTS OF EACH ANTIBIOTIC MAY BE INCREASED. RESULT: Possible permanent hearing loss and kidney damage. Aminoglycoside brand names are listed in the *Brand Names* section.

AMINOGLYCOSIDE....BIRTH CONTROL PILLS (oral contraceptives)

THE EFFECT OF THE BIRTH CONTROL PILL MAY BE DECREASED. RESULT: Increased risk of pregnancy unless another form of contraception is used. Breakthrough bleeding is a symptom of a possible interaction. Birth control pill brand names:

Brevicon	Nordette
Demulen	Norinyl
Enovid	Norlestrin
Loestrin	Ortho-Novum
Lo-Ovral	Ovcon
Micronor	Ovral
Modicon	Ovrette
Nor-Q.D.	Ovulen

AMINOGLYCOSIDE....CEPHALOSPORIN ANTIBIOTICS

THE ADVERSE SIDE EFFECTS OF EACH DRUG MAY BE INCREASED. RESULT: Possible kidney damage. Report symptoms such as unusual decrease in urine output, blood in the urine, excessive thirst, appetite loss, weakness, dizziness, drowsiness, nausea. Cephalosporin brand names are listed in the *Brand Names* section.

AMINOGLYCOSIDE....DIGOXIN (Lanoxin)

THE EFFECT OF DIGOXIN MAY BE DECREASED. Digoxin is used for congestive heart failure and to restore irregular heart beats to normal rhythm. RESULT: The heart disorder may not be controlled properly. NOTE: Only the aminoglycoside neomycin (Mycifradin, Neobiotic) interacts.

AMINOGLYCOSIDE....ESTROGENS (female hormones)

THE EFFECT OF THE ESTROGEN MAY BE DE-CREASED. Estrogens are prescribed for estrogen deficiency during menopause and after hysterectomy (surgical removal of the uterus), to prevent painful swelling of the breasts after pregnancy in women choosing not to nurse, and to treat amenorrhea (failure to menstruate). RESULT: The conditions treated may not be controlled properly. Estrogen brand names:

Amen	Menrium
Aygestin	Milprem
DES	Norlutate
Estinyl	Norlutin
Estrace	Ogen
Estratab	PMB
Estrovis	Premarin
Evex	Provera
Feminone	Tace
Menest	

AMINOGLYCOSIDE....VANCOMYCIN (Vancocin)

THE ADVERSE SIDE EFFECTS OF EACH DRUG MAY BE INCREASED. RESULT: Possible permanent hearing loss and kidney damage. Vancomycin is an antibiotic prescribed for enterocolitis (inflammation of the large and small intestines).

CEPHALOSPORIN....AMINOGLYCOSIDE ANTIBIOTICS

THE ADVERSE EFFECTS OF EACH DRUG MAY BE INCREASED. RESULT: Possible kidney damage. Report symptoms such as unusual decrease in urine output, blood in the urine, excessive thirst, appetite loss, weakness, dizziness, drowsiness, nausea. Aminoglycoside brand names are listed in the *Brand Names* section.

CEPHALOSPORIN ....CHLORAMPHENICOL (Chloromycetin, Mychel)

THIS COMBINATION MAY CAUSE EXCESSIVE BONE MARROW DEPRESSION. Report symptoms such as sore throat, fever, chills, mouth ulcers, bleeding or bruising anywhere on the body, black or tarry stools, unusual loss of energy. Chloramphenicol is prescribed for serious infections for which less potentially dangerous antibiotics are ineffective.

CEPHALOSPORIN....PROBENECID (Benemid, ColBenemid)

THE EFFECT OF THE CEPHALOSPORIN ANTIBIOTIC MAY BE INCREASED. RESULT: Increased risk of kidney damage. Report symptoms such as unusual decrease in urine output, blood in the urine, excessive thirst, appetite loss, weakness, dizziness, drowsiness, nausea. Probenecid is used in gout treatment.

CHLORAMPHENICOL....ANTICOAGULANT DRUGS

THE EFFECT OF THE ANTICOAGULANT MAY BE INCREASED. The anticoagulants are used to thin the blood and prevent it from clotting. RESULT: Increased risk of hemorrhage. Report bruising or bleeding anywhere on the body, black or tarry stools. NOTE: The anticoagulant dicumarol is the most likely to interact. Anticoagulant brand names (generic names in parentheses):

Athrombin-K (warfarin)
Coufarin (warfarin)
Coumadin (warfarin)
dicumarol (various companies)
Hedulin (phenindione)
Miradon (anisindione)
Panwarfin (warfarin)

CHLORAMPHENICOL....BIRTH CONTROL PILLS (oral contraceptives)

THE EFFECT OF THE BIRTH CONTROL PILL MAY BE DECREASED. RESULT: Increased risk of pregnancy unless another form of contraception is used. Breakthrough bleeding is a symptom of a possible interaction. Birth control pill brand names:

Brevicon   Loestrin
Demulen   Lo-Ovral
Enovid   Micronor

Modicon
Nor-Q.D.
Nordette
Norinyl
Norlestrin

Ortho-Novum
Ovcon
Ovral
Ovrette
Ovulen

CHLORAMPHENICOL....CANCER DRUGS

THIS COMBINATION CAN CAUSE EXCESSIVE BONE MARROW DEPRESSION. Report symptoms such as sore throat, fever, chills, mouth ulcers, bleeding or bruising anywhere on the body, black or tarry stools, unusual loss of energy. Cancer drug brand names:

Adriamycin
Adrucil
Alkeran
BCNU
Cosmegen
Cytoxan
Efudex
Elspar
Imuran

Leukeran
Mexate
Mutamycin
Myleran
Oncovin
Platinol
Purinethol
Velban
5-FU

CHLORAMPHENICOL....CEPHALOSPORIN ANTIBIOTICS

THIS COMBINATION CAN CAUSE EXCESSIVE BONE MARROW DEPRESSION. Report symptoms such as sore throat, fever, chills, mouth ulcers, bleeding or bruising anywhere on the body, black or tarry stools, unusual loss of energy. Cephalosporin brand names are listed in the *Brand Names* section.

CHLORAMPHENICOL....CLINDAMYCIN (Cleocin) or LINCOMYCIN (Lincocin)

THE EFFECT OF BOTH ANTIBIOTICS MAY BE DE-CREASED. RESULT: The infection may not respond to treatment properly.

CHLORAMPHENICOL....DIABETES DRUGS (ORAL)

THE EFFECT OF THE DIABETES DRUGS MAY BE INCREASED. The diabetes drugs are used to lower the blood

sugar level in diabetics. RESULT: The blood sugar level may fall
too low. Report symptoms of hypoglycemia (low blood sugar):
sweating, weakness, faintness, heart palpitations, tachycardia
(rapid heart beat), headache, confusion, visual disturbances, loss
of coordination. Diabetes drug brand names (generic names in
parentheses):

> Diabinese (chlorpropamide)
> Dymelor (acetohexamide)
> Orinase (tolbutamide)
> Tolinase (tolazamide)

CHLORAMPHENICOL....ESTROGENS (female hormones)

THE EFFECT OF THE ESTROGEN MAY BE DE-
CREASED. Estrogens are prescribed for estrogen deficiency
during menopause and after hysterectomy (surgical removal of
the uterus), to prevent painful swelling of the breasts after
pregnancy in women choosing not to nurse, and to treat amenorrhea (failure to menstruate). RESULT: The coonditions treated
may not be controlled properly. Estrogen brand names:

Amen	Menrium
Aygestin	Milprem
DES	Norlutate
Estinyl	Norlutin
Estrace	Ogen
Estratab	PMB
Estrovis	Premarin
Evex	Provera
Feminone	Tace
Menest	

CHLORAMPHENICOL....GRISEOFULVIN

THIS COMBINATION CAN CAUSE EXCESSIVE BONE
MARROW DEPRESSION. Report symptoms such as sore throat,
fever, chills, mouth ulcers, bleeding or bruising anywhere on the
body, black or tarry stools, unusual loss of energy. Griseofulvin is
prescribed orally for fungal infections of the hair, skin, fingernails, and toenails. Griseofulvin brand names:

> Fulvicin P/G
> Fulvicin U/F

Gifulvin V
Grisactin
Gris-PEG

CHLORAMPHENICOL....PENICILLIN ANTIBIOTICS

THE EFFECT OF PENICILLIN MAY BE DECREASED. RESULT: The infection treated may not respond to treatment properly. Penicillin brand names are listed in the *Brand Names* section.

CHLORAMPHENICOL....PHENYTOIN (Dilantin)

THE EFFECT OF PHENYTOIN MAY BE INCREASED. Phenytoin is an anticonvulsant used to control seizures in disorders such as epilepsy. RESULT: Possible adverse side effects caused by too much phenytoin. Report loss of coordination, visual disturbances.

*CLINDAMYCIN/LINCOMYCIN....ADSORBENTS (used in diarrhea products)

THE EFFECTS OF CLINDAMYCIN AND LINCOMYCIN MAY BE DECREASED. RESULT: The infections treated may not be controlled properly. Adsorbents are used in diarrhea products. Adsorbent-containing diarrhea products:

Diar-Aid   Kaopectate
Digestalin   Parepectolin
Donnagel   Pepto-Bismol
Donnagel-PG   Polymagma

CLINDAMYCIN/LINCOMYCIN....CHLORAMPHENICOL (Chloromycetin, Mychel)

THE EFFECT OF BOTH ANTIBIOTICS MAY BE DECREASED. RESULT: The infection may not respond to treatment properly.

CLINDAMYCIN/LINCOMYCIN....ERYTHROMYCIN ANTIBIOTICS

THE EFFECT OF CLINDAMYCIN AND LINCOMYCIN MAY BE DECREASED. RESULT: The infection treated may not be controlled properly. Erythromycin brand names:

Bristamycin
E.E.S.
E-Mycin
Ery-Tab
Eryc
Erypar
EryPed

Ethril
Ilosone
Ilotycin
Pedamycin
Robimycin
Wyamycin S

ERYTHROMYCIN....ASTHMA DRUGS (THEOPHYLLINE FAMILY)

THE EFFECT OF THE ASTHMA DRUG MAY BE IN-CREASED. Asthma drugs are used to open lung air passaages and make breathing easier in asthmatic conditions. RESULT: Adverse side effects caused by too much asthma drug. Report symptoms such as nausea, headache, dizziness, irritability, trem-ors, insomnia, cardiac arrhythmias (heart beat irregularities), tachycardia (rapid heart beat); possible seizures. Theophylline asthma drug brand names (generic names in parentheses):

Accurbron (theophylline)
Bronkodyl (theophylline)
Choledyl (oxtriphylline)
Dilor (dyphylline)
Elixicon (theophylline)
Elixophyllin (theophylline)
LaBID (theophylline)
Lufyllin (diphylline)
Quibron-T (theophylline)
Respbid (theophylline)
Slo-Phyllin (theophylline)
Somophyllin (aminophylline)
Somophyllin-T (theophylline)

Sustaire (theophylline)
Theobid (theophylline)
Theodur (theophylline)
Theolair (theophylline)
Theophyl (theophylline)
Theovent (theophylline)
Multi-ingredient products
containing theophylline:
Amesec, Asbron G,
Brondecon, Marax,
Mudrane, Quibron, Tedral
SA

ERYTHROMYCIN....CARBAMAZEPINE (Tegretol)

THE EFFECT OF CARBAMAZEPINE MAY BE IN-CREASED. Carbamazepine is an anticonvulsant used to control seizures in disorders such as epilepsy. RESULT: Adverse side effects caused by too much carbamazepine. Report symptoms such as dizziness, nausea, abdominal pain, loss of coordination.

ERYTHROMYCIN....DIGOXIN (Lanoxin)

THE EFFECT OF DIGOXIN MAY BE INCREASED. Digoxin is used for congestive heart failure and to restore irregular heart beats to normal rhythm. RESULT: Possible adverse side effects from too much digoxin. Report symptoms such as nausea, visual disturbances, confusion, headache, loss of energy, appetite loss, cardiac arrhythmias (heart beat irregularities), tachycardia (rapid heart beat) or bradycardia (slow heart beat).

ERYTHROMYCIN....CLINDAMYCIN (Cleocin) or LINCOMYCIN (Lincocin)

THE EFFECT OF THE ANTIBIOTICS CLINDAMYCIN AND LINCOMYCIN MAY BE DECREASED. RESULT: The infection treated may not be controlled properly.

ERYTHROMYCIN....PENICILLIN ANTIBIOTICS

THE EFFECT OF EITHER ANTIBIOTIC MAY BE INCREASED OR DECREASED. Since results are unpredictable, this combination should probably be avoided. Penicilllin brand names are listed in the *Brand Names* section.

*GRISEOFULVIN....ANTICOAGULANTS

THE EFFECT OF THE ANTICOAGULANT MAY BE DECREASED. The anticoagulants are used to thin the blood and prevent it from clotting. RESULT: The blood may clot despite anticoagulant treatment. Anticoagulant brand names (generic names in parentheses):

Athrombin-K (warfarin)
Coufarin (warfarin)
Coumadin (warfarin)
dicumarol (various companies)
Hedulin (phenindione)
Miradon (anisindione)
Panwarfin (warfarin)

GRISEOFULVIN....BARBITURATES

THE EFFECT OF GRISEOFULVIN MAY BE DECREASED. RESULT: The fungal infection treated may not be controlled properly. Barbiturates are used as sedatives or sleeping pills. Barbiturate brand names:

phenobarbital	Luminal
Alurate	Mebaral
Amytal	Nembutal
Butisol	Seconal
Buticap	Sedadrops
Carbrital	Solfoton
Eskabarb	Tuinal
Lotusate	

GRISEOFULVIN....CHLORAMPHENICOL (Chloromycetin, Mychel)

THIS COMBINATION CAN CAUSE EXCESSIVE BONE MARROW DEPRESSION. Report symptoms such as sore throat, fever, chills, mouth ulcers, bleeding or bruising anywhere on the body, black or tarry stools, unusual loss of energy. Chloramphenicol is prescribed for serious infections for which less potentially dangerous antibiotics are ineffective.

GRISEOFULVIN....PRIMIDONE (Mysoline)

THE EFFECT OF GRISEOFULVIN MAY BE DECREASED. RESULT: The fungal infection treated may not be controlled properly. Primidone is an anticonvulsant used to treat seizure disorders such as epilepsy.

KETOCONAZOLE....ANTACIDS (ALL)

THE EFFECT OF KETOCONAZOLE MAY BE DECREASED. RESULT: The fungal infection treated may not be controlled properly. This interaction is prevented by taking ketoconazole at least two hours prior to taking the antacid. Antacid brand names:

Alka-Seltzer	Maalox
AllternaGel	Mylanta
Delcid	Riopan
Di-Gel	Rolaids
Gelusil	Tums
Kudrox	WinGel

KETOCONAZOLE....CIMETIDINE (Tagamet)

THE EFFECT OF KETOCONAZOLE MAY BE DE-CREASED. RESULT: The fungal infection treated may not be controlled properly. Cimetidine is used in stomach ulcer treatment. This interaction is prevented by taking ketoconazole at least two hours prior to taking cimetidine.

METRONIDAZOLE....ALCOHOL (beer, liquor, wine, etc.)

THIS COMBINATION CAN CAUSE A REACTION SIMI-LAR TO THAT CAUSED BY DISULFIRAM. Disulfiram (Antabuse) discourages alcoholics from drinking by reacting with alcohol to cause severe adverse side effects. Metronidazole interacts similarly, but not quite so severely. Symptoms include dizziness, flushing, headache, shortness of breath.

*METRONIDAZOLE....ANTICOAGULANTS

THE EFFECT OF THE ANTICOAGULANT MAY BE INCREASED. The anticoagulants are used to thin the blood and prevent it from clotting. RESULT: Increased risk of hemorrhage. Report bruising or bleeding anywhere on the body, black or tarry stools. Anticoagulant brand names (generic names in parentheses):

Athrombin-K (warfarin)
Coufarin (warfarin)
Coumadin (warfarin)
dicumarol (various companies)
Hedulin (phenindione)
Miradon (anisindione)
Panwarfin (warfarin)

METRONIDAZOLE
....CHLORAMPHENICOL (Chloromycetin, Mychel)

THIS COMBINATION CAN CAUSE EXCESSIVE BONE MARROW DEPRESSION. Report symptoms such as sore throat, fever, chills, mouth ulcers, bleeding or bruising anywhere on the body, black or tarry stools, unusual loss of energy. Chloramphenicol is prescribed for serious infections for which less potentially dangerous antibiotics are ineffective.

METRONIDAZOLE....DISULFIRAM (Antabuse)

THIS COMBINATION MAY CAUSE CONFUSION AND PSYCHOTIC OR ABERRANT BEHAVIOR. Disulfiram is used in alcoholism.

PENICILLIN (AMPICILLIN, BACAMPICILLIN ONLY)....ALLOPURINOL (Zyloprim)

THE RISK OF AN ANTIBIOTIC-CAUSED SKIN RASH IS INCREASED. Allopurinol is used to treat gout.

PENICILLIN....BIRTH CONTROL PILLS (oral contraceptives)

THE EFFECT OF THE BIRTH CONTROL PILL MAY BE DECREASED. RESULT: Increased risk of pregnancy unless another form of contraception is used. Breakthrough bleeding is a symptom of a possible interaction. Birth control pill brand names:

Brevicon	Nordette
Demulen	Norinyl
Enovid	Norlestrin
Loestrin	Ortho-Novum
Lo-Ovral	Ovcon
Micronor	Ovral
Modicon	Ovret
Nor-Q.D.	Ovulen

PENICILLIN....CHLORAMPHENICOL (Chloromycetin, Mychel)

THE EFFECT OF PENICILLIN MAY BE DECREASED. RESULT: The infection treated may not be controlled properly. Chloramphenicol is prescribed for serious infections for which less potentially dangerous antibiotics are ineffective.

PENICILLIN....ERYTHROMYCIN ANTIBIOTICS

THE EFFECT OF EITHER ANTIBIOTIC MAY BE IN-CREASED OR DECREASED. Since results are unpredictable, this combination should probably be avoided. Erythromycin brand names are listed in the *Brand Names* section.

PENICILLIN....ESTROGENS (female hormones)

THE EFFECT OF THE ESTROGEN MAY BE DE-CREASED. Estrogens are prescribed for estrogen deficiency during menopause and after hysterectomy (surgical removal of the uterus), to prevent painful swelling of the breasts after pregnancy in women choosing not to nurse, and to treat amenorrhea (failure to menstruate). RESULT: The conditions treated may not be controlled properly. Estrogen brand names:

Amen	Menrium
Aygestin	Milprem
DES	Norlutate
Estinyl	Norlutin
Estrace	Ogen
Estratab	PMB
Estrovis	Premarin
Evex	Provera
Feminone	Tace
Menest	

PENICILLIN....TETRACYCLINE ANTIBIOTICS

THE EFFECT OF PENICILLIN MAY BE DECREASED. RESULT: The infection treated may not be controlled properly. Tetracycline brand names are listed in the *Brand Names* section.

*SULFONAMIDE....ANTICOAGULANTS

THE EFFECT OF THE ANTICOAGULANT MAY BE INCREASED. The anticoagulants are used to thin the blood and prevent it from clotting. RESULT: Increased risk of hemorrhage. Report bruising or bleeding anywhere on the body, black or tarry stools. NOTE: The anticoagulant dicumarol is the most likely to interact. Anticoagulant brand names (generic names in parentheses):

Athrombin-K (warfarin)
Coufarin (warfarin)
Coumadin (warfarin)
dicumarol (various companies)
Hedulin (phenindione)
Miradon (anisindione)
Panwarfin (warfarin)

SULFONAMIDE....BIRTH CONTROL PILLS (oral contraceptives)

THE EFFECT OF THE BIRTH CONTROL PILL MAY BE DECREASED. RESULT: Increased risk of pregnancy unless another form of contraception is used. Breakthrough bleeding is a symptom of a possible interaction. Birth control pill brand names:

Brevicon	Nordette
Demulen	Norinyl
Enovid	Norlestrin
Loestrin	Ortho-Novum
Lo-Ovral	Ovcon
Micronor	Ovral
Modicon	Ovrette
Nor-Q.D.	Ovulen

SULFONAMIDE....CHLORAMPHENICOL (Chloromycetin, Mychel)

THIS COMBINATION CAN CAUSE EXCESSIVE BONE MARROW DEPRESSION. Report symptoms such as sore throat, fever, chills, mouth ulcers, bleeding or bruising anywhere on the body, black or tarry stools, unusual loss of energy. Chloramphenicol is prescribed for serious infections for which less potentially dangerous antibiotics are ineffective.

SULFONAMIDE....DIABETES DRUGS

THE EFFECT OF THE DIABETES DRUGS MAY BE INCREASED. The diabetes drugs are used to lower the blood sugar level in diabetics. RESULT: The blood sugar level may fall too low. Report symptoms of hypoglycemia (low blood sugar): sweating, weakness, faintness, heart palpitations, tachycardia (rapid heart beat), headache, confusion, visual disturbances, loss of coordination. Diabetes drug brand names (generic names in parentheses):

Diabinese (chlorpropamide)
Dymelor (acetohexamide)
Orinase (tolbutamide)
Tolinase (tolazamide)

SULFONAMIDE....ESTROGENS (female hormones)

THE EFFECT OF THE ESTROGEN MAY BE DE-CREASED. Estrogens are prescribed for estrogen deficiency during menopauuse and after hysterectomy (surgical removal of the uterus), to prevent painful swelling of the breasts after pregnancy in women choosing not to nurse, and to treat amenor-rhea (failure to menstruate). RESULT: The conditions trated may not be controlled properly. Estrogen brand names:

Amen	Menrium
Aygestin	Milprem
DES	Norlutate
Estinyl	Norlutin
Estrace	Ogen
Estratab	PMB
Estrovis	Premarin
Evex	Provera
Feminone	Tace
Menest	

SULFONAMIDE....METHENAMINE (Hiprex, Mandelamine)

THIS COMBINATION MAY CAUSE CRYSTALLURIA (CRYSTALS IN THE URINE). Methenamine is an antibiotic used in urinary tract infections.

SULFONAMIDE....METHOTREXATE (Mexate)

THE EFFECT OF METHOTREXATE MAY BE IN-CREASED. RESULT: Adverse side effects from too much methotrexate. Symptoms include nausea, bleeding anywhere on the body, black or tarry stools, diarrhea, skin rash, skin or mouth ulcers, hair loss, sore throat, fever, chills, loss of energy. Methotre-xate is used in cancer treatment.

SULFONAMIDE....PHENYTOIN (Dilantin)

THE EFFECT OF PHENYTOIN MAY BE INCREASED. Phenytoin is an anticonvulsant used to control seizures in disor-ders such as epilepsy. RESULT: Possible adverse side effects caused by too much phenytoin. Report loss of coordination, visual disturbances.

*TETRACYCLINES (ALL)....ANTACIDS

THE EFFECT OF THE TETRACYCLINE MAY BE DE-CREASED. RESULT: The infection may not respond to the tetracycline treatment. To prevent this interaction, do not take these medications within two hours of each other. Antacid brand names:

AlternaGel	Maalox
Delcid	Mylanta
Di-Gel	Riopan
Gelusil	WinGel
Kudrox	

TETRACYCLINES (ALL)....ANTICOAGULANTS

THE EFFECT OF THE ANTICOAGULANT MAY BE INCREASED. Anticoagulants are used to thin the blood and prevent it from clotting. RESULT: Increased risk of hemorrhage. Report symptoms such as black or tarry stools, bleeding or bruising anywhere on the body. DOXYCYCLINE (Doxychel, Vibramycin, Vibratab) is the tetracycline most likely to cause this interaction. Coumadin is the most widely used anticoagulant drug. Anticoagulant brand names:

Athrombin-K (warfarin)
Coufarin (warfarin)
Coumadin (warfarin)
dicumarol (various companies)
Hedulin (phenindione)
Miradon (anisindione)
Panwarfin (warfarin)

TETRACYCLINE (DOXYCYCLINE ONLY) ....BARBITURATES

THE EFFECT OF DOXYCYCLINE MAY BE DECREASED. RESULT: The infection may not respond to the doxycycline treatment unless the dosage is raised. Barbiturates are prescribed as sedatives or sleeping pills. NOTE: Only doxycycline (Doxychel, Vibramycin, Vibratab) interacts. Brand names of barbiturates:

phenobarbital	Amytal
Alurate	Butisol

Buticap
Carbrital
Eskabarb
Lotusate
Luminal
Mebaral

Nembutal
Seconal
Sedadrops
Solfoton
Tuinal

TETRACYCLINES (ALL)....BIRTH CONTROL PILLS (oral contraceptives)

THE EFFECT OF BIRTH CONTROL PILLS MAY BE DECREASED. RESULT: Increased risk of pregnancy unless an alternate method of contraception is used during the antibiotic treatment regimen. Breakthrough bleeding is a symptom of a possible interaction. Birth control pill brand names:

Brevicon
Demulen
Enovid
Loestrin
Lo-Ovral
Micronor
Modicon
Nor-Q.D.

Nordette
Norinyl
Norlestrin
Ortho-Novum
Ovcon
Ovral
Ovrette
Ovulen

TETRACYCLINE (DOXYCYCLINE ONLY) ....CARBAMAZEPINE (Tegretol)

THE EFFECT OF DOXYCYCLINE MAY BE DECREASED. RESULT: The infection treated may not respond to the doxycycline treatment unless the dosage is raised. Carbamazepine is prescribed to control seizures in disorders such as epilepsy.

TETRACYCLINES (ALL)....DIGOXIN (Lanoxin)

THE EFFECT OF DIGOXIN MAY BE INCREASED. Digoxin is used to treat congestive heart failure or to restore irregular heart beats to normal rhythm. RESULT: Possible adverse side effects caused by too much digoxin. Report symptoms such as nausea, visual disturbances, confusion, loss of energy, headache, heart irregularities.

TETRACYCLINES (ALL)....ESTROGENS (female hormones)

THE EFFECT OF ESTROGENS MAY BE DECREASED. Estrogens are prescribed for estrogen deficiency during menopause and after hysterectomy (surgical removal of the uterus), to prevent painful swelling of the breasts after pregnancy in women choosing not to nurse, and to treat amenorrhea (failure to menstruate). RESULT: The conditions may not be controlled properly during antibiotic treatment. Estrogen brand names:

Amen	Menrium
Aygestin	Milprem
DES	Norlutate
Estinyl	Norlutin
Estrace	Ogen
Estratab	PMB
Estrovis	Premarin
Evex	Provera
Feminone	Tace
Menest	

TETRACYCLINES (ALL)....IRON

THE EFFECT OF THE TETRACYCLINE MAY BE DE-CREASED. RESULT: The infection may not respond to the tetracycline treatment. To prevent this interaction, do not take within two hours of each other. IRON is listed on vitamin-mineral supplement labels as ferrous sulfate or ferrous gluconate.

TETRACYCLINES (ALL)....LAXATIVES

(only those containing magnesium: citrate of magnesia, epsom salts, milk of magnesia)

THE EFFECT OF THE TETRACYCLINE MAY BE DE-CREASED. RESULT: The infection may not respond to the tetracycline treatment. To prevent this interaction, do not take these medications within two hours of each other.

*TETRACYCLINES (ALL)....MILK, DAIRY PRODUCTS

THE EFFECT OF THE TETRACYCLINE MAY BE DE-CREASED. NOTE: This interaction applies to all tetracyclines except DOXYCYCLINE and MINOCYCLINE. RESULT: The infection may not respond to the tetracycline treatment. To prevent this interaction, do not take within two hours of each other. Note: All food will decrease the absorption of tetracycline to a degree, so it is best to take this antibiotic between meals.

TETRACYCLINES (ALL)....PENICILLIN ANTIBIOTICS

THE EFFECT OF PENICILLIN MAY BE DECREASED. Penicillin is an antibiotic used to treat a wide variety of infections. RESULT: The infection may not respond properly to treatment. Penicillin brand names are listed in the *Brand Names* section.

TETRACYCLINE (DOXYCYCLINE ONLY) ....PHENYTOIN (Dilantin)

THE EFFECT OF DOXYCYCLINE MAY BE DECREASED. RESULT: The infection may not respond to the doxycycline treatment unless the dosage is raised. Phenytoin is prescribed to control seizures in disorders such as epilepsy. NOTE: Only doxycycline (Doxychel, Vibramycin, Vibratab) interacts.

TETRACYCLINE (DOXYCYCLINE ONLY) ....PRIMIDONE (Mysoline)

THE EFFECT OF DOXYCYCLINE MAY BE DECREASED. RESULT: The infection may not respond to the doxycycline treatment unless the dosage is raised. Primidone is prescribed to control seizures in disorders such as epilepsy. NOTE: Only doxycycline (Doxychel, Vibramycin, Vibratab) interacts.

TETRACYCLINES (ALL)....VITAMIN A

THIS COMBINATION MAY CAUSE PRESSURE WITHIN THE SKULL with symptoms such as severe headache, nausea, visual disturbances. Avoid taking a vitamin supplement containing vitamin A during extended tetracycline treatment.

TETRACYCLINES (ALL)....ZINC

THE EFFECT OF THE TETRACYCLINE MAY BE DECREASED. NOTE: This interaction applies to all tetracyclines except DOXYCYCLINE and MINOCYCLINE. RESULT: The infection may not respond to the tetracycline treatment. To prevent this interaction, do not take within two hours of each other. ZINC is a mineral found in many vitamin-mineral supplements.

TROLEANDOMYCIN
....ASTHMA DRUGS (THEOPHYLLINE FAMILY)

THE EFFECT OF THE ASTHMA DRUG MAY BE IN-CREASED. Asthma drugs are used to open lung air passages and make breathing easier in asthmatic conditions. RESULT: Adverse side effects caused by too much asthma drug. Report symptoms such as nausea, headache, dizziness, irritability, tremors, insomnia, cardiac arrhythmias (heart beat irregularities), tachycardia (rapid heart beat); possible seizures. Theophylline asthma drug brand names (generic names in parentheses):

Accurbron (theophylline)
Bronkodyl (theophylline)
Choledyl (oxtriphylline)
Dilor (dyphylline)
Elixicon (theophylline)
Elixophyllin (theophylline)
LaBID (theophylline)
Lufyllin (diphylline)
Quibron-T (theophylline)
Respbid (theophylline)
Slo-Phyllin (theophylline)
Somophyllin (aminophylline)
Somophyllin-T (theophylline)

Sustaire (theophylline)
Theobid (theophylline)
Theodur (theophylline)
Theolair (theophylline)
Theophyl (theophylline)
Theovent (theophylline)
Multi-ingredient products
  containing theophylline:
  Amesec, Asbron G,
  Brondecon, Marax,
  Mudrane, Quibron, Tedral
  SA

TROLEANDOMYCIN....BIRTH CONTROL PILLS (oral contraceptives)

THIS COMBINATION CAN CAUSE CHOLESTATIC JAUNDICE. Jaundice symptoms include a yellow discoloration of the skin and eyes. The physician should avoid prescribing this antibiotic to women taking birth control pills. Birth control pill brand names:

Brevicon
Demulen
Enovid
Loestrin
Lo-Ovral

Micronor
Modicon
Nor-Q.D.
Nordette
Norinyl

Norlestrin	Ovral
Ortho-Novum	Ovrette
Ovcon	Ovulen

TROLEANDOMYCIN....CARBAMAZEPINE (Tegretol)

THE EFFECT OF CARBAMAZEPINE MAY BE IN-CREASED. Carbamazepine is an anticonvulsant used to control seizures in disorders such as epilepsy. RESULT: Adverse side effects caused by too much carbamazepine. Report symptoms such as dizziness, nausea, abdominal pain, loss of coordination.

TROLEANDOMYCIN....ESTROGENS (female hormones)

THIS COMBINATION CAN CAUSE CHOLESTATIC JAUNDICE. Jaundice symptoms include a yellow discoloration of the skin and eyes. Estrogens are prescribed for estrogen deficiency during menopause and after hysterectomy (surgical removal of the uterus), to prevent painful swelling of the breasts after pregnancy in women choosing not to nurse, and to treat amenorrhea (failur to menstruate). The physician should avoid prescribing this antibiotic to women taking estrogens. Brand names of estrogens:

Amen	Menrium
Aygestin	Milprem
DES	Norlutate
Estinyl	Norlutin
Estrace	Ogen
Estratab	PMB
Estrovis	Premarin
Evex	Provera
Feminone	Tace
Menest	

18

Drug Interactions in Treatment of Insomnia

Almost everyone experiences occasional insomnia (sleeplessness), especially during periods of unusual tension or upset. Physicians may prescribe a sedative or sleeping pill for short-term use.

The two types or families of prescription-only sleeping pills are *barbiturates* and *non-barbiturates*. Nonprescription sleeping pills contain *antihistamines*, which produce drowsiness as a side effect (in this case the side effect is *desirable*).

BRAND NAMES

I. BARBITURATE SLEEPING PILLS:

phenobarbital
Alurate
Amytal
Butisol
Buticap
Carbrital
Eskabarb
Lotusate

Luminal
Mebaral
Nembutal
Seconal
Sedadrops
Solfoton
Tuinal

II. NON-BARBITURATE SLEEPING PILLS:

Ativan (lorazepam)—also
  prescribed as a daytime
  tranquilizer
Dalmane (flurazepam)
Doriden (glutethimide)

Halcion (triazolam)
Noctec (chloral hydrate)
Noludar (methyprylon)
Parest (methaqualone)
Placidyl (ethchlorvynol)

Quaalude (methaqalone)
Restoril (temazepam)
Somnos (chloral hydrate)

Triclos (triclofos)
Valmid (ethinamate)

III. ANTIHISTAMINE-CONTAINING SLEEPING PILLS (NONPRESCRIPTION):

Compoz (diphenhydramine)
Nervine (pyrilamine)
Nytol (pyrilamine)
Nytol with DPH
  (diphenhydramine)
Quiet World (pyrilamine)

Sleep-Eze (pyrilamine)
Sominex (pyrilamine)
Sominex Formula 2
  (diphenhydramine)
Unisom (doxylamine)

DRUG INTERACTIONS

SLEEPING PILLS....OTHER DEPRESSANTS DRUGS

Sleeping pills are central nervous system depressants. They depress or impair functions such as coordination and alertness. Excessive depression and impairment can occur when a sleeping pill is taken with any other central nervous system depressant. RESULT: Drowsiness, dizziness, loss of muscle coordination and mental alertness; in severe cases, failure of blood circulation and breathing functions causing coma and death. The physician should monitor the patient carefully and adjust the dosages to minimize the excessive depressant effects. Interacting depressant categories and brand names:

ALCOHOL (beer, liquor, wine, etc.)
ANTICHOLINERGICS—Uses and brand names:
  Those used to control tremors resulting from Parkinson's disease or from treatment with antipsychotic drugs:
    Akineton, Artane, Cogentin, Kemadrin, Pagitane
  Others:
    Norflex (a muscle relaxant)
    Robinul (used for stomach, digestive tract disorders)
    Transderm-Scop (used for motion sickness)
ANTICONVULSANTS (Used to control seizures in disorders such as epilepsy). Brand names: Depakene, Dilantin, Messantoin, Mysoline, Peganone, Tegretol, Tridione, Zarontin
ANTIDEPRESSANTS (CYCLIC TYPE)—Used to alleviate mental depression. Brand names: Adapin, Asendin, Aventyl, Desyrel, Elavil, Endep, Etrafon, Limbitrol, Ludiomil, Norpramin, Pamelor, Pertofrane, Sinequan, Surmontil, Tofranil, Tofranil-PM, Triavil, Vivactil

ANTIHISTAMINES (Used for allergies, colds). Brand names: Actidil, Antivert, Atarax, Benadryl, Bendectin, Bonine, Chlor-Trimeton, Clistin, Decapryn, Dimetane, Dramamine, Histadyl, Inhiston, Marezine, Optimine, PBZ, Periactin, Polaramine, Pyronil, Travist, Teldrin, Triten, Vistaril

ANTIPSYCHOTICS (Used for severe mental disorders)

Antipsychotic brand names: Compazine, Haldol, Loxitane, Mellaril, Moban, Navane, Proketazine, Prolixin, Quide, Serentil, Sparine, Stelazine, Taractan, Thorazine, Tindal, Trilafon, Vesprin

FENFLURAMINE (Pondimin) (a diet pill)

HIGH BLOOD PRESSURE DRUGS (brand names in parentheses):

clonidine (Catapres, Combipres)

guanabenz (Wytensin)

methyldopa (Aldoclor, Aldomet, Aldoril)

reserpine-type drugs:

deserpidine (Enduronyl, Harmonyl, Oreticyl)

rauwolfia (Raudixin, Rauzide)

reserpine (Diupres, Diutensen-R, Hydropres, Rau-Sed, Regroton, Renese-R, Reserpoid, Salutensin, Sandril, Ser-Ap-Es, Serpasil, Serpasil-Apresoline, Serpasil-Esidrix)

MUSCLE RELAXANTS

Dantrium, Flexeril, Lioresal, Norflex, Norgesic, Norgesic Forte, Paraflex, Parafon Forte, Quinamm, Rela, Robaxin, Robaxisal, Skelaxin, Soma, Soma Compound, Valium

NARCOTICS

Codeine products:

Ascriptin w/Codeine, Bancap w/Codeine, Bufferin w/Codeine, Empirin w/Codeine, Empracet w/Codeine, Fiorinaal w/Codeine, Phenaphen w/Codeine, Tylenol w/Codeine

Other narcotic or narcotic-like products:

Demerol, Dilaudid, Dolophene, morphine, Merpergan Fortis, Norcet, Numorphan, Percocet, Percodan, Synalgos-DC, Talwin, Talwin Compound, Tylox, Vicodan, Zactane, Zactirin

PROPOXYPHENE (pain reliever):

Darvocet-N, Darvon, Dolene, Wygesic

TRANQUILIZERS

Benzodiazepine tranquilizers:

Ativan, Centrax, Librium, Limbitrol (also an antidepressant), Paxipam, Serax, SK-Lygen, Tranxene, Valium, Xanax

Non-Benzodiazepine tranquilizers:

Atarax, Equanil, meprobamate, Meprospan, Meprotab, Miltown, Trancopal, Tybatran, Vistaril

I. BARBITURATE SLEEPING PILL INTERACTIONS

*BARBITURATE....ANTICOAGULANTS

THE EFFECT OF THE ANTICOAGULANT MAY BE DECREASED. Anticoagulants are used to thin the blood and prevent it from clotting. RESULT: The blood may clot despite anticoagulant treatment. Anticoagulant brand names (generic names in parentheses):

Athrombin-K (warfarin)
Coufarin (warfarin)
Coumadin (warfarin)
dicumarol (various companies)
Hedulin (phenindione)
Miradon (anisindione)
Panwarfin (warfarin).

BARBITURATE....ANTIDEPRESSANTS (CYCLIC TYPE)

THE EFFECT OF THE ANTIDEPRESSANT MAY BE DECREASED. Antidepressants are used to alleviate mental depression and elevate the mood. RESULT: The depression may not be controlled properly. NOTE: The antidepressant trazadone (Desyrel) may not interact except in the following part of the interaction: Since both drugs are central system depressants, excessive "physical" depression can occur with associated symptoms—drowsiness, dizziness, loss of muscle coordination and mental alertness; in severe cases, failure of blood circulation and breathing functions, causing coma and death. Antidepressant brand names (generic names in parenthesis):

Adapin (doxepin)
Asendin (amoxapine)
Aventyl (nortriptyline)
Desyrel (trazadone)
Elavil (amitriptyline)
Endep (amitriptyline)
Etrafon (amitriptyline/
  perphenazine)
Limbitrol (amitriptyline/
  chlordiazepoxide)
Ludiomil (maprotiline)

Norpramin (desipramine)
Pamelor (nortriptyline)
Pertofrane (desipramine)
Sinequan (doxepin)
Surmontil (trimipramine)
Tofranil, Tofranil-PM
  (imipramine)
Triavil (amitriptyline/
  perphenazine)
Vivactil (protriptyline)

BARBITURATE.... .ASTHMA DRUGS (THEOPHYLLINE FAMILY)

THE EFFECT OF THE ASTHMA DRUG MAY BE DE-CREASED. Asthma drugs open lung air passages to ease breathing in asthmatics. RESULT: The asthma episode may not be relieved properly. Theophylline family asthma drug brand names (generic names in parentheses):

Accurbron (theophylline)
Bronkodyl (theophylline)
Choledyl (oxtriphylline)
Dilor (dyphylline)
Elixicon (theophylline)
Elixophyllin (theophylline)
LaBID (theophylline)
Lufyllin (dyphylline)
Quibron-T (theophylline)
Respbid (theophylline)
Slo-Phyllin (theophylline)
Somophyllin (aminophylline)
Somophyllin-T (theophylline)

Sustaire (theophylline)
Theobid (theophylline)
Theodur (theophylline)
Theolair (theophylline)
Theophyl (theophylline)
Theovent (theophylline)
   Multi-ingredient products
   containing theophylline:
   Amesec, Asbron G,
   Brondecon, Marax,
   Mudrane, Quibron, Tedral
SA

BARBITURATE....BETA BLOCKER HEART DRUGS

THE EFFECT OF THE BETA BLOCKER MAY BE DE-CREASED. Beta blocker heart drugs are used to prevent angina, to restore irregular heart beats to normal rhythm, and to lower blood pressure. RESULT: The condition treated may not be controlled properly. Beta blocker brand names (generic names in parentheses):

Blocadren (timolol)
Corgard (nadolol)
Inderal (propranolol)
Lopressor (metoprolol)
Tenormin (atenolol)
Visken (pindolol)

BARBITURATE....BIRTH CONTROL PILLS (oral contraceptives)

THE EFFECT OF THE BIRTH CONTROL PILL MAY BE DECREASED. RESULT: Approximately twenty-five times increased risk of pregnancy unless an alternate method of contraception is used. Breakthrough bleeding is a symptom of a possible interaction. Birth control pill brand names:

Brevicon
Demulen
Enovid
Leostrin
Lo-Ovral
Micronor
Modicon
Nor-Q.D.

Nordette
Norinyl
Norlestrin
Ortho-Novum
Ovcon
Ovral
Ovrette
Ovulen

BARBITURATE....CORTICOSTEROIDS

THE EFFECT OF THE CORTICOSTEROID MAY BE DECREASED. Corticosteroids are prescribed for arthritis, severe allergies, asthma, endocrine disorders, leukemia, colitis and enteritis (innflammation of the intestinal tract), and various skin, lung, and eye diseases. RESULT: The conditions treated may not be controlled properly. Corticosteroid brand names (generic names in parentheses):

Aristocort (triamcinolone)
Celestone (betamethasone)
Cortef (hydrocortisone)
Decadron (dexamethasone)
Delta-Cortef (prednisolone)
Deltasone (prednisone)
hydrocortisone (various
    companies)

Kenacort (triamcinolone)
Medrol (methylprednisolone)
Meticorten (prednisone)
Orasone (prednisone)
prednisone (various companies)

BARBITURATE....DIGITOXIN (Crystodigin, Purodigin)

THE EFFECT OF DIGITOXIN MAY BE DECREASED. Digitoxin is used for congestive heart failure and to restore irregular heart beats to normal rhythm. RESULT: The heart disorder may not be controlled properly.

BARBITURATE....DOXYCYCLINE (Doxychel, Vibramycin, Vibratab)

THE EFFECT OF DOXYCYCLINE MAY BE DECREASED. Doxycycline is an antibiotic used to combat infection. RESULT: The infection may not be controlled properly.

BARBITURATE....ESTROGENS (female hormones)

THE EFFECT OF THE ESTROGEN MAY BE DE-CREASED. Estrogens are prescribed for estrogen deficiency during menopause and after hysterectomy (surgical removal of the uterus), to prevent painful swelling of the breasts after pregnancy in women choosing not to nurse, and to treat amenorrhea (failure to menstruate). RESULT: The conditions treated may not be controlled properly. Estrogen brand names:

Amen	Menrium
Aygestin	Milprem
DES	Norlutate
Estinyl	Norlutin
Estrace	Ogen
Estratab	PMB
Estrovis	Premarin
Evex	Provera
Feminone	Tace
Menest	

BARBITURATE....FOLIC ACID (Vitamin B₉)

THE EFFECT OF FOLIC ACID MAY BE DECREASED. Folic acid is one of the B-complex vitamins. RESULT: Possible folic acid deficiency with associated symptoms: loss of energy, uncommon memory lapses, pale complexion, nervousness and irritability, digestive tract symptoms. To counter the effects of this interaction, take a vitamin supplement containing folic acid or eat a fresh fruit and a green leafy vegetable daily.

BARBITURATE....GRISEOFULVIN

THE EFFECT OF GRISEOFULVIN MAY BE DE-CREASED. Griseofulvin is given orally to combat fungal infections of the hair, skin, fingernails, and toenails. RESULT: The infection may not be controlled properly. Griseofulvin brand names:

Fulvicin P/G
Fulvicin U/F
Grifulvin
Grisactin
Gris-PEG

BARBITURATE....METHADONE (Dolophine)

THE EFFECT OF METHADONE MAY BE DECREASED. Methadone is a narcotic pain reliever used to help free addicts from their dependence on heroin or other narcotics. RESULT: The addiction may not be controlled properly.

BARBITURATE....PHENYTOIN (Dilantin)

THE EFFECT OF PHENYTOIN MAY BE DECREASED. Phenytoin is an anticonvulsant prescribed to control seizures in disorders such as epilepsy. RESULT: The seizure disorder may not be controlled properly. Since physicians often prescribe the barbiturate phenobarbital along with phenytoin for seizure control, blood levels should be monitored to determine the proper doses for each individual patient. Other interacting phenytoin-like drugs are Mesantoin (mephenytoin) and Peganone (ethotoin).

BARBITURATE....QUINIDINE

THE EFFECT OF QUINIDINE MAY BE DECREASED. Quinidine is an antiarrhythmic drug used to restore irregular heart beats to normal rhythm. RESULT: The heart beat irregularity may not be controlled properly. Quinidine brand names:

Cardioquin
Duraquin
Quinaglute Dura-Tabs
Quinidex
Extentabs
Quinora

BARBITURATE....QUININE (Coco-quinine, Quinamm, Quine)

THE EFFECT OF QUININE MAY BE DECREASED. Quinine is a nonprescription drug used for malaria and to relieve nighttime leg cramps. RESULT: The conditions treated may not be controlled properly.

BARBITURATE....RIFAMPIN (Rifadin, Rimactane)

THE EFFECT OF THE BARBITURATE MAY BE DECREASED. RESULT: The insomnia may not be relieved properly.

Rifampin is used to treat tuberculosis and may be given to suspected meningitis carriers.

BARBITURATE (phenobarbital only)
....VALPROIC ACID (Depakene)

THE EFFECT OF PHENOBARBITAL MAY BE INCREASED. RESULT: Since both drugs are central nervous system depressants, be alert for symptoms of excessive depression: drowsiness, dizziness, loss of coordination and mental alertness. Valproic acid is an anticonvulsant used to prevent seizures in disorders such as epilepsy.

II. NON-BARBITURATE SLEEPING PILL INTERACTIONS

CHLORAL HYDRATE (Noctec, Somnos)....ALCOHOL (beer, liquor, wine, etc.)

THIS COMBINATION MAY CAUSE A REACTION SIMILAR TO THAT CAUSED BY DISULFIRAM. Disulfiram (Antabuse) is a drug given to alcoholics to discourage them from drinking—it reacts with alcohol to cause severe adverse side effects. Chloral hydrate interacts similarly and causes the same symptoms: dizziness, flushing, headache, shortness of breath.

CHLORAL HYDRATE (Noctec, Somnos)
....ANTICOAGULANTS

THE EFFECT OF THE ANTICOAGULANT MAY BE INCREASED. Anticoagulants are used to thin the blood and prevent it from clotting. RESULT: Increased risk of hemorrhage. Report symptoms such as bruising or bleeding anywhere on the body, black or tarry stools. Anticoagulant brand names (generic names in parentheses):

Athrombin-K (warfarin)   Hedulin (phenindione)
Coufarin (warfarin)   Liquamar (phenprocoumon)
Coumadin (warfarin)   Miradon (anisindione)
dicamarul (various companies)   Panwarfin (warfarin)

ETHCHLORVYNOL (Placidyl)....ANTICOAGULANTS

THE EFFECT OF THE ANTICOAGULANT MAY BE DECREASED. Anticoagulants are used to thin the blood and prevent it from clotting. RESULT: The blood may clot despite anticoagulant treatment. Anticoagulant brand names (generic names in parentheses):

Athrombin-K (warfarin)
Coufarin (warfarin)
Coumadin (warfarin)
dicumarol (various companies)
Hedulin (phenindione)
Miradon (anisindione)
Panwarfin (warfarin)

ETHINAMATE (Valmid)

See SLEEPING PILLS....OTHER DEPRESSANTS interaction at beginning of *Drug Interactions* section.

FLURAZEPAM (Dalmane)....ANTIDEPRESSANTS (CYCLIC TYPE)

THE EFFECT OF THE ANTIDEPRESSANT MAY BE DECREASED. Antidepressants are used to alleviate mental depression and elevate the mood. RESULT: The depression may not be controlled properly. NOTE: The antidepressant trazadone (Desyrel) may not interact except in the following part of the interaction: Since both drugs are central nervous system depressants, excessive *physical* depression can occur with associated symptoms—drowsiness, dizziness, loss of muscle coordination and mental alertness; in severe cases, failure of blood circulation and breathing functions causing coma and death. Antidepressant brand names (generic names in parentheses):

Adapin (doxepin)
Asendin (amoxapine)
Aventyl (nortriptyline)
Desyrel (trazadone)
Elavil (amitriptyline)
Endep (amitriptyline)
Etrafon (amitriptyline/
  perphenazine)
Limbitrol (amitriptyline/
  chlordiazepoxide)
Ludiomil (maprotiline)

Norpramin (desipramine)
Pamelor (nortriptyline)
Pertofrane (desipramine)
Sinequan (doxepin)
Surmontil (trimipramine)
Tofranil, Tofranil-PM
  (imipramine)
Triavil (amitriptyline/
  perphenazine)
Vivactil (protriptyline)

FLURAZEPAM (Dalmane)
....ASTHMA DRUGS (THEOPHYLLINE FAMILY)

THE EFFECT OF THE ASTHMA DRUG MAY BE DE-CREASED. Asthma drugs open lung air passages to ease breathing in asthmatics. RESULT: The asthma episode may not be relieved properly. Theophylline family asthma drug brand names (generic names in parentheses):

Accurbron (theophylline)
Bronkodyl (theophylline)
Choledyl (oxtriphylline)
Dilor (dyphylline)
Elixicon (theophylline)
Elixophyllin (theophylline)
LaBID (theophylline)
Lufyllin (dyphylline)
Quibron-T (theophylline)
Respbid (theophylline)
Slo-Phyllin (theophylline)
Somophyllin (aminophylline)
Somophyllin-T (theophylline)

Sustaire (theophylline)
Theobid (theophylline)
Theodur (theophylline)
Theolair (theophylline)
Theophyl (theophylline)
Theovent (theophylline)
   Multi-ingredient products
   containing theophylline:
   Amesec, Asbron G,
   Brondecon, Marax,
   Mudrane, Quibron, Tedral
   SA

FLURAZEPAM (Dalmane)....BIRTH CONTROL PILLS

THE EFFECT OF THE BIRTH CONTROL PILL MAY BE DECREASED. RESULT: Approximately twenty-five times increased risk of pregnancy unless an alternate method of contraception is used. Breakthrough bleeding is a symptom of a possible interaction. Birth control pill brand names:

Brevicon
Demulen
Enovid
Loestrin
Lo-Ovral
Micronor
Modicon
Nor-Q.D.

Nordette
Norinyl
Norlestrin
Ortho-Novum
Ovcon
Ovral
Ovrette
Ovulen

FLURAZEPAM (Dalmane)....CIMETIDINE (Tagamet)

THE EFFECT OF FLURAZEPAM MAY BE INCREASED. RESULT: Excessive sedation and central nervous system depression with associated symptoms: dizziness, drowsiness, loss of coordination; in severe cases, failure of blood circulation and breathing functions causing coma and death. Cimetidine is used to treat peptic and duodenal ulcers.

FLURAZEPAM (Dalmane)....ESTROGENS (female hormones)

THE EFFECT OF THE ESTROGEN MAY BE DE-CREASED. Estrogens are prescribed for estrogen deficiency during menopause and after hysterectomy (surgical removal of the uterus), to prevent painful swelling of the breasts after pregnancy in women choosing not to nurse, and to treat amenorrhea (failure to menstruate). RESULT: The conditions treated may not be controlled properly. Estrogen brand names:

Amen	Menrium
Aygestin	Milprem
DES	Norlutate
Estinyl	Norlutin
Estrace	Ogen
Estratab	PMB
Estrovis	Premarin
Evex	Provera
Feminone	Tace
Menest	

FLURAZEPAM (Dalmane)....LEVODOPA (Dopar, Larodopa, Sinemet)

THE EFFECT OF LEVODOPA MAY BE DECREASED. Levodopa is used to treat Parkinson's disease. RESULT: The condition may not be controlled properly.

FLURAZEPAM (Dalmane)....RIFAMPIN (Rifadin, Rimactane)

THE EFFECT OF FLURAZEPAM MAY BE DECREASED. RESULT: The insomnia may not be relieved properly. Rifampin is used to treat tuberculosis and may be given to suspected meningitis carriers.

*GLUTETHIMIDE (Doriden)....ANTICOAGULANTS

THE EFFECT OF THE ANTICOAGULANT MAY BE DECREASED. Anticoagulants are used to thin the blood and prevent it from clotting. RESULT: The blood may clot despite anticoagulant treatment. Anticoagulant brand names (generic names in parentheses):

Athrombin-K (warfarin)
Coufarin (warfarin)
dicumarol (various companies)
Hedulin (phenindione)
Miradon (anisindione)
Panwarfin (warfarin)

TRIAZOLAM (Halcion)

See *Flurazepam* interactions.

LORAZEPAM (Ativan)

See *Flurazepam* interactions.

METHAQUALONE (Parest, Quaalude)

See *Sleeping Pills....Other Depressants* interaction at beginning of *Drug Interactions* section.

METHYPRYLON (Noludar)

See *Sleeping Pills....Other Depressants* interaction at beginning of *Drug Interactions* section.

TEMAZEPAM (Restoril)

See *Flurazepam* interactions.

TRICLOFOS (Triclos)....ALCOHOL (beer, liquor, wine)

THIS COMBINATION MAY CAUSE A REACTION SIMILAR TO THAT CAUSED BY DISULFIRAM. Disulfiram (Antabuse) is a drug given to alcoholics to discourage them from drinking—it reacts with alcohol to cause severe adverse side effects. Triclofos interacts similarly and causes the same symptoms: dizziness, flushing, headache, shortness of breath.

III. FOR NONPRESCRIPTION ANTIHISTAMINE-SLEEPING PILL INTERACTIONS IN DETAIL, see the *Allergy* chapter—
all antihistamine interactions listed there apply.

19

Drug Interactions in Treatment of Nervousness and Anxiety (Tranquilizer Interactions)

Drugs used to alleviate nervousness, anxiety, and tension are called *tranquilizers*. They are prescribed for anxiety disorders and for short-term relief of nervousness and anxiety.

TRANQUILIZER DRUGS:

    benzodiazepine family
    chlormezanone
    hydroxyzine
    meprobamate
    tybamate

By far the most frequently used tranquilizers are the benzodiazepine drugs, with Valium as the most often prescribed. Hydroxyzine is an antihistamine with relaxing or calming side effects. Meprobamate, once the most popular tranquilizer, has fallen into disuse since the development of the newer Valium-type benzodiazepine tranquilizers.

BRAND NAMES

BENZODIAZEPINE TRANQUILIZERS:

Ativan (lorazepam)
Centrax (prazepam)
Dalmane (flurazepam)—
  prescribed as a sleeping pill

Halcion (triazolam)—prescribed
  as a sleeping pill
Librium (chlordiazepoxide)
Limbitrol (chlordiazepoxide/

amitriptyline)
Paxipam (halazepam)
Restoril (temazepam)—prescribed
as a sleeping pill
Serax (oxazepam)

SK-Lygen (chlordiazepoxide)
Tranxene (clorazepate)
Valium (diazepam)
Xanax (alprazolam)

OTHERS:

Atarax (hydroxyzine)
Equanil (meprobamate)
meprobamate (various
companies)
Meprospan (meprobamate)
Meprotab (meprobamate)

Miltown (meprobamate)
Trancopal (chlormezanone)
Tybatran (tybamate)
Vistaril (hydroxyzine)

DRUG INTERACTIONS

TRANQUILIZERS (ALL)....OTHER DEPRESSANT DRUGS

The tranquilizers are central nervous system depressants. They depress or impair functions such as coordination and alertness. Excessive depression or impairment can occur when a tranquilizer is taken with any other central nervous system depressant. RESULT: drowsiness, dizziness, loss of muscle coordination and mental alertness; in severe cases, failure of blood circulation and breathing functions causing coma and death. The physician should monitor the patient carefully and adjust the dosages to minimize the excessive depressant effects. Interacting depressant categories and brand names:

ALCOHOL (beer, liquor, wine, etc.)
ANTICHOLINERGICS—Uses and brand names:
Those used to control tremors resulting from Parkinson's disease or from treatment with antipsychotic drugs: Akineton, Artane, Cogentin, Kemadrin, Pagitane

Others:
Benadryl (an antihistamine)
Norflex (a muscle relaxant)
Robinul (used for stomach, digestive tract disorders)
Transderm-Scop (used for motion sickness)
ANTICONVULSANTS (Used to control seizures in disorders such as epilepsy). Brand names: Depakene, Dilantin, Mesantoin, Mysoline, Peganone, Tegretol, Tridione, Zarontin

ANTIDEPRESSANTS (CYCLIC TYPE)—Used to alleviate mental depression. Brand names: Adapin, Asendin, Aventyl, Desyrel, Elavil, Endep, Etrafon, Limbitrol, Ludiomil, Norpramin, Pamelor, Pertofrane, Sinequan, Surmontil, Tofranil, Tofranil-PM, Triavil, Vivactil

ANTIHISTAMINES (Used for allergies, colds). Brand names: Actidil, Antivert, Atarax, Benadryl, Bendectin, Bonine, Chlor-Trimeton, Clistin, Decapryn, Dimetane, Dramamine, Histadyl, Inhiston, Marezine, Optimine, PBZ, Periactin, Polaramine, Pyronil, Tavist, Teldrin, Triten, Vistaril

ANTIPSYCHOTICS (Used for severe mental disorders). Brand names: Compazine, Haldol, Loxitane, Mellaril, Moban, Navane, Proketazine, Prolixin, Quide, Serentil, Sparine, Stelazine, Taractan, Thorazine, Tindal, Trilafon, Vesprin

FENFLURAMINE (Pondimin)—a diet pill

HIGH BLOOD PRESSURE DRUGS (brand names in parentheses):

clonidine (Catapres, Combipres)

guanabenz (Wytensin)

methyldopa (Aldoclor, Aldomet, Aldoril)

reserpine-type drugs:

deserpidine (Enduronyl, Harmonyl, Oreticyl)

rauwolfia (Raudixin, Rauzide)

reserpine (Diupres, Diutensen-R, Hydropres, Rau-Sed, Regroton, Renese-R, Reserpoid, Salutensin, Sandril, Ser-Ap-Es, Serpasil, Serpasil-Apresoline, Serpasil-Esidrix)

MUSCLE RELAXANTS

Dantrium, Flexeril, Lioresal, Norflex, Norgesic, Norgesic Forte, Paraflex, Parafon Forte, Quinamm, Rela, Robaxin, Robaxisal, Skelaxin, Soma, Soma Compound, Valium

NARCOTICS

Codeine products:

Ascriptin w/Codeine, Bancap w/Codeine, Bufferin w/Codeine, Empirin w/Codeine, Empracet w/Codeine, Fiorinal w/Codeine, Phenaphen w/Codeine, Tylenol w/Codeine

Other narcotic or narcotic-like products:

Demerol, Dilaudid, Dolophene, morphine, Merpergan Fortis, Norcet, Numorphan, Percocet, Percodan, Synalgos-DC, Talwin, Talwin Compound, Tylox, Vicodan, Zactane, Zactirin

PROPOXYPHENE (pain reliever): Darvocet-N, Darvon, Dolene, Wygesic

SLEEPING PILLS

Barbiturate sleeping pills:

phenobarbital, Alurate, Amytal, Butisol, Buticap, Carbrital, Eskabarb, Lotusate, Luminal, Mebaral, Nembutal, Seconal, Sedadrops, Solfoton, Tuinal

Non-Barbiturate sleeping pills:

Ativan (also used as a tranquilizer), Dalmane, Doriden, Halcion, Noctec, Noludar, Parest, Placidyl, Quaalude, Restoril, Somnos, Triclos, Valmid

I. BENZODIAZEPINE INTERACTIONS

BENZODIAZEPINE TRANQUILIZER ....ASTHMA DRUGS (THEOPHYLLINE FAMILY)

THE EFFECT OF THE ASTHMA DRUG MAY BE DECREASED. Asthma drugs are used to open lung air passages to make breathing easier in asthmatics. RESULT: The asthma episode may not be relieved properly. Theophylline-type asthma drug brand names (generic names in parentheses):

Accurbron (theophylline)
Bronkodyl (theophylline)
Choledyl (oxtriphylline)
Dilor (dyphylline)
Elixicon (theophylline)
Elixophyllin (theophylline)
LaBID (theophylline)
Lufyllin (dyphylline)
Quibron-T (theophylline)
Respbid (theophylline)
Slo-Phyllin (theophylline)

Somophyllin (aminophylline)
Somophyllin-T (theophylline)
Sustaire (theophylline)
Theobid (theophylline)
Theodur (theophylline)
Theolair (theophylline)
Theophyl (theophylline)
Theovent (theophylline)
Multi-ingredient products
containing theophylline:
Amesec, Asbron G,
Brondecon, Marax,
Mudrane, Quibron, Tedral
SA

BENZODIAZEPINE TRANQUILIZER....BIRTH CONTROL PILLS

A. THE EFFECT OF THE BIRTH CONTROL PILL MAY BE DECREASED. RESULT: Possible increased risk of pregnancy unless an alternate method of contraception is used. Breakthrough bleeding is a symptom of a possible interaction.

B. THE EFFECT OF CERTAIN TRANQUILIZERS MAY BE INCREASED (Librium, Limbitrol, SK-Lygen, Valium); THE EFFECT OF OTHER BENZODIAZEPINE TRANQUILIZERS MAY BE DECREASED. Birth control pill brand names:

Brevicon
Demulen
Enovid
Loestrin
Lo-Ovral
Micronor
Modicon
Nor-Q.D.
Nordette

Norinyl
Norlestrin
Ortho-Novum
Ovcon
Ovral
Ovrette
Ovulen

BENZODIAZEPINE TRANQUILIZER
....CIMETIDINE (Tagamet)

THE EFFECT OF THE TRANQUILIZER MAY BE IN-CREASED. RESULT: Adverse side effects from too much tranquilizer drug. Report symptoms such as excessive sedation, drowsiness, dizziness, loss of coordination and mental alertness; in severe cases, failure of blood circulation and breathing functions causing coma and death. NOTE: The tranquilizers Ativan (lorazepam) and Serax (oxazepam) do not interact. Cimetidine is used to treat peptic and duodenal ulcers.

BENZODIAZEPINE TRANQUILIZER
....ESTROGENS (female hormones)

A. THE EFFECT OF THE ESTROGEN MAY BE DE-CREASED. Estrogens are prescribed for estrogen deficiency during menopause and after hysterectomy (surgical removal of the uterus), to prevent painful swelling of the breasts after pregnancy in women choosing not to nurse, and to treat amenor-rhea (failure to menstruate). RESULT: The conditions treated may not be controlled properly.

B. THE EFFECT OF CERTAIN TRANQUILIZERS MAY BE INCREASED (Librium, Limbitrol, SK-Lygen, Valium); THE EFFECT OF OTHER BENZODIAZEPINE TRANQUILIZERS MAY BE DECREASED. Estrogen brand names:

Amen
Aygestin
DES
Estinyl
Estrace
Estratab
Estrovis

Evex
Feminone
Menest
Menrium
Milprem
Norlutate
Norlutin

Ogen	Provera
PMB	Tace
Premarin	

BENZODIAZEPINE TRANQUILIZER
....LEVODOPA (Dopar, Larodopa, Sinemet)

THE EFFECT OF LEVODOPA MAY BE DECREASED. Levodopa is prescribed for Parkinson's disease. RESULT: The condition may not be controlled properly. NOTE: This interaction has been documented only with the tranquilizer diazepam (Valium), but the other benzodiazepines *may* interact similarly.

BENZODIAZEPINE TRANQUILIZER
....RIFAMPIN (Rifadin, Rimactane)

THE EFFECT OF THE TRANQUILIZER MAY BE DECREASED. RESULT: The nervousness and anxiety may not be relieved properly. NOTE: The tranquilizers Ativan (lorazepam) and Serax (oxazepam) may not interact. Rifampin is used to treat tuberculosis and may be given to suspected carriers of meningitis.

II. INTERACTIONS OF THE OTHER TRANQUILIZER DRUGS

CHLORMEZANONE (Trancopal)

See *Tranquilizers (All)....Other Depressant Drugs* interaction at beginning of *Drug Interactions* section.

HYDROXYZINE (Atarax, Vistaril)....ANTICHOLINERGIC DRUGS

A. THIS COMBINATION CAUSES EXCESSIVE ANTICHOLINERGIC SIDE EFFECTS. RESULT: Blurred vision, dry mouth, constipation, heart palpitations, slurred speech, difficulty in urination, stomach irritation, possible toxic psychosis (agitation, disorientation, delirium).

B. CERTAIN ANTICHOLINERGIC DRUGS CAN CAUSE EXCESSIVE DEPRESSANT SIDE EFFECTS. RESULT: Drowsiness, dizziness, loss of muscle coordination and mental alertness making it hazardous to drive or do other things requiring complete alertness; in severe cases, failure of blood circulation and breathing functions causing coma and death. The anticholinergic products causing this interaction include Akineton, Artane,

Cogentin, Kemadrin, Norflex, Pagitane, Robinul, and Trans-derm-Scop. Brand names and uses of antocholinergic drugs:

> Those used to control tremors resulting from Parkinson's disease or from treatment with antipsychotic drugs: Akineton, Artane, Cogentin, Kemadrin, Pagitane
>
> Those used in stomach, digestive tract disorders: Bentyl, Combid, Donnatal, Probanthine, Robinul
>
> Others: Benadryl (an antihistamine), Norflex (a muscle relaxant), Transderm-Scop (used for motion sickness)

MEPROBAMATE

See *Tranquilizers (All)....Other Depressant Drugs* interaction at beginning of *Drug Interactions* section.

TYBAMATE (Tybatron)

See *Tranquilizers (All)....Other Depressant Drugs* interaction at beginning of *Drug Interactions* section.

20

Drug Interactions in Treatment of Overweight (Diet Pill Interactions)

With today's emphasis on looks and fitness, many overweight people turn to appetite suppressants, or diet pills, to help them shed a few pounds—or a *lot* of pounds in some cases. By curbing the appetite, these drugs serve as temporary help while one develops the proper eating habits needed over the long term.

The drugs used in diet pills are *amphetamines* and *non-amphetamines*, both of which are prescription-only. The amphetamines have fallen into disfavor for this use because of their high abuse potential. Nonprescription products contain *phenylpropanolamine*—the same nasal decongestant drug used in cold/cough products—because of its side effect to suppress the appetite.

BRAND NAMES

AMPHETAMINE PRODUCTS:

Benzedrine
Biphetamine
Delcobese
Desoxyn
Dexedrine
Didrex (benzphetamine)
Obetrol

NON-AMPHETAMINE PRODUCTS:

Adipex
Fastin
Ionamin
Mazanor
Melfiat
Plegine
Pondimin
Pre-Sate

Preludin
Sanorex
Tenuate
Tenuate Dospan
Tepanil
Tepanil Ten-Tab
Unifast
Voranil

PHENYLPROPANOLAMINE PRODUCTS (NONPRESCRIPTION):

Anorexin
Appedrine
Appress
Ayds (capsule, droplets)
Coffee-Break
Control
Dex-A-Diet II
Dexatrim
Diadax
Diet Gard
Dietac

E-Z Trim
P.P.A.
P.V.M.
Permathene-12
Pro Dax 21
Prolamine
Resolution
Super Odrinex
Ultra-Lean
Vita-Slim

DRUG INTERACTIONS

DIET PILL....OTHER STIMULANT DRUGS

The appetite suppressants are central nervous system stimulants. Excessive stimulation can occur when an appetite suppressant is taken with any other central nervous system stimulant. RESULT: nervousness, agitation, tremors, tachycardia (rapid heart beat), heart palpitations, fever, loss of muscle coordination, rapid, shallow breathing, insomnia; in severe cases, a dangerous rise in blood pressure can occur, indicated by headache, visual disturbances, or confusion. The physician should monitor the patient carefully and adjust the dosages to minimize the additive stimulant effects. NOTE: The one exception to this interaction is the non-amphetamine diet pill fenfluramine (Pondimin), the only diet pill which is a *depressant* instead of a stimulant. Interacting stimulant categories and brand names:

> *ANTIDEPRESSANTS (MAOI type)—The MAOI antidepressants, prescribed for mental depression, are not used as much now that the safer cyclic antidepressants such as Elavil and Sinequan are available. Brand names of the MAOI type: Eutonyl, Marplan, Nardil, Parnate
>
> ASTHMA DRUGS (EPINEPHRINE FAMILY)—Used to open air passages and make breathing easier in asthmatics. Brand names: Aerolone, Alupent, AsthmaNefrin, Brethine, Bricanyl, Bronitin, Bronkaid, Dispos-a-Med, Duo-Medihaler, Ephedrine, Isuprel, Medihaler-Epi, Medihaler-Iso, Metaprel, Norisodrine, Primatene Proventil, Vapo-Iso-Solution, Ventolin
>
> ASTHMA DRUGS (THEOPHYLLINE FAMILY)—Used to open air passages and make breathing easier in asthmatics. Brand names: Accurbron, Amesec, Asbron G, Brondecon, Bronkodyl, Choledyl, Dilor, Elixicon, Elixophyllin, LaBID, Lufyllin, Marax, Mudrane, Quibron, Quibron-T, Quinamm, Respbid, Slo-Phyllin, Somophyllin, Somophyllin-T, Sustaire, Tedral SA, Theobid, Theodur, Theolair, Theophyl, Theovent
>
> CAFFEINE—The stimulant in coffee, tea, cola beverages, in some nonprescription diet pills, products for cold and cough, pain, and menstrual discomfort.
>
> COLD/COUGH PRODUCTS CONTAINING DECONGESTANT DRUGS—Decongestant drugs listed on nonprescription product labels (the same drugs are used in prescription-only products):
>> ORAL drugs (tablet, capsule, liquid):
>>> ephedrine
>>> methoxyphenamine
>>> phenylephrine
>>> phenylpropanolamine
>>> pseudoephedrine
>>
>> NASAL drugs (drops, spray, inhaler):
>>> oxymetazoline
>>> phenylephrine
>>> propylhexadrine
>>> xylometazoline
>
> DEANOL (Deaner)—Used in hyperkinetic behavior and learning disorders.
>
> METHYLPHENIDATE (Ritalin)—Used in hyperkinetic behavior and learning disorders in children; narcolepsy (uncontrollable desire to sleep); mild depression; apathetic or withdrawn senile behavior.

PEMOLINE (Cylert)—Used in hyperkinetic behavior and learning disorders in children.

PENTYLENETETRAZOL (Metrazol)—Used to enhance mental and physical activity in the elderly.

I. AMPHETAMINE DRUG INTERACTIONS

AMPHETAMINE or PHENYLPROPANOLAMINE .....ANTIDEPRESSANTS (CYCLIC TYPE)

THIS COMBINATION CAN CAUSE EXCESSIVE CENTRAL NERVOUS SYSTEM STIMULATION. RESULT: nervousness, agitation, tremors, tachycardia (rapid heart beat), heart palpitations, fever, loss of muscle coordination, rapid, shallow breathing, insomnia; in severe cases, a dangerous rise in blood pressure can occur, indicated by headache, visual disturbances, or confusion. NOTE: The antidepressant trazadone (Desyrel) may not interact. Antidepressants are used to alleviate mental depression and elevate the mood. Antidepressant brand names (generic names in parentheses):

Adapin (doxepin)
Asendin (amoxapine)
Aventyl (nortriptyline)
Desyrel (trazadone)
Elavil (amitriptyline)
Endep (amitriptyline)
Etrafon (amitriptyline/
  perphenazine)
Limbitrol (amitriptyline/
  chlordiazepoxide)
Ludiomil (maprotiline)

Norpramin (desipramine)
Pamelor (nortriptyline)
Pertofrane (desipramine)
Sinequan (doxepin)
Surmontil (trimipramine)
Tofranil, Tofranil-PM
  (imipramine)
Triavil (amitriptyline/
  perphenazine)
Vivactil (protriptyline)

AMPHETAMINE or PHENYLPROPANOLAMINE....BETA BLOCKER HEART DRUGS

THE EFFECT OF THE BETA BLOCKER MAY BE ANTAGONIZED. Beta blockers are used to prevent angina, to restore irregular heart beats to normal rhythm, and to lower high blood pressure. RESULT: The condition treated may not be controlled properly. This combination can also cause a paradoxical marked rise in blood pressure accompanied by severe headache, confusion, and visual disturbances. Beta blocker brand names (generic names in parentheses):

Blocadren (timolol)
Corgard (nadolol)
Inderal (propranolol)
Lopressor (metoprolol)
tenormin (atenolol)
Visken (pindolol)

AMPHETAMINE or
PHENYLPROPANOLAMINE....DIABETES DRUGS

THE EFFECT OF THE DIABETES DRUG MAY BE AN-
TAGONIZED. Diabetes drugs are used to lower the blood sugar
level in diabetics. RESULT: The blood sugar level may remain too
high. Report symptoms of hyperglycemia (high blood sugar):
excessive thirst or hunger, large urine output, weight loss, lethargy, drowsiness, loss of coordination. Diabetes drug brand names
(generic names in parentheses):

Diabinese (chlorpropamide)
Dymelor (acetohexamide)
Orinase (tolbutamide)
Tolinase (tolazamide)

AMPHETAMINE or
PHENYLPROPANOLAMINE....DIGITALIS HEART DRUGS

THIS COMBINATION MAY CAUSE HEART BEAT IR-
REGULARITIES. Digitalis is used for congestive heart failure
and to restore irregular heart beats to normal rhythm. Digitalis
family brand names (generic names in parentheses):

Crystodigin (digitoxin)
Digifortis (digitalis)
Lanoxin (digoxin)
Purodigin (digitoxin)

AMPHETAMINE or
PHENYLPROPANOLAMINE....DIURETICS

THE EFFECT OF THE DIURETIC ON BLOOD PRES-
SURE MAY BE ANTAGONIZED. Diuretics lower blood pressure
by removing excess fluid from the body. RESULT: The blood
pressure may not be controlled properly. Diuretic brand names
(generic names in parentheses):

Aldactazide (spironolactone, hydrochlorothiazide)
Aldactone (spironolactone)
Anhydron (cyclothiazide)
Aquatag (benzthiazide)
Aquatensin (methyclothiazide)
Diucardin (hydroflumethiazide)
Diulo (metolazone)
Diuril (chlorothiazide)
Dyazide (triamterene, hydrochlorothiazide)
Dyrenium (triamterene)
Edecrin (ethacrynic acid)
Enduron (methyclothiazide)
Esidrix (hydrochlorothiazide)
Exna (benzthiazide)

Hydrodiuril (hydrochlorothiazide)
Hydromox (quinethazone)
Hygroton (chlorthalidone)
Lasix (furosemide)
Metahydrin (trichlormethiazide)
Midamor (amiloride)
Moduretic (amiloride, hydrochlorothiazide)
Naqua (trichlormethiazide)
Naturetin (bendroflumethiazide)
Oretic (hydrochlorothiazide)
Renese (polythiazide)
Saluron (hydroflumethiazide)
Zaroxolyn (metolazone)

AMPHETAMINE or PHENYLPROPANOLAMINE....HIGH BLOOD PRESSURE DRUGS

THE EFFECT OF THE HIGH BLOOD PRESSURE DRUG MAY BE ANTAGONIZED. RESULT: The blood pressure may not be controlled properly. High blood pressure drugs (brand names in parentheses):

clonidine (Catapres, Combipres)
guanabenz (Wytensin)
guanethidine (Esimil, Ismelin)
hydralazine (Apresazide, Apresoline, Apresoline-Esidrix, Dralserp, Dralzine, Ser-Ap-Es, Serpasil-Apresoline, Unipres)
methyldopa (Aldoclor, Aldomet, Aldoril)
minoxidil (Loniten)
prazosin (Minipress)
reserpine-type drugs:
    deserpidine (Enduronyl, Harmonyl, Oreticyl)
    rauwolfia (Raudixin, Rauzide)
    reserpine (Diupres, Diutensen-R, Hydropres, Rau-Sed, Regroton, Renese-R, Reserpoid, Salutensin, Sandril, Ser-Ap-Es, Serpasil, Serpasil-Apresoline, Serpasil-Esidrix)

AMPHETAMINE....ACETAZOLAMIDE (Diamox)

THE EFFECT OF AMPHETAMINE MAY BE INCREASED. RESULT: Possible adverse side effects from too much amphetamine with associated symptoms: dizziness, nervousness and irritability, blurred vision, dry mouth, heart palpitations or arrhythmias (heart beat irregularities), rise in blood pressure, exaggerated movements. Acetazolamide is used primarily to treat glaucoma.

AMPHETAMINE....ANTACIDS

THE EFFECT OF AMPHETAMINE MAY BE IN-CREASED. RESULT: Possible adverse side effects from too much amphetamine with associated symptoms: dizziness, nervousness and irritability, blurred vision, dry mouth, heart palpitations or arrhythmias (heart beat irregularities), rise in blood pressure, exaggerated movements. Antacid brand names:

Alka-Seltzer	Kudrox
AlternaGel	Maalox
Delcid	Mylanta
Di-Gel	Riopan
Gelusil	WinGel

AMPHETAMINE
....ANTIPSYCHOTICS (PHENOTHIAZINE FAMILY)

THE APPETITE SUPPRESSION EFFECT OF AMPHETAMINE MAY BE DECREASED. RESULT: The appetite may not be controlled properly. Antipsychotics are "major" tranquilizers used to treat severe mental disorders such as schizophrenia. Phenothiazine antipsychotic brand names (generic names in parentheses):

Compazine (prochlorperazine)	Sparine (promazine)
Mellaril (thioridazine)	Stelazine (trifluoperazine)
Proketazine (carphenazine)	Thorazine (chlorpromazine)
Prolixin (fluphenazine)	Tindal (acetophenazine)
Quide (piperacetazine)	Trilafon (perphenazine)
Serentil (mesoridazine)	Vesprin (triflupromazine)

AMPHETAMINE....HALOPERIDOL (Haldol)

THE APPETITE SUPPRESSION EFFECT OF AMPHETAMINE MAY BE DECREASED. RESULT: The appetite may not be controlled properly. Haloperidol is a major tranquilizer used to treat severe mental disorders such as schizophrenia.

AMPHETAMINE....MILK OF MAGNESIA

THE EFFECT OF AMPHETAMINE MAY BE IN-
CREASED. RESULT: Possible adverse side effects from too much
amphetamine with associated symptoms: dizziness, nervousness
and irritability, blurred vision, dry mouth, heart palpitations or
arrhythmias (heart beat irregularities), rise in blood pressure,
exaggerated movements. Milk of magnesia is a laxative.

II. NON-AMPHETAMINE DRUG INTERACTIONS

NON-AMPHETAMINE DIET PILLS

See *Diet Pills....Other Stimulant Drugs* interaction at beginning
of *Drug Interactions* section.

FENFLURAMINE (Pondimin)....CENTRAL NERVOUS
SYSTEM DEPRESSANTS

THIS COMBINATION CAN CAUSE EXCESSIVE CEN-
TRAL NERVOUS SYSTEM DEPRESSION. RESULT:
Drowsiness, dizziness, loss of muscle coordination and mental
alertness; in severe cases, failure of blood circulation and
breathing functions causing coma and death. For a detailed look
at which drugs are central nervous system depressants, see *Allergy*
chapter.

III. PHENYLPROPANOLAMINE INTERACTION

PHENYLPROPANOLAMINE DIET
PILL....INDOMETHACIN (Indocin)

THIS COMBINATION CAN CAUSE THE BLOOD PRES-
SURE TO RISE TOO HIGH. RESULT: Headache, visual
disturbances. Indomethacin is a non-corticosteroid drug used to
alleviate pain and inflammation in arthritic conditions.

21

Drug Interactions in Treatment of Pain

Pain can be a symptom of almost any ailment. Though sometimes excruciating, it is invaluable as both a diagnostic aid and a sensory warning signal that something is wrong.

Pain is categorized as superficial, visceral, or somatic. *Superficial* pain comes from skin or mucous membranes and is usually sharp and localized. *Visceral* pain is deeper, originating in an organ system such as the stomach or kidneys. *Somatic* pain comes from skeletal muscles, joints, or ligaments and is usually dull, aching, and not sharply localized—for example, headache, toothache, and arthritic and muscular aches. Pain relieving drugs are divided into two classes: non-narcotics and narcotics.

BRAND NAMES

NON-NARCOTIC PAIN RELIEVERS:

Acetaminophen
   Anacin-3
   Bromo Seltzer
   Datril
   Excedrin PM
   Febrinol
   Fendon
   Liquiprin
   Percogesic
   Phenaphen
   Tapar
   Tempra
   Tylenol

Valadol
Aspirin
  Alka-Seltzer
  Anacin
  A.S.A.
  Ascriptin
  Ascriptin A/D
  B.C.
  Bayer
  Bufferin
  Cama
  Ecotrin
  Empirin
  Measurin
  Momentum
  Pabirin
  Persistin
  St. Joseph Aspirin
  Stanback
  Other aspirin-like products: Arthralgen, Arthropan, Calurin, Disalcid, Dolobid, Magan, Mobidin, Pabalate, Salrin, Uracel, Uromide
Combination acetaminophen/aspirin products:
  Capron
  Dolor
  Duradyne
  Gemnisyn
  Excedrin
  Goody's Headache Powders
  Nilain
  Trigesic
  Vanquish

NON-CORTICOSTEROID PRODUCTS (prescription-only):

Anaprox (naproxen)
Clinoril (sulindac)
Feldene (piroxicam)
Meclomen (meclofenamate)
Motrin (ibuprofen)

Nalfon (fenoprofen)
Naprosyn (naproxen)
Rufen (ibuprofen)
Tolectin (tolmetin)
Zomaz (zomepirac)

NARCOTIC PAIN RELIEVERS:

Codeine products
  Ascriptin w/Codeine
  Bancap w/Codeine

Bufferin w/Codeine
Empracet w/Codeine
Fiorinal w/Codeine
Phenaphen w/Codeine
Tylenol w/Codeine
Meperidine products
  Demerol
  Mepergan Fortis
Oxycodone products
  Percocet
  Percodan
  Tylox
Pentazocine products
  Talwin Nx
  Talwin Compound
Propoxyphene products
  Darvocet-N
  Darvon
  Dolene
  Wygesic
Other narcotic products
  Dicodid (hydrocodone)
  Dilaudid (hydromorphone)
  Dolophine (methadone)
  Levo-Dromoran (levorphanol)
  morphine (various companies)
  Norcet (hydrocodone)
  Numorphan (oxymorphone)
  Synalgos-DC (dihydrocodeine)
  Vicodin (hydrocodone)
  Zactane (ethoheptazine)
  Zactirin (ethoheptazine)

DRUG INTERACTIONS

I. NON-NARCOTIC DRUG INTERACTIONS

ACETAMINOPHEN....ALCOHOL (beer, liquor, wine, etc.)

THIS COMBINATION CAN CAUSE LIVER DAMAGE.
This interaction is probably significant only to those who *regularly*
ingest large amounts of alcohol and large amounts of an acetaminophen product.

ASPIRIN....ANTACIDS

THE EFFECT OF ASPIRIN MAY BE DECREASED. Antacid brand names: AlternaGel, Delcid, Di-Gel, Gelusil, Kudrox, Maalox, Mylanta, Riopan, WinGel, etc.

*ASPIRIN....ANTICOAGULANT DRUGS

THE EFFECT OF THE ANTICOAGULANT MAY BE INCREASED. Anticoagulants are used to thin the blood and prevent it from clotting. RESULT: Increased risk of hemorrhage. Aspirin can cause stomach irritation/ulceration, which may be worsened by this drug interaction. Report symptoms such as black or tarry stools, bleeding or bruising, abdominal pain (especially after eating), unusual loss of energy. Coumadin is the most widely used anticoagulant drug. Anticoagulant drug brand names (generic names in parentheses):

Athrombin-K (warfarin)
Coufarin (warfarin)
Coumadin (warfarin)
dicumarol (various companies)
Hedulin (phenindione)
Miradon (anisindione)
Panwarfin (warfarin)

ASPIRIN....CORTICOSTEROID DRUGS

THE EFFECT OF ASPIRIN MAY BE DECREASED. RESULT: The symptoms may not be controlled properly unless the dose of aspirin is raised to higher than normal levels. There is also an increased risk of stomach bleeding and ulceration with this combination. Corticosteroids are prescribed for arthritis, severe allergies, asthma, endocrine disorders, leukemia, colitis and enteritis (inflammation of the intestinal tract), and various skin, lung, and eye diseases. Corticosteroid brand names (generic names in parentheses):

Aristocort (triamcinolone)
Celestone (betamethasone)
Cortef (hydrocortisone)
Decadron (dexamethasone)
Delta-Cortef (prednisolone)
Deltasone (prednisone)
hydrocortisone (various companies)

Kenacort (triamcinolone)   Orasone (prednisone)
Medrol (methylprednisolone)   prednisone (various companies)
Meticorten (prednisone)

*ASPIRIN....METHOTREXATE (Mexate)

THE EFFECT OF METHOTREXATE MAY BE IN-
CREASED. Methotrexate is used in cancer treatment. RESULT:
Possible adverse side effects from too much methotrexate. Report
symptoms such as nausea, diarrhea, black or tarry stools, skin
rash, mouth ulcers.

*ASPIRIN....PROBENECID (Benemid, ColBenemid)

THE EFFECT OF PROBENECID MAY BE DECREASED.
Probenecid is used to treat gout. RESULT: The condition may not
be controlled properly, especially if aspirin is taken in the larger
doses required for arthritic conditions.

*ASPIRIN....SULFINPYRAZONE (Anturane)

THE EFFECT OF SULFINPYRAZONE MAY BE DE-
CREASED. Sulfinpyrazone is used to treat gout. RESULT: The
condition may not be controlled properly, especially if aspirin is
taken in the larger doses required for arthritic conditions. There
is also an increased risk of stomach irritation and bleeding. In
addition, the aspirin blood level may increase to toxic concentrations causing *salicylism.* Report symptoms such as tinnitus
(ringing in the ears), deafness, dizziness or nausea, restlessness,
delirium, rapid breathing, burning sensations.

ASPIRIN....VITAMIN C

THE EFFECT OF VITAMIN C MAY BE DECREASED.
Vitamin C prevents scurvy. RESULT: Possible vitamin C deficiency and symptoms of scurvy: bleeding gums, tongue sores,
pain in muscles or joints, weight loss, lethargy. NOTE: High doses
of vitamin C (over 2000 mg a day) can raise aspirin blood levels to
toxic concentrations causing *salicylism.* Be alert for symptoms such
as tinnitus (ringing in the ears), deafness, dizziness or nausea,
restlessness, delirium, rapid breathing, burning sensations.

NON-CORTICOSTEROID DRUGS (ALL)....BETA BLOCKER HEART DRUGS

THE EFFECT OF THE BETA BLOCKER DRUG MAY BE DECREASED. Beta blockers are used to treat angina, irregular heart beats, and high blood pressure. RESULT: The condition treated may not be controlled properly. Beta blocker brand names (generic names in parentheses):

Blocadren (timolol)
Corgard (nadolol)
Inderal (propranolol)
Lopressor (metoprolol)
Tenormin (atenolol)
Visken (pindolol)

NON-CORTICOSTEROID DRUGS (ALL)....DIURETIC DRUGS

THE EFFECT OF THE DIURETIC DRUG MAY BE DECREASED. The diuretics remove excess body fluid (edema) and are used to treat congestive heart failure and high blood pressure. RESULT: The condition treated may not be controlled properly. Diuretic drug brand names (generic names in parentheses):

Aldactazide (hydrochlorothiazide/ spironolactone)
Anhydron (cyclothiazide)
Aquatag (benzthiazide)
Aquatensin (methyclothiazide)
Diucardin (hydroflumethiazide)
Diulo (metolazone)
Diuril (chlorothiazide)
Dyazide (hydrochlorothiazide/ triamterene)
Edecrin (ethacrynic acid)
Enduron (methyclothiazide)
Esidrix (hydrochlorothiazide)
Exna (benzthiazide)
Hydrodiuril (hydrochlorothiazide)
Hydromox (quinethazone)
Hygroton (chlorthalidone)
Lasix (furosemide)
Metahydrin (trichlormethiazide)
Moduretic (hydrochlorothiazide/ amiloride)
Naqua (trichlormethiazide)
Naturetin (bendroflumethiazide)
Oretic (hydrochlorothiazide)
Renese (polythiazide)
Saluron (hydroflumethiazide)
Zaroxolyn (metolazone)

NON-CORTICOSTEROID DRUGS (ALL)....LITHIUM

THE EFFECT OF LITHIUM MAY BE INCREASED. Lithium is an antipsychotic drug used to treat manic depressive disorders. RESULT: Possible adverse side effects from too much lithium. Report symptoms such as weakness, lethargy, dry mouth, loss of appetite, abdominal pain, dizziness, nausea, confusion, lack of muscle coordination, slurred speech. Lithium brand names:

>Eskalith
>Lithane
>Lithobid
>Lithonate
>Lithotab

NON-CORTICOSTEROID DRUG (SULINDAC only)....ANTICOAGULANT DRUGS

THE EFFECT OF THE ANTICOAGULANT MAY BE INCREASED. Anticoagulants are used to thin the blood and prevent it from clotting. RESULT: Increased risk of hemorrhage. Report symptoms such as black or tarry stools, bleeding or bruising, unusual loss of energy. Coumadin is the most widely used anticoagulant drug. Anticoagulant drug brand names (generic names in parentheses):

>Athrombin-K (warfarin)
>Coufarin (warfarin)
>Coumadin (warfarin)
>dicumarol (various companies)
>Hedulin (phenindione)
>Miradon (anisindione)
>Panwarfin (warfarin)

II. NARCOTIC DRUG INTERACTIONS

NARCOTIC DRUGS (ALL)....OTHER DEPRESSANT DRUGS

The narcotics are central nervous system depressants. They depress or impair functions such as coordination and alertness. Excessive depression or impairment can occur when a tranquilizer is taken with any other central nervous system depressant. RESULT: drowsiness, dizziness, loss of muscle coordination and mental alertness; in severe cases, failure of blood circulation and breathing functions causing coma and death. The physician should monitor the patient carefully and adjust the dosages to minimize the excessive depressant effects. Interacting depressant categories and brand names:

ALCOHOL (beer, liquor, wine, etc.)

ANTICHOLINERGICS—Uses and brand names:
  Those used to control tremors resulting from Parkinson's disease or treatment with antipsychotic drugs: Akineton, Artane, Cogentin, Kemadrin, Pagitane

Others:
  Disipal (used for stomach, digestive tract disorders)
  Norflex (a muscle relaxant)
  Robinul (used for stomach, digestive tract disorders)
  Transderm-Scop (used for motion sickness)

ANTICONVULSANTS (Used to control seizures in disorders such as epilepsy). Brand names: Depakene, Dilantin, Mesantoin, Mysoline, Peganone, Tegretol, Tridione, Zarontin

ANTIDEPRESSANTS (CYCLIC TYPE)—Used to alleviate mental depression. Brand names: Adapin, Asendin, Aventyl, Desyrel, Elavil, Endep, Etrafon, Limbitrol, Ludiomil, Norpramin, Pamelor, Pertofrane, Sinequan, Surmontil, Tofranil, Tofranil-PM, Triavil, Vivactil

ANTIHISTAMINES (Used for allergies, colds). Brand names: Actidil, Antivert, Atarax, Benadryl, Bendectin, Bonine, Chlor-Trimeton, Clistin, Decapryn, Dimetane, Dramamine, Histadyl, Inhiston, Marezine, Optimine, PBZ, Periactin, Polaramine, Pyronil, Tavist, Teldrin, Triten, Vistaril

ANTIPSYCHOTICS (Used for severe mental disorders).
  Antipsychotic brand names: Compazine, Haldol, Loxitane, Mellaril, Moban, Navane, Proketazine, Prolixin, Quide, Serentil, Sparine, Stelazine, Taractan, Thorazine, Tindal, Trilafon, Vesprin

FENFLURAMINE (Pondimin)—a diet pill

HIGH BLOOD PRESSURE DRUGS (brand names in parentheses):
  clonidine (Catapres, Combipres)
  guanabenz (Wytensin)
  methyldopa (Aldoclor, Aldomet, Aldoril)
  reserpine-type drugs:
    deserpidine (Enduronyl, Harmonyl, Oreticyl)
    rauwolfia (Raudixin, Rauzide)
    reserpine (Diupres, Diutensen-R, Hydropres, Rau-Sed, Regroton, Renese-R, Reserpoid, Salutensin, Sandril, Ser-Ap-Es, Serpasil, Serpasil-Apresoline, Serpasil-Esidrix)

MUSCLE RELAXANTS
  Dantrium, Flexeril, Lioresal, Norflex, Norgesic, Norgesic Forte,
  Paraflex, Parafon Forte, Quinamm, Rela, Robaxin, Robaxisal,
  Skelaxin, Soma, Soma Compound, Valium
SLEEPING PILLS
  Barbiturate sleeping pills:
    phenobarbital, Alurate, Amytal, Butisol, Buticap,
    Carbrital, Eskabarb, Lotusate, Luminal, Mebaral,
    Nembutal, Seconal, Sedadrops, Solfoton, Tuinal
  Non-Barbiturate sleeping pills:
    Ativan (also used as a tranquilizer), Dalmane, Doriden,
    Halcion, Noctec, Noludar, Parest, Placidyl, Quaalude,
    Restoril, Somnos, Triclos, Valmid
TRANQUILIZERS
  Benzodiazepine tranquilizers:
    Ativan, Centrax, Librium, Limbitrol (also an antidepressant),
      Paxipam, Serax, SK-Lygen, Tranxene, Valium, Xanax
  Non-Benzodiazepine tranquilizers:
    Atarax, Equanil, meprobamate, Meprospan, Meprotab, Mil-
    town, Trancopal, Tybatran, Vistaril

MEPERIDINE (Demerol, Mepergan Fortis)....
ANTIDEPRESSANTS (MAOI TYPE)

THIS COMBINATION CAN CAUSE SEVERE ADVERSE
SIDE EFFECTS with symptoms such as high fever, hyperexcitability, sweating, body rigidity, breathing difficulties, low blood
pressure, loss of consciousness. Antidepressants are used to alleviate mental depression and elevate the mood. The MAOI type
antidepressants are not used much now that the safer tricyclic
antidepressants such as Elavil and Sinequan are available. MAOI
antidepressant brand names (generic names in parentheses):

  Eutonyl (pargyline)
  Marplan (isocarboxazid)
  Nardil (phenelzine)
  Parnate (tranylcypromine)

*PROPOXYPHENE (Darvocet-N, Darvon, Dolene, Wygesic)....
ALCOHOL

THIS COMBINATION CAN CAUSE EXCESSIVE CEN-
TRAL NERVOUS SYSTEM DEPRESSION. RESULT:

drowsiness, dizziness, loss of muscle coordination and mental alertness; in severe cases, failure of blood circulation and breathing functions causing coma and death. NOTE: THIS COMBINATION HAS RESULTED IN SEVERAL FATALITIES AND SHOULD BE AVOIDED.

*PROPOXYPHENE (Darvocet-N, Darvon, Dolene, Wygesic)....CARBAMAZEPINE (Tegretol)

THE EFFECT OF CARBAMAZEPINE MAY BE IN-CREASED. Carbamazepine is an anticonvulsant used to prevent seizures in disorders such as epilepsy. RESULT: Possible adverse side effects from too much carbamazepine. Report symptoms such as dizziness, nausea, loss of coordination, stomach pain. Also, since both drugs are central nervous system depressants, possible excessive depression with associated symptoms: drowsiness, dizziness, loss of muscle coordination and mental alertness; in severe cases, failure of blood circulation and breathing functions causing coma and death.

METHADONE (Dolophine)....BARBITURATES

THE EFFECT OF METHADONE MAY BE DECREASED. Methadone is used to help free addicts from their dependence on heroin or other narcotics. RESULT: The addiction may not be controlled properly. Barbiturates are used as sedatives or sleeping pills. Barbiturate brand names:

phenobarbital	Luminal
Alurate	Mebaral
Amytal	Nembutal
Butisol	Seconal
Buticap	Sedadrops
Carbrital	Solfoton
Eskabarb	Tuinal
Lotusate	

METHADONE (Dolophine)....CARBAMAZEPINE (Tegretol)

THE EFFECT OF METHADONE MAY BE DECREASED. Methadone is used to help free addicts from their dependence on heroin or other narcotics. RESULT: The addiction may not be controlled properly. Carbamazepine is an anticonvulsant used to prevent seizures in disorders such as epilepsy.

METHADONE (Dolophine)....PHENYTOIN (Dilantin)

THE EFFECT OF METHADONE MAY BE DECREASED. Methadone is used to help free addicts from their dependence on heroin or other narcotics. RESULT: The addiction may not be controlled properly. Phenytoin is an anticonvulsant used to prevent seizures in disorders such as epilepsy. Other interacting phenytoin-like drugs are Mesantoin (mephenytoin) and Peganone (ethotoin).

METHADONE (Dolophine)....PRIMIDONE (Mysoline)

THE EFFECT OF METHADONE MAY BE DECREASED. Methadone is used to help free addicts from their dependence on heroin or other narcotics. RESULT: The addiction may not be controlled properly. Primidone is an anticonvulsant used to prevent seizures in disorders such as epilepsy.

METHADONE (Dolophine)....RIFAMPIN (Rifadin, Rimactane)

THE EFFECT OF METHADONE MAY BE DECREASED. Methadone is used to help free addicts from their dependence on heroin or other narcotics. RESULT: The addiction may not be controlled properly. Rifampin is used to treat tuberculosis and may be given to suspected carriers of meningitis.

22

Drug Interactions in Treatment of Psychosis (Mental Illness)

A psychosis is a severe mental illness such as schizophrenia, paranoia, or manic-depressive disorder.

Schizophrenia is the most common psychosis. The sufferer exhibits an inability to relate to other people, and usually has delusions, hallucinations, and a loss of contact with reality.

Paranoia causes one to believe it is his supreme purpose to undertake some irrational (to him totally rational and justified) act, and that others are trying to prevent him from completing his self-appointed task.

In *manic-depression*, the mood swings to and fro like a pendulum—from abject depression to unbridled optimism—totally out of proportion to the situation.

Until research uncovers the specific genetic, physical, or chemical causes for this type of illness, treatment is aimed at controlling the symptoms so that the patient can function in society without harming himself or others.

The drugs used to treat psychoses are called *antipsychotics*. The three types are phenothiazines, non-phenothiazines, and lithium.

BRAND NAMES

PHENOTHIAZINE ANTIPSYCHOTIC DRUGS

Compazine (prochlorperazine)
Mellaril (thioridazine)

Proketazine (carphenazine)
Prolixin (fluphenazine)

Quide (piperacetazine)   Thorazine (chlorpromazine)
Serentil (mesoridazine)   Tindal (acetophenazine)
Sparine (promazine)   Trilafon (perphenazine)
Stelazine (trifluoperazine)   Vesprin (triflupromazine)

NON-PHENOTHIAZINE ANTIPSYCHOTIC DRUGS

Haldol (haloperidol)   Navane (thiothixene)
Loxitane (loxapine)   Taractan (chlorprothixene)
Moban (molindone)

LITHIUM

Eskalith   Lithonate
Lithane   Lithonate-S
Lithobid   Lithotabs

DRUG INTERACTIONS

I. ANTIPSYCHOTIC DRUG INTERACTIONS

ANTIPSYCHOTIC DRUGS (ALL except lithium)....OTHER DEPRESSANTS

The antipsychotics are central nervous system depressants. They depress or impair functions such as coordination and alertness. Excessive depression or impairment can occur when an antipsychotic is taken with any other central nervous system depressant. RESULT: drowsiness, dizziness, loss of muscle coordination and mental alertness; in severe cases, failure of blood circulation and breathing functions causing coma and death. The physician should monitor the patient carefully and adjust the dosages to minimize the excessive depressant effects. Interacting depressant categories and brand names:

ALCOHOL (beer, liquor, wine, etc.)
ANTICHOLINERGICS—These can also cause increased anticholinergic side effects: blurry vision, dry mouth, constipation, difficult urination, heart palpitations; possible toxic psychosis (agitation, disorientation, delirium). Those used to control tremors resulting from Parkinson's disease or treatment with antipsychotic drugs:
Akineton, Artane, Cogentin, Kemadrin, Pagitane
Others:
Benadryl (an antihistamine)
Norflex (a muscle relaxant)

Robinul (used for stomach, digestive tract disorders)

Transderm-Scop (used for motion sickness)

ANTICONVULSANTS (Used to control seizures in disorders such as epilepsy). Brand names: Depakene, Dilantin, Mesantoin, Mysoline, Peganone, Tegretol, Tridione, Zarontin

ANTIDEPRESSANTS (CYCLIC TYPE) (Used to alleviate mental depression). Brand names: Adapin, Asendin, Aventyl, Desyrel, Elavil, Endep, Etrafon, Limbitrol, Ludiomil, Norpramin, Pamelor, Pertofrane, Sinequan, Surmontil Tofranil, Tofranil-PM, Triavil, Vivactil

ANTIHISTAMINES (Used for allergies, colds). Brand names: Actidil, Antivert, Antarax, Benadryl, Bendectin, Bonine, Chlor-Trimeton, Clistin, Decapryn, Dimetane, Dramamine, Histadyl, Inhiston, Marezine, Optimine, PBZ, Periactin, Polaramine, Pyronil, Tavist, Teldrin, Triten, Vistaril

FENFLURAMINE (Pondimin)—a diet pill

HIGH BLOOD PRESSURE DRUGS (brand names in parentheses):

clonidine (Catapres, Combipres)

guanabenz (Wytensin)

methyldopa (Aldoclor, Aldomet, Aldoril)

reserpine-type drugs:

deserpidine (Enduronyl, Harmonyl, Oreticyl)

rauwolfia (Raudixin, Rauzide)

reserpine (Diupres, Diutensen-R, Hydropres, Rau-Sed, Regroton, Renese-R, Reserpoid, Salutensin, Sandril, Ser-Ap-Es, Serpasil, Serpasil-Apresoline, Serpasil-Esidrix)

MUSCLE RELAXANTS

Dantrium, Flexeril, Lioresal, Norflex, Norgesic, Norgesic Forte, Paraflex, Parafon Forte, Quinamm, Rela, Robaxin, Robaxisal, Skelaxin, Soma, Soma Compound, Valium

NARCOTICS

Codeine products:

Ascriptin w/Codeine, Bancap w/Codeine, Bufferin w/Codeine, Empirin w/Codeine, Empracet w/Codeine, Fiorinal w/Codeine, Phenaphen w/Codeine, Tylenol w/Codeine

Other narcotic or narcotic-like products:

Demerol, Dilaudid, Dolophene, morphine, Merpergan Fortis, Norcet, Numorphan, Percocet, Percodan, Synalgos-DC,Talwin, Talwin Compound, Tylox, Vicodan, Zactane, Zactirin

PROPOXYPHENE (pain reliever):

Darvocet-N, Darvon, Dolene, Wygesic

SLEEPING PILLS

Barbiturate sleeping pills:

phenobarbital, Alurate, Amytal, Butisol, Buticap, Carbrital,
Eskabarb, Lotusate, Luminal, Mebaral, Nembutal, Seconal,
Sedadrops, Solfoton, Tuinal
Non-Barbiturate sleeping pills:
     Ativan (also used as a tranquilizer), Dalmane, Doriden,
     Halcion, Noctec, Noludar, Parest, Placidyl, Quaalude, Re-
7x54   storil, Somnos, Triclos, Valmid
TRANQUILIZERS
  Benzodiazepine tranquilizers:
     Ativan, Centrax, Librium, Limbitrol (also an antidepressant),
     Paxipam, Serax, SK-Lygen, Tranxene, Valium, Xanax
  Non-Benzodiazepine tranquilizers:
     Atarax, Equanil, meprobamate, Meprospan, Meprotab, Mil-
     town, Trancopal, Tybatran, Vistaril

ANTIPSYCHOTICS (ALL)....ANTICONVULSANTS

THE EFFECT OF THE ANTICONVULSANT MAY BE
DECREASED. Anticonvulsants are used to prevent seizures in
disorders such as epilepsy. RESULT: The disorder may not be
controlled properly. Also, since both drugs are central nervous
system depressants, possible excessive depressant effects with
associated symptoms: drowsiness, dizziness, loss of muscle coordination and mental alertness; in severe cases, failure of blood
circulation and breathing functions causing coma and death.
Anticonvulsant brand names (generic names in parentheses):

Depakene (valproic acid)	Peganone (ethotoin)
Dilantin (phenytoin)	Tegretol (carbamazepine)
Mesantoin (mephenytoin)	Tridione (trimethadione)
Mysoline (primidone)	Zarontin (ethosuximide)

ANTIPSYCHOTICS (ALL)....ANTICHOLINERGICS

A. THIS COMBINATION MAY CAUSE EXCESSIVE
ANTICHOLINERGIC SIDE EFFECTS. RESULT: Blurred vi-
sion, dry mouth, constipation, heart palpitations, slurred speech,
difficulty in urination, stomach irritation, possible toxic psychosis
(agitation, disorientation, delirium).
     B. CERTAIN ANTICHOLINERGIC DRUGS CAN CAUSE
EXCESSIVE DEPRESSANT SIDE EFFECTS. RESULT: Drowsiness, dizziness, loss of muscle coordination and mental alertness
making it hazardous to drive or do other things requiring
complete alertness; in severe cases, failure of blood circulation and

breathing functions causing coma and death. The anticholinergic products causing this interaction include Akineton, Artane, Benadryl, Cogentin, Kemadrin, Norflex, Pagitane, Robinul, and Transderm-Scop. Brand names and uses of anticholinergic drugs:

> Those used to control tremors resulting from Parkinson's disease or from treatment with antipsychotic drugs: Akineton, Artane, Cogentin, Kemadrin, Pagitane
> Those used in stomach, digestive tract disorders: Bentyl, Combid, Donnatal, Probanthine, Robinul
> Others:
> Benadryl (an antihistamine), Norflex (a muscle relaxant), Transderm-Scop (used for motion sickness)

ANTIPSYCHOTICS (ALL)
....ASTHMA DRUGS (EPINEPHRINE FAMILY)

THIS COMBINATION CAN CAUSE A SEVERE DROP IN BLOOD PRESSURE. RESULT: dizziness, weakness, faintness; possible seizures and shock. Asthma drugs open lung air passages and make breathing easier in asthmatics. Epinephrine-type asthma drug brand names (generic names in parentheses):

Aerolone (isoproterenol)
Alupent (metaproterenol)
AsthmaNefrin (epinephrine)
Brethine (terbutaline)
Bricanyl (terbutaline)
Bronitin (epinephrine)
Bronkaid (epinephrine)
Dispos-a-Med (isoproterenol)
Duo-Medihaler (isoproterenol)
Ephedrine (various companies)

Isuprel (isoproterenol)
Medihaler-Epi (epinephrine)
Medihaler-Iso (isoproterenol)
Metaprel (metaproterenol)
Norisodrine (isoproterenol)
Primatene (epinephrine)
Proventil (albuterol)
Vapo-Iso-Solution (isoproterenol)
Ventolin (albuterol)

ANTIPSYCHOTICS (ALL)....BETA BLOCKER HEART DRUGS

THE EFFECT OF THE BETA BLOCKER MAY BE INCREASED. Beta blockers are used for angina, to restore irregular heart beats to normal rhythm, and to treat high blood pressure. RESULT: The blood pressure may drop too low (with dizziness, weakness, faintness); other adverse side effects: bradycardia (slow heart beat), fatigue, cardiac arrhythmias (heart beat irregularities), asthma-like wheezing or difficulty breathing. Beta blocker brand names (generic names in parentheses):

Blocadren (timolol)
Corgard (nadolol)
Inderal (propranolol)
Lopressor (metoprolol)
Tenormin (atenolol)
Visken (pindolol)

ANTIPSYCHOTICS (ALL)....CAFFEINE

THE EFFECT OF CAFFEINE MAY BE INCREASED. Caffeine is a stimulant. RESULT: Possible adverse side effects from too much caffeine with associated symptoms: *caffeinism* (nervousness and irritability, headache, trembling, rapid breathing, insomnia); also, caffeine may antagonize the effects of the antipsychotic drug, resulting in less control of the mental disorder treated. Caffeine sources: coffee, tea, cola beverages and other soft drinks, chocolate, some nonprescription diet pills, and products for cold/cough, pain, and menstrual discomfort—read product label list of ingredients.

ANTIPSYCHOTICS (ALL)....DIURETIC DRUGS

THIS COMBINATION MAY CAUSE THE BLOOD PRESSURE TO DROP TOO LOW. RESULT: dizziness, weakness, faintness, possible shock. Diuretics remove excess body fluid (edema) and are used to treat high blood pressure and congestive heart failure. Diuretic brand names (generic names in parentheses):

Aldactazide (spironolactone, hydrochlorothiazide)
Aldactone (spironolactone)
Anhydron (cyclothiazide)
Aquatag (benzthiazide)
Aquatensin (methyclothiazide)
Diucardin (hydroflumethiazide)
Diulo (metolazone)
Diuril (chlorothiazide)
Dyazide (triamterene, hydrochlorothiazide)
Dyrenium (triamterene)
Edecrin (ethacrynic acid)
Enduron (methyclothiazide)
Esidrix (hydrochlorothiazide)

Exna (benzthiazide)
Hydrodiuril (hydrochlorothiazide)
Hydromox (quinethazone)
Hygroton (chlorthalidone)
Lasix (furosemide)
Metahydrin (trichlormethiazide)
Midamor (amiloride)
Moduretic (amiloride, hydrochlorothiazide)
Naqua (trichlormethiazide)
Naturetin (bendroflumethiazide)
Oretic (hydrochlorothiazide)
Renese (polythiazide)
Saluron (hydroflumethiazide)
Zaroxolyn (metolazone)

ANTIPSYCHOTICS (ALL)....GUANETHIDINE (Esimil, Ismelin)

THE EFFECT OF GUANETHIDINE MAY BE DE-CREASED. Guanethidine is used to lower high blood pressure. RESULT: The blood pressure may not be controlled properly.

ANTIPSYCHOTICS (ALL)....VASODILATOR BLOOD PRESSURE DRUGS

THIS COMBINATION MAY CAUSE THE BLOOD PRES-SURE TO DROP TOO LOW. RESULT: dizziness, weakness, faintness, possible shock. Vasodilators dilate blood vessels and allow blood to flow more easily. Vasodilator brand names (generic names in parentheses):

Apresoline (hydralazine)
Other products containing hydralazine: Apresazide, Apresoline-Esidrix, Dralserp, Dralzine, Ser-Ap-Es, Serpasil-Apresoline, Unipres
Loniten (minoxidil)

PHENOTHIAZINE ANTIPSYCHOTICS....AMPHETAMINES

THE APPETITE SUPPRESSION EFFECT OF AMPHETAMINE MAY BE DECREASED. Amphetamine is used as a diet pill (this use is in disfavor); for behavior problems in children; and for narcolepsy (uncontrollable desire to sleep). RESULT: If the amphetamine is used to control the appetite, it may not work as well. Amphetamine brand names:

Benzedrine
Biphetamine
Delcobese
Desoxyn
Dexedrine
Didrex
Obetrol

PHENOTHIAZINE ANTIPSYCHOTICS....ANTACIDS

THE EFFECT OF THE PHENOTHIAZINE ANTIPSY-CHOTIC MAY BE DECREASED. RESULT: The mental disorder may not be controlled properly. All antacids interact except sodium bicaronate antacids such as Alka-Seltzer. Antacid brand names:

AlternaGel

Delcid

Di-Gel

Gelusil

Kudrox

Maalox

Mylanta

Riopan

WinG el

PHENOTHIAZINE ANTIPSYCHOTICS
....LEVODOPA (Dopar, Larodopa, Sinemet)

THE EFFECT OF BOTH DRUGS MAY BE DECREASED. Levodopa is used to control the tremors of Parkinson's disease. RESULT: The conditions treated by either drug may not be controlled properly.

PHENOTHIAZINE ANTIPSYCHOTICS....LITHIUM

THE EFFECT OF THE PHENOTHIAZINE ANTIPSY-CHOTIC MAY BE DECREASED. RESULT: The mental disorder may not be controlled properly. Lithium is used to treat manic-depressive disorders. NOTE: Lithium combined with the phenothiazine antipsychotic thiordiazine (mellaril) has caused severe nervous system toxicity. Lithium brand names:

Eskalith

Lithane

Lithonate

Lithobid

Lithonate-S,

Lithotabs

II. NON-PHENOTHIAZINE ANTIPSYCHOTIC DRUG INTERACTIONS

HALOPERIDOL (Haldol)....LITHIUM

THE EFFECT OF HALOPERIDOL MAY BE INCREASED. RESULT: Possible adverse side effects from too much haloperidol with associated symptoms: aberrant or psychotic behavior, tremors, confusion, insomnia, toxic psychosis (agitation, disorientation, delirium). Lithium is used to treat manic-depressive disorders. Lithium brand names:

Eskalith
Lithane
Lithonate
Lithobid
Lithonate-S
Lithotabs

HALOPERIDOL (Haldol)....METHYLDOPA (Aldoclor, Aldomet, Aldoril)

THE EFFECT OF HALOPERIDOL MAY BE INCREASED. RESULT: Possible adverse side effects from too much haloperidol with associated symptoms: aberrant or psychotic behavior, tremors, confusion, insomnia, toxic psychosis (agitation, disorientation, delirium). Methyldopa is used to treat high blood pressure.

III LITHIUM DRUG INTERACTIONS

LITHIUM.... ASTHMA DRUGS (THEOPHYLLINE FAMILY)

THE EFFECT OF LITHIUM MAY BE DECREASED. Lithium is an antipsychotic drug used to treat manic-depressive disorders. RESULT: The condition treated may not be controlled properly. Theophylline family asthma drug brand names (generic names in parentheses):

Accurbron (theophylline)
Bronkodyl (theophylline)
Choledyl (oxtriphylline)
Dilor (diphylline)
Elixicon (theophylline)
Elixophyllin (theophylline)
LaBID (theophylline)
Lufyllin (diphylline)
Quibron-T (theophylline)
Respbid (theophylline)
Slo-Phyllin (theophylline)
Somophyllin (aminophylline)
Somophyllin-T (theophylline)

Sustaire (theophylline)
Theobid (theophylline)
Theodur (theophylline)
Theolair (theophylline)
Theophyl (theophylline)
Theovent (theophylline)
Multi-ingredient products
   containing theophylline:
Amesec, Asbron G, Brondecon,
   Marax, Mudrane, Quibron,
   Tedral SA

LITHIUM....DIURETICS

THE EFFECT OF LITHIUM MAY BE INCREASED. RESULT: Possible adverse side effects from too much lithium.

Report symptoms such as dizziness, nausea, confusion, weakness, lethargy, dry mouth, appetite loss, stomach or abdominal pain, loss of coordination. Diuretics remove excess body fluid and are used to treat high blood pressure and congestive heart failure. Interacting diuretics are the "potassium-losing" diuretics listed below (generic names in parentheses):

Anhydron (cyclothiazide)
Aquatag (benzthiazide)
Aquatensin (methyclothiazide)
Diucardin (hydroflumethiazide)
Diulo (metolazone)
Diuril (chlorothiazide)
Edecrin (ethacrynic acid)
Enduron (methyclothiazide)
Esidrix (hydrochlorothiazide)
Exna (benzthiazide)
Hydrodiuril (hydrochlorothiazide)

Hydromox (quinethazone)
Hygroton (chlorthalidone)
Lasix (furosemide)
Metahydrin (trichlormethiazide)
Naqua (trichlormethiazide)
Naturetin (bendroflumethiazide)
Oretic (hydrochlorothiazide)
Renese (polythiazide)
Saluron (hydroflumethiazide)
Zaroxolyn (metolazone)

NOTE: The following diuretic products contain a "potassium-sparing" ingredient along with the "potassium-losing" diuretic, so they may not interact as significantly:

Aldactazide (spironolactone, hydrochlorothiazide)
Dyazide (triamterene, hydrochlorothiazide)
Moduretic (amiloride, hydrochlorothiazide)

LITHIUM....HALOPERIDOL (Haldol)

THE EFFECT OF HALOPERIDOL MAY BE INCREASED. RESULT: Possible adverse side effects from too much haloperidol with associated symptoms: aberrant or psychotic behavior, tremors, confusion, insomnia, toxic psychosis (agitation, disorientation, delirium). Haloperidol is an antipsychotic drug used to treat severe mental disorders.

LITHIUM....IODINE-CONTAINING PRODUCTS

THIS COMBINATION MAY CAUSE HYPOTHYROIDISM. RESULT: Insufficient function of the thyroid gland. Products containing iodine:

Expectorants (agents which help remove phlegm):
    hydriodic acid syrup
    Iodo-Niacin

Pima
SSKI (saturated solution of potassium iodide)
Others:
    Combid—used in stomach, digestive tract disorders
    Darbid—used in stomach, digestive tract disorders

LITHIUM....NON-CORTICOSTEROID PAIN RELIEVERS

THE EFFECT OF LITHIUM MAY BE INCREASED. RE-SULT: Possible adverse side effects from too much lithium. Report symptoms such as dizziness, nausea, confusion, weakness, lethargy, dry mouth, appetite loss, stomach or abdominal pain, loss of coordination. Non-corticosteroids are used to relieve the pain and inflammation of arthritic conditions and some are used as general pain relievers. Non-corticosteroid brand names (generic names in parentheses):

aspirin (Anacin, Ascriptin, Aspergum, Bayer, Bufferin, CAMA, Ecotrin, Empirin, Measurin, Momentum, Pabirin, Persistin, St. Joseph Aspirin; other aspirin-like pain relievers which interact similarly to aspirin: Arthralgen, Arthropan, Calurin, Disalcid, Dolobid, Magan, Mobidin, Pabalate, Salrin, Uracel, Uromide)
Anaprox (naproxen)
Butazolidin (phenylbutazone)
Clinoril (sulindac)
Feldene (prioxicam)
Indocin (indomethacin)
Meclomen (meclofenamate)
Motrin (ibuprofen)
Nalfon (fenoprofen)
Naprosyn (naproxen)
Ponstel (mefenamic acid)
Rufen (ibuprofen)
Tandearil (oxyphenbutazone)
Tolectin (tolmetin)
Zomax (zomepirac)

LITHIUM....PHENOTHIAZINE ANTIPSYCHOTICS

THE EFFECT OF THE PHENOTHIAZINE ANTIPSY-CHOTIC MAY BE DECREASED. RESULT: The mental disorder may not be controlled properly. NOTE: Lithium combined with the phenothiazine antipsychotic thiordiazine (mellaril) has caused severe nervous system toxicity. Phenothiazine antipsychotic brand names (generic names in parentheses):

Compazine (prochlorperazine)
Mellaril (thioridazine)
Proketazine (carphenazine)
Prolixin (fluphenazine)
Quide (piperacetazine)
Serentil (mesoridazine)

Sparine (promazine)
Stelazine (trifluoperazine)
Thorazine (chlorpromazine)
Tindal (acetophenazine)
Trilafon (perphenazine)
Vesprin (triflupromazine)

LITHIUM....SALT (sodium chloride)

THE EFFECT OF LITHIUM MAY BE INCREASED. RE-SULT: Possible adverse side effects from too much lithium. Report symptoms such as dizziness, nausea, confusion, weakness, lethargy, dry mouth, appetite loss, stomach or abdominal pain, loss of coordination. Salt sources:

table salt
antacids containing sodium (check product label)

23

Drug Interactions in Treatment of Thyroid Disorders

The thyroid gland, located on the neck, plays an important role in body metabolism. A person with *hyperthyroidism* produces too much thyroid hormone, which causes overactivity, anxiety, hand tremors, weight loss, and perhaps bulging of the eyes. *Hypothyroidism*, or lack of enough thyroid hormone, may cause the thyroid gland to enlarge in an effort to produce more hormone, causing a goiter. Associated symptoms include weight gain, dry coarse hair, and face puffiness. Newborn infants with a congenital thyroid deficiency suffer from what is called *cretinism*. In adults, severe cases of hypothyroidism are called *myxedema*.

Hypothyroidism and goiter are treated with replacement *thyroid drugs*. Hyperthyroidism is treated with the antithyroid drugs *propylthiouracil* and *methimazole*.

BRAND NAMES

THYROID DRUGS:

Armour Thyroid (thyroid)
Cytomel (liothyronine)
Euthroid (liotrix)
Levothroid (levothyroxine)

Proloid (thyroglobulin)
Synthroid (levothyroxine)
Thyrar (thyroid)
Thyrolar (liotrix)

ANTITHYROID DRUGS:

propylthiouracil (various companies)
Tapazole (methimazole)

DRUG INTERACTIONS

I. THYROID DRUG INTERACTIONS

*THYROID DRUG....ANTICOAGULANTS

THE EFFECT OF THE ANTICOAGULANT MAY BE INCREASED. Anticoagulants are used to thin the blood and prevent it from clotting. RESULT: Increased risk of hemorrhage. Report symptoms such as bruising or bleeding anywhere on the body, black or tarry stools. This interaction occurs only when patients already stabilized on an anticoagulant are given thyroid. If the patient has been taking the thyroid before anticoagulant therapy is begun, this interaction has not been found to occur. Anticoagulant brand names (generic names in parentheses):

Athrombin-K (warfarin)
Coufarin (warfarin)
Coumadin (warfarin)
dicumarol (various companies)
Hedulin (phenindione)
Miradon (anisindione)
Panwarfin (warfarin)

THYROID DRUG....DIABETES DRUGS

THE EFFECT OF THE DIABETES DRUG MAY BE ANTAGONIZED. Diabetes drugs lower the blood sugar level in diabetics. RESULT: The blood sugar level may remain too high. Report symptoms of hyperglycemia (high blood sugar): excessive thirst and hunger, large urine output, weight loss, drowsiness, loss of energy, loss of coordination.

Diabinese (chlorpropamide)
Dymelor (acetohexamide)
Orinase (tolbutamide)
Tolinase (tolazamide)

THYROID DRUG....CHOLESTYRAMINE (Cuemid, Questran)

THE EFFECT OF THE THYROID DRUG MAY BE DECREASED. RESULT: The hypothyroidism may not be corrected properly. Cholestyramine is used in patients with elevated cholesterol blood levels. Take the thyroid drug one hour before or four hours after cholestyramine to prevent this interaction.

THYROID DRUG....CHOLESTIPOL (Colestid)

THE EFFECT OF THE THYROID DRUG MAY BE DE-CREASED. RESULT: The hypothyroidism may not be corrected properly. Cholestipol is used in patients with elevated cholesterol blood levels. Take the thyroid drug one hour before or four hours after colestipol to prevent this interaction.

II. ANTITHYROID DRUG INTERACTIONS

METHIMAZOLE (Tapazole)....ANTICOAGULANTS

THE EFFECT OF THE ANTICOAGULANT MAY BE INCREASED. Anticoagulants are used to thin the blood and prevent it from clotting. RESULT: Increased risk of hemorrhage. Report symptoms such as bruising or bleeding anywhere on the body, black or tarry stools. Anticoagulant brand names (generic names in parentheses):

Athrombin-K (warfarin)	Hedulin (phenindione)
Coufarin (warfarin)	heparin (various companies)
Coumadin (warfarin)	Miradon (anisindione)
dicumarol (various companies)	Panwarfin (warfarin)

PROPYLTHIOURACIL... .ANTICOAGULANTS

THE EFFECT OF THE ANTICOAGULANT MAY BE INCREASED. Anticoagulants are used to thin the blood and prevent it from clotting. RESULT: Increased risk of hemorrhage. Report symptoms such as bruising or bleeding anywhere on the body, black or tarry stools. Anticoagulant brand names (generic names in parentheses):

Athrombin-K (warfarin)	Hedulin (phenindione)
Coufarin (warfarin)	heparin (various companies)
Coumadin (warfarin)	Miradon (anisindione)
dicumarol (various companies)	Panwarfin (warfarin)

24

Drug Interactions
in Treatment of
Ulcers

A *gastric* ulcer is an erosion in the lining of the stomach. A *duodenal* ulcer occurs in the duodenum (the first part of the small intestine, which the stomach content empties into). The usual symptom of an ulcer is pain or "heartburn" in the upper abdomen or lower chest, especially after eating irritating foods or ingesting alcohol or coffee. Bleeding from the ulcer may cause the stool to look black or tarry, and general weakness and fatigue may occur due to loss of blood.

The current medical trend is away from requiring special diets for ulcer patients. There is little evidence showing that bland diets help to heal ulcers. Patients should determine individually what foods (if any) cause discomfort, and avoid them. Nevertheless, it's still a sound idea for ulcer patients to avoid alcohol, coffee, colas, and other beverages containing caffeine, which increases stomach acid secretion.

There are four kinds of drugs used to treat ulcers. *Antacids* work by neutralizing the acid secreted by the stomach. *Anticholinergics* reduce acid secretion and reduce "motility" or movement of the smooth muscle in the stomach and intestine. *Histamine* H_2 *antagonists* inhibit stomach acid secretion. *Sucralfate* works by forming a sort of "bandage" around the ulcer, protecting it from irritating acid.

BRAND NAMES

ANTACIDS

Alkets
AlternaGel

Aludrox
BiSoDol

Camalox
Creamalin
Delcid
Di-Gel
Gaviscon
Gelusil
Kolantyl
Kudrox
Maalox

Magnatril
Mylanta
Riopan
Rolaids
Silain-Gel
Simeco
Tums
WinGel

ANTICHOLINERGICS

Anaspaz
Barbidonna
Belladenal
Bellergal
Bentyl
Butibel
Cantil
Chardonna
Combid
Cystospaz
Daricon
Donnatal
Enarax

Kinesed
Levsin
Levsinex
Librax
Milpath
Pamine
Pathibamate
Pathilon
Probanthine
Sidonna
Valpin
Vistrax

HISTAMINE H$_2$ ANTAGONISTS

Tagamet (cimetidine)
Zantac (ranitidine)

SUCRALFATE

Carafate

DRUG INTERACTIONS

ANTACIDS

See *Indigestion* chapter—all antacid interactions are discussed in detail there.

ANTICHOLINERGICS (ALL)....AMANTADINE (Symmetrel)

THIS COMBINATION MAY CAUSE EXCESSIVE ANTI-CHOLINERGIC SIDE EFFECTS. RESULT: dry mouth, blurred vision, dizziness, constipation, difficult urination, stomach irritation, slurred speech, loss of coordination, heart palpitations, possible toxic psychosis (disorientation, agitation, delirium). Amantadine is used to treat Parkinson's disease.

ANTICHOLINERGICS (ALL)....ANTACIDS

THE EFFECT OF THE ANTICHOLINERGIC MAY BE DECREASED. RESULT: The anticholinergic may not work as well as expected. To prevent this interaction, separate the dose of each drug by at least an hour.

ANTICHOLINERGICS (ALL) ....ANTIDEPRESSANTS (CYCLIC TYPE)

THIS COMBINATION MAY CAUSE EXCESSIVE ANTICHOLINERGIC SIDE EFFECTS. RESULT: dry mouth, blurred vision, dizziness, constipation, difficult urination, stomach irritation, slurred speech, loss of coordination, heart palpitations, possible toxic psychosis (disorientation, agitation, delirium). Antidepressants are used to alleviate mental depression and elevate the mood. NOTE: The antidepressant trazadone (Desyrel) may not interact. Antidepressant brand names (generic names in parentheses):

Adapin (doxepin)
Asendin (amoxapine)
Aventyl (nortriptyline)
Desyrel (trazadone)
Elavil (amitriptyline)
Endep (amitriptyline)
Etrafon (amitriptyline/
    perphenazine)
Limbitrol (amitriptyline/
    chlordiazepoxide)
Ludiomil (maprotiline)

Norpramin (desipramine)
Pamelor (nortriptyline)
Pertofrane (desipramine)
Sinequan (doxepin)
Surmontil (trimipramine)
Tofranil, Tofranil-PM
    (imipramine)
Triavil (amitriptyline/
    perphenazine)
Vivactil (protriptyline)

ANTICHOLINERGICS (ALL)....ANTIDYSKINETICS

THIS COMBINATION MAY CAUSE EXCESSIVE ANTICHOLINERGIC SIDE EFFECTS. RESULT: dry mouth, blurred vision, dizziness, constipation, difficult urination, stomach irritation, slurred speech, loss of coordination, heart palpitations, possible toxic psychosis (disorientation, agitation, delirium). Antidyskinetics are used to alleviate the shaking and tremors of Parkinson's disease. Antidyskinetic brand names (generic names in parentheses):

Akineton (biperiden)
Artane (trihexpyhenidyl)
Cogentin (benztropine)
Kemadrin (procyclidine)
Pagitane (cycrimine)

ANTICHOLINERGICS (ALL)....ANTIHISTAMINES

THIS COMBINATION MAY CAUSE EXCESSIVE ANTI-CHOLINERGIC SIDE EFFECTS. RESULT: dry mouth, blurred vision, dizziness, constipation, difficult urination, stomach irritation, slurred speech, loss of coordination, heart palpitations, possible toxic psychosis (disorientation, agitation, delirium). Antihistamines are used in a variety of products for allergies, cold and cough, and in nonprescription sleep aids—read product label list of ingredients and consult the *Allergy* chapter for names of antihistamines.

ANTICHOLINERGICS (ALL)....ANTIPSYCHOTICS

THIS COMBINATION MAY CAUSE EXCESSIVE ANTI-CHOLINERGIC SIDE EFFECTS. RESULT: dry mouth, blurred vision, dizziness, constipation, difficult urination, stomach irritation, slurred speech, loss of coordination, heart palpitations, possible toxic psychosis (disorientation, agitation, delirium). Antipsychotics are used in severe mental disorders such as schizophrenia. Most antipsychotics are of the phenothiazine family. Antipsychotic brand names (generic names in parentheses):

PHENOTHIAZINES
Compazine (prochlorperazine)
Mellaril (thioridazine)
Proketazine (carphenazine)
Prolixin (fluphenazine)
Quide (piperacetazine)
Serentil (mesoridazine)
Sparine (promazine)
Stelazine (trifluoperazine)
Thorazine (chlorpromazine)
Tindal (acetophenazine)

Trilafon (perphenazine)
Vesprin (triflupromazine)
OTHERS
Haldol (haloperidol)
Loxitane (loxapine)
Moban (molindone)
Navane (thiothixene)
Taractan (chlorprothixene)

ANTICHOLINERGICS (ALL)....DIGOXIN (Lanoxin)

THE EFFECT OF DIGOXIN MAY BE INCREASED. Digoxin is used to treat congestive heart failure and to restore irregular heart beats to normal rhythm. RESULT: Possible adverse side effects from too much digoxin with associated symptoms: nausea, visual disturbances, confusion, appetite loss, loss of energy, headache, heart beat irregularities.

ANTICHOLINERGICS (ALL)
....DISOPYRAMIDE (Norpace)

THIS COMBINATION MAY CAUSE EXCESSIVE ANTICHOLINERGIC SIDE EFFECTS. RESULT: dry mouth, blurred vision, dizziness, constipation, difficult urination, stomach irritation, slurred speech, loss of coordination, heart palpitations, possible toxic psychosis (disorientation, agitation, delirium). Disopyramide is used to restore irregular heart beats to normal rhythm.

ANTICHOLINERGICS (ALL)....LEVODOPA (Dopar, Larodopa, Sinemet)

A. THE EFFECT OF LEVODOPA MAY BE DECREASED. Levodopa is used to alleviate the symptoms of Parkinson's disease. RESULT: The disease may not be controlled properly.
B. THIS COMBINATION MAY ALSO CAUSE EXCESSIVE "ANTICHOLINERGIC" SIDE EFFECTS. RESULT: dry mouth, blurred vision, dizziness, constipation, difficult urination, stomach irritation, slurred speech, loss of coordination, heart palpitations, possible toxic psychosis (disorientation, agitation, delirium).

ANICHOLINERGICS (ALL)....QUINIDINE

THIS COMBINATION MAY CAUSE EXCESSIVE ANTI-CHOLINERGIC SIDE EFFECTS. RESULT: dry mouth, blurred vision, dizziness, constipation, difficult urination, stomach irritation, slurred speech, loss of coordination, heart palpitations, possible toxic psychosis (disorientation, agitation, delirium). Quinidine is used to restore irregular heart beats to normal rhythm. Quinidine brand names:

Cardioquin
Duraquin
Quinaglute Dura-Tabs
Quinidex
Extentabs
Quinora

ANTICHOLINERGICS (ALL)....QUININE (Coco-Quinine, Quinamm, Quine)

THIS COMBINATION MAY CAUSE EXCESSIVE ANTI-CHOLINERGIC SIDE EFFECTS. RESULT: dry mouth, blurred vision, dizziness, constipation, difficult urination, stomach irritation, slurred speech, loss of coordination, heart palpitations, possible toxic psychosis (disorientation, agitation, delirium). Quinine is a nonprescription drug used to treat malaria and to prevent nighttime leg cramps.

CIMETIDINE (Tagamet)....ANTACIDS

THE EFFECT OF CIMETIDINE MAY BE DECREASED. RESULT: The ulcer may not be controlled properly. It's especially important to be aware of this interaction, since both drugs are routinely used together in ulcer treatment. To prevent the interaction, separate doses by at least an hour.

CIMETIDINE (Tagamet)....ANTICOAGULANTS

THE EFFECT OF THE ANTICOAGULANT MAY BE INCREASED. Anticoagulants are used to thin the blood and prevent it from clotting. RESULT: Increased risk of hemorrhage. Interacting anticoagulant brand names (generic names in parentheses):

Athrombin-K (warfarin)
Coufarin (warfarin)
Coumadin (warfarin)
dicumarol (various companies)
Panwarfarin (warfarin)

CIMETIDINE (Tagamet)
....ASTHMA DRUGS (THEOPHYLLINE FAMILY)

THE EFFECT OF THE ASTHMA DRUG MAY BE IN-
CREASED. Asthma drugs are used to open lung air passages and
make breathing easier in asthmatics. RESULT: Possible adverse
side effects from too much theophylline with associated symptoms: nausea, dizziness, headache, irritability, insomnia, tachycardia (rapid heart beat), heart beat irregularities, tremors, possible
seizures. Theophylline-type asthma drug brand names (generic
names in parentheses):

Accurbron (theophylline)
Bronkodyl (theophylline)
Choledyl (oxtriphylline)
Dilor (dyphylline)
Elixicon (theophylline)
Elixophyllin (theophylline)
LaBID (theophylline)
Lufyllin (dyphylline)
Quibron-T (theophylline)
Respbid (theophylline)
Slo-Phyllin (theophylline)
Somophyllin (aminophylline)
Somophyllin-T (theophylline)

Sustaire (theophylline)
Theobid (theophylline)
Theodur (theophylline)
Theolair (theophylline)
Theophyl (theophylline)
Theovent (theophylline)
   Multi-ingredient products
   containing theophylline:
   Amesec, Asbron G,
   Brondecon, Marax,
   Mudrane, Quibron, Tedral
   SA

CIMETIDINE (Tagamet)....BETA BLOCKER HEART
DRUGS

THE EFFECT OF THE BETA BLOCKER MAY BE IN-
CREASED. Beta blockers are used for angina, to restore irregular
heart beats to normal rhythm, and to treat high blood pressure.
RESULT: Adverse side effects from too much beta blocker with
associated symptoms: bradycardia (slow heart beat), fatigue, heart
beat irregularities, asthma-like wheezing or difficulty breathing,
low blood pressure (with dizziness, weakness, faintness). The beta
blocker drugs atenolol (Tenormin) and nadolol (Corgard) may

not interact significantly. Beta blocker brand names (generic names in parentheses):

Blocadren (timolol)
Corgard (nadolol)
Inderal (propranolol)
Lopressor (metoprolol)
Tenormin (atenolol)
Visken (pindolol)

CIMETIDINE (Tagamet)....CAFFEINE

THE EFFECT OF CAFFEINE MAY BE INCREASED. Caffeine is a stimulant. RESULT: Possible "caffeinism" with associated symptoms: nervousness and irritability, headache, tremors, rapid breathing, insomnia. Caffeine sources:

coffee
tea
colas and other soft drinks
chocolate
cocoa
some nonprescription diet pills
products for cold/cough, pain, and menstrual discomfort—read product label list of ingredients.

CIMETIDINE (Tagamet)....PHENYTOIN (Dilantin)

THE EFFECT OF PHENYTOIN MAY BE INCREASED. Phenytoin is an anticonvulsant used to control seizures in disorders such as epilepsy. RESULT: Possible adverse side effects from too much phenytoin with associated symptoms: visual disturbances, loss of coordination.

CIMETIDINE (Tagamet)....SUCRALFATE (Carafate)

THE EFFECT OF SUCRALFATE MAY BE DECREASED. RESULT: The ulcer may not be controlled properly. It's especially important to be aware of this interaction, since both drugs are prescribed for ulcer treatment. This combination probably should not be used together.

CIMETIDINE (Tagamet)....TRANQUILIZERS

THE EFFECT OF THE TRANQUILIZER MAY BE IN-CREASED. Tranquilizers are used to alleviate nervousness and anxiety. RESULT: Adverse side effects from too much tranquilizer with associated symptoms: excessive sedation, drowsiness, loss of coordination and mental alertness; in severe cases, failure of breathing and blood circulation functions causing coma and death. NOTE: The tranquilizers Ativan (lorazepam) and Serax (oxazepam) do not interact. Interacting tranquilizers are of the benzodiazepine family:

Ativan (lorazepam)
Centrax (prazepam)
Dalmane (flurazepam)—
   prescribed as a sleeping pill
Halcion (triazolam)—prescribed
   as a sleeping pill
Librium (chlordiazepoxide)
Limbitrol (chlordiazepoxide/
   amitriptyline)

Paxipam (halazepam)
Restoril (temazepam)—prescribed
   as a sleeping pill
Serax (oxazepam)
SK-Lygen (chlordiazepoxide)
Tranxene (clorazepate)
Valium (diazepam)
Xanax (alprazolam)

RANITIDINE (Zantac) is a drug similar to cimetidine (Tagamet), but without the interaction potential of cimetidine. Currently, no adverse drug interactions have been reported with ranitidine.

SUCRALFATE (Carafate)....CIMETIDINE (Tagamet)

THE EFFECT OF SUCRALFATE MAY BE DECREASED. RESULT: The ulcer may not be controlled properly. It's especially important to be aware of this interaction, since both drugs are prescribed for ulcer treatment. This combination probably should not be used together.

Appendix

FOOD INCREASES THE EFFECT OF SOME DRUGS.

Drugs whose effect may be increased by food and as a rule should be taken with food for consistency of effect:

beta blocker heart drugs—
> Used to prevent angina, to restore irregular heart beats to normal rhythm, and to treat high blood pressure. Beta blocker brand names: Blocadren, Corgard, Inderal, Lopressor, Tenormin, Visken

carbamazepine (Tegretol)—An anticonvulsant used to prevent seizures

diazepam (Valium)—A tranquilizer

diuretics—Used to treat high blood pressure and congestive heart failure. Interacting diuretic brand names: Anhydron, Aquatag, Aquatensin, Diucardin, Diulo, Diuril, Enduron, Esidrix, Exna, Hydrodiuril, Hydromox, Hygroton, Metahydrin, Naqua, Naturetin, Oretic, Renese, Saluron, Zaroxolyn

hydralazine (Apresoline)—Used to treat high blood pressure

nitrofurantoin (Furadantin, Macrodantin)—An antibiotic used to combat urinary tract infections

phenytoin (Dilantin)—An anticonvulsant used to prevent seizures

spironolactone (Aldactazide, Aldactone)—A diuretic used to treat high blood pressure and congestive heart failure

FOOD DECREASES THE EFFECT OF SOME DRUGS.

Give these drugs one hour before or two hours after meals to avoid an interaction which may decrease their effects:

Captopril (Capoten)—Used to treat high blood pressure and congestive heart failure
Antibiotics (see INFECTION chapter for brand names)
  EXCEPTIONS—antibiotics which are unaffected by food:
    amoxicillin (Amoxil, Larotid, Polymox, Robamox, Trimox, Wymox)
    bacampacillin (Spectrobid)
    doxycycline (Doxychel, Vibramycin, Vibratab)
    hetacillin (Versapen)
    erythromycin estolate (Ilosone)
    erythromycin enteric-coated (E-Mycin, Ery-Tab, Eryc, Ilotycin, Robimycin)
    minocycline (Minocin)

ALKALINIZING FOODS....METHENAMINE (Hiprex, Mandelamine, Urex)

THE EFFECT OF METHENAMINE MAY BE DE-CREASED. Methenamine is used to combat urinary tract (bladder and kidney) infections. RESULT: The infection may not be controlled properly. Avoid alkalinizing foods such as:

almonds, buttermilk, chestnuts, citrus juices (e.g., orange, grapefruit), coconut, cream, fruit (except cranberries, plums, prunes), milk, vegetables (except corn, lentils).

ALKALINIZING FOODS....QUINIDINE

(Cardioquin, Duraquin, Quinaglute Dura-Tabs, Quinidex Extentabs, Quinora)

THE EFFECT OF QUINIDINE MAY BE INCREASED. Quinidine is used to restore irregular heart beats to normal rhythm. RESULT: Possible adverse side effects from too much quinidine with associated symptoms: heart palpitations or heart beat irregularities, dizziness, headache, ringing in the ears, visual disturbances. Avoid alkalinizing foods such as:

almonds, buttermilk, chestnuts, citrus juices (e.g., orange, grapefruit), coconut, cream, fruit (except cranberries, plums, prunes), milk, vegetables (except corn, lentils).

ALKALINIZING FOODS....QUININE (Coco-Quinine, Quinamm, Quine)

THE EFFECT OF QUININE MAY BE INCREASED. Quinine is a nonprescription drug used for malaria and for nighttime leg cramps. RESULT: Possible adverse side effects from too much quinine with associated symptoms: dizziness, headache, ringing in the ears, visual disturbances. Avoid alkalinizing foods such as:

> almonds, buttermilk, chestnuts, citrus juices (e.g., orange, grapefruit), coconut, cream, fruit (except cranberries, plums, prunes), milk, vegetables (except corn, lentils).

CAFFEINE-CONTAINING FOODS....ASTHMA DRUGS (THEOPHYLLINE FAMILY)

THE EFFECT OF THE ASTHMA DRUG MAY BE IN-CREASED. Asthma drugs open lung air passages and make breathing easier in asthmatics. RESULT: Possible adverse side effects from too much theophylline with associated symptoms: nausea, dizziness, headache, irritability, tremors, insomnia, tachycardia (rapid heart beat), heart beat irregularities, possible seizures. NOTE: For theophylline-type asthma drug brand names, see *Asthma* chapter. Caffeine sources are:

> coffee, tea, colas and other soft drinks, chocolate, cocoa, some nonprescription diet pills, products for cold/cough, pain, and menstrual discomfort—read product label list of ingredients.

CARBOHYDRATE FOODS....ACETAMINOPHEN

THE EFFECT OF ACETAMINOPHEN MAY BE DE-CREASED. Acetaminophen is a popular nonprescription pain and fever reliever. RESULT: The pain or fever may not be relieved properly. Carbohydrate sources: bread, crackers, dates, jelly, etc. Acetaminophen brand names are:

> Anacin-3, Bromo Seltzer, Datril, Excedrin PM, Febrinol, Liquiprin, Percogesic, Phenaphen, Tapar, Tempra, Tylenol, Valadol.

CHARCOAL-BROILED BEEF OR HAMBURGER....ASTHMA DRUGS (THEOPHYLLINE FAMILY)

THE EFFECT OF THE ASTHMA DRUG MAY BE DE-CREASED. Asthma drugs open lung air passages and make breathing easier in asthmatics. RESULT: The asthma may not be controlled properly. NOTE: For theophylline-type asthma drug brand names, see *Asthma* chapter.

FATTY FOODS....GRISEOFULVIN (Fulvicin P/G, Fulvicin U/F, Grifulvin V, Grisactin, Gris-PEG)

THE EFFECT OF GRISEOFULVIN MAY BE INCREASED. Griseofulvin is given orally to combat fungal infections of the hair, skin, fingernails, and toenails. This is a *beneficial* interaction and griseofulvin should be taken at meal time with fatty foods such as:

avocados, beef, butter, cake, cream, chicken salad, French fries, fried chicken, etc.

HIGH FIBER FOODS....DIGOXIN (Lanoxin)

THE EFFECT OF DIGOXIN MAY BE DECREASED. Digoxin is used for congestive heart failure and to restore irregular heart beats to normal rhythm. RESULT: The condition treated may not be controlled properly. Give digoxin one hour before or two hours after high fiber foods such as:

prune juice, bran cereal, whole wheat foods, grains, raw vegetables, cooked leafy vegetables, fruits.

HIGH PROTEIN FOODS (meat, dairy products).... LEVODOPA (Dopar, Larodopa, Sinemet)

THE EFFECT OF LEVODOPA MAY BE DECREASED. Levodopa is used to control the tremors of Parkinson's disease. RESULT: The condition may not be controlled properly. Avoid or minimize high protein foods.

LEAFY GREEN VEGETABLES....THYROID (Armour Thyroid, Cytomel, Euthroid, Levothroid, Proloid, Synthroid, Thyrar, Thyrolar)

THE EFFECT OF THE THYROID DRUG MAY BE ANTAGONIZED. Thyroid is prescribed to correct hypothyroidism (insufficient function of the thyroid gland) and goiter (enlargement of the thyroid gland). RESULT: The thyroid disorder may not be controlled properly. Avoid or minimize servings of leafy green vegetables such as:

asparagus, broccoli, Brussels sprouts, cabbage, kale, lettuce, peas, spinach, turnip greens, watercress.

LICORICE....HIGH BLOOD PRESSURE DRUGS (ALL)

THE EFFECT OF THE HIGH BLOOD PRESSURE DRUG MAY BE ANTAGONIZED. RESULT: The blood pressure may not be controlled properly. Avoid *natural* licorice—the synthetic kind is okay. NOTE: See *High Blood Pressure* chapter for blood pressure drug brand names.

LICORICE....DIGITALIS HEART DRUGS (Crystodigin, Digifortis, Lanoxin, Purodigin)

THE EFFECT OF DIGITALIS MAY BE INCREASED. Digitalis is used for congestive heart failure and to restore irregular heart beats to normal rhythm. RESULT: Possible adverse side effects from too much digitalis drug with associated symptoms: nausea, confusion, visual disturbances, headache, loss of energy, appetite loss, heart beat irregularities. Avoid *natural* licorice—the synthetic kind is okay.

MILK AND DAIRY PRODUCTS....TETRACYCLINE ANTIBIOTICS

THE EFFECT OF TETRACYCLINE MAY BE DE-CREASED. Tetracycline is an antibiotic used to combat infection. RESULT: The infection treated may not be controlled properly. To prevent this interaction, take tetracycline one hour before or two hours after ingesting milk or dairy products. EXCEPTIONS: doxycycline (Doxychel, Vibramycin, Vibratab) and minocycline (Minocin). NOTE: For tetracycline brand names, see *Infection* chapter.

SALT....LITHIUM (Eskalith, Lithane, Lithonate, Lithobid, Lithonate-S, Lithotabs)

A LOW SALT DIET INCREASES THE EFFECT OF LITHIUM; A HIGH SALT DIET DECREASES THE EFFECT OF LITHIUM. Lithium is used to treat certain severe mental disorders. RESULT:

A. A diet containing too little salt may cause lithium toxicity with associated symptoms: dizziness, dry mouth, weakness, confusion, loss of energy, appetite loss, nausea, stomach or abdominal pain, loss of coordination, slurred speech.

B. If the diet contains too much salt, the condition treated may not be controlled properly.

Sodium chloride (table salt) is found in a variety of foods.

TYRAMINE-CONTAINING FOODS....ANTIDEPRESSANTS —MAOI TYPE (Eutonyl, Marplan, Nardil, Parnate)

THIS COMBINATION CAN CAUSE A MARKED RISE IN BLOOD PRESSURE. RESULT: Severe headache, fever, visual disturbances, confusion which may be followed by brain hemorrhage. Tyramine is a central nervous system stimulant. Antidepressants are used to alleviate mental depression and elevate the mood. This type of antidepressant—with the imposing name MAOI (MonoAmine Oxidase Inhibitor)—is not used much now that safer antidepressants such as Elavil, Sinequan, and Desyrel are available.

Avoid foods containing tyramine, such as:

avocados, baked potatoes, bananas, bean pods, beer, bologna, Brie, broad beans, caviar, cheeses, chicken liver, chocolate, coffee, cola beverages, figs (canned), meat tenderizers, nuts, packet soups, pepperoni, pickled herring, raspberries, salami, sauerkraut, summer sausage, sour cream, soy sauce, wines, yeast, yogurt.

VITAMIN B₆ (PYRIDOXINE)-CONTAINING FOODS.... LEVODOPA (Dopar, Larodopa, Sinemet)

THE EFFECT OF LEVODOPA MAY BE DECREASED. Levodopa is used to control the tremors of Parkinson's disease. RESULT: The condition may not be controlled properly.

Avoid or minimize these foods, high in vitamin B₆:

avocados, bacon, baker's yeast, Brewer's yeast, bran products, beef kidney, beef liver, dry skim milk, kidney beans, lentils, lima beans, malted milk, molasses, navy beans, oatmeal, pork, potatoes (sweet), salmon (fresh), soy beans, split peas, tuna, walnuts, wheat germ, yams (NOTE: many vitamin supplements contain vitamin B₆).

VITAMIN-K RICH FOODS....ANTICOAGULANTS

(Athrombin-K, Coufarin, Coumadin, dicumarol, Hedulin, Miradon, Panwarfin)

THE EFFECT OF THE ANTICOAGULANT MAY BE DECREASED. Anticoagulants are used to thin the blood and prevent it from clotting. RESULT: The blood may clot despite anticoagulant treatment. To minimize this interaction, don't overdo it on these vitamin K-containing foods:

liver, leafy vegetables (asparagus, broccoli, Brussels sprouts, cabbage, cauliflower, kale, lettuce, peas, spinach, turnip greens, watercress).

ALCOHOL↔DRUG INTERACTIONS

ALCOHOL....OTHER DEPRESSANTS

Alcohol (beer, liquor, wine, etc.) is a central nervous system depressant. It depresses or impairs functions such as coordination and alertness. Excessive depression or impairment can occur when alcohol is taken with any other central nervous system depressant. RESULT: drowsiness, dizziness, loss of muscle coordination and mental alertness; in severe cases, failure of blood circulation and breathing functions causing coma and death. Interacting depressant categories and brand names:

ANTICHOLINERGICS—Uses and brand names:
    Those used to control tremors resulting from Parkinson's disease or treatment with antipsychotic drugs:
    Akineton, Artane, Cogentin, Kemadrin, Pagitane
    Others:
    Norflex (a muscle relaxant)
    Robinul (used for stomach, digestive tract disorders)
    Transderm-Scop (used for motion sickness)
ANTICONVULSANTS (Used to control seizures in disorders such as epilepsy). Brand names: Depakene, Dilantin, Mesantoin, Mysoline, Peganone, Tegretol, Tridione, Zarontin
ANTIDEPRESSANTS (CYCLIC TYPE)—Used to alleviate mental depression. Brand names: Adapin, Asendin, Aventyl, Desyrel, Elavil, Endep, Etrafon, Limbitrol, Ludiomil, Norpramin, Pam-

elor, Pertofrane, Sinequan, Surmontil, Tofranil, Tofranil-PM, Triavil, Vivactil.

ANTIHISTAMINES (Used for allergies, colds). Brand names: Actidil, Antivert, Atarax, Benadryl, Bendectin, Bonine, Chlor-Trimeton, Clistin, Decapryn, Dimetane, Dramamine, Histadyl, Inhiston, Marezine, Optimine, PBZ, Periactin, Polaramine, Pyronil, Tavist, Teldrin, Triten, Vistaril.

ANTIPSYCHOTICS (Used for severe mental disorders). Antipsychotic brand names: Compazine, Haldol, Loxitane, Mellaril, Moban, Navane, Proketazine, Prolixin, Quide, Serentil, Sparine, Stelazine, Taractan, Thorazine, Tindal, Trilafon, Vesprin.

FENFLURAMINE (Pondimin)—A diet pill

HIGH BLOOD PRESSURE DRUGS (brand names in parentheses):
clonidine (Catapres, Combipres)
guanabenz (Wytensin)
methyldopa (Aldoclor, Aldomet, Aldoril)
reserpine-type drugs:
  deserpidine (Enduronyl, Harmonyl, Oreticyl)
  rauwolfia (Raudixin, Rauzide)
  reserpine (Diupres, Diutensen-R, Hydropres, Rau-Sed, Re-groton, Renese-R, Reserpoid, Salutensin, Sandril, Ser-Ap-Es, Serpasil, Serpasil-Apresoline, Serpasil-Esidrix)

MUSCLE RELAXANTS
Dantrium, Flexeril, Lioresal, Norflex, Norgesic, Norgesic Forte, Paraflex, Parafon Forte, Quinamm, Rela, Robaxin, Robaxisal, Skelaxin, Soma, Soma Compound, Valium

NARCOTICS
Codeine products:
  Ascriptin w/Codeine, Bancap w/Codeine, Bufferin w/Codeine, Empirin w/Codeine, Empracet w/Codeine, Fiorinal w/Codeine, Phenaphen w/Codeine, Tylenol w/Codeine
Other narcotic or narcotic-like products:
  Demerol, Dilaudid, Dolphene, morphine, Merpergan Fortis, Norcet, Numorphan, Percocet, Percodan, Synalgos-DC, Talwin, Talwin Compound, Tylox, Vicodan, Zactane, Zactirin

*PROPOXYPHENE (pain reliever): Darvocet-N, Darvon, Dolene, Wygesic

SLEEPING PILLS
Barbiturate sleeping pills:
  phenobarbital, Alurate, Amytal, Butisol, Buticap, Carbrital, Eskabarb, Lotusate, Luminal, Mebaral, Nembutal, Seconal, Sedadrops, Solfoton, Tuinal

Non-Barbiturate sleeping pills:
   Ativan (also used as a tranquilizer), Dalmane, Doriden, Halcion, Noctec, Noludar, Parest, Placidyl, Quaalude, Restoril, Somnos, Triclos, Valmid
TRANQUILIZERS
Benzodiazepine tranquilizers:
   Ativan, Centrax, Librium, Limbitrol (also an antidepressant), Paxipam, Serax, SK-Lygen, Tranxene, Valium, Xanax
Non-Benzodiazepine tranquilizers:
   Atarax, Equanil, meprobamate, Meprospan, Meprotab, Miltown, Trancopal, Tybatran, Vistaril

ALCOHOL....ACETAMINOPHEN

THIS COMBINATION MAY DAMAGE THE LIVER. Acetaminophen is a popular nonprescription pain and fever reliever. This interaction is most significant to those who drink large amounts of alcohol and use large doses of acetaminophen. Acetaminophen brand names are:

Anacin-3, Bromo Seltzer, Datril, Excedrin PM, Febrinol, Liquiprin, Percogesic, Phenaphen, Tapar, Tempra, Tylenol, Valnadol.

ALCOHOL....ANGINA HEART DRUGS

THIS COMBINATION CAN CAUSE THE BLOOD PRESSURE TO DROP TOO LOW. RESULT: Postural hypotension (sudden drop in blood pressure when changing positions, especially when rising after sitting or lying down) with associated symptoms: dizziness, weakness, faintness; a severe drop in blood pressure may cause seizures or shock. Limiting alcohol ingestion to small amounts minimizes this interaction. Angina drugs are used to relieve angina pain. Angina drug brand names are):

Cardilate, Duotrate, Isordil, Nitro-BID, Nitro-Dur, Nitrodisc, nitroglycerine (various companies), Nitroglyn, Nitrol ointment, Nitrospan, Nitrostat, Pentritol, Peritrate, Persantine, Sorbitrate, Susadrin, Transderm-Nitro.

ALCOHOL....ANTICOAGULANTS

THE EFFECT OF THE ANTICOAGULANT MAY BE INCREASED. Anticoagulants are used to thin the blood and prevent it from clotting. RESULT: Increased risk of hemorrhage. Limiting alcohol ingestion to small amounts minimizes this interaction. However, chronic alcohol use even in moderate amounts may *decrease* the effect of the anticoagulant, which would require a dosage adjustment. The most widely used anticoagulant is warfarin in the Coumadin brand name. Anticoagulant brand names are:

> Athrombin-K, Coufarin, Coumadin, dicumarol, Hedulin, Miradon, Panwarfin.

ALCOHOL....ASPIRIN

THIS COMBINATION MAY INCREASE THE RISK OF STOMACH BLEEDING AND ULCERATION. Aspirin brand names are:

> Anacin, Ascriptin, Aspergum, Bayer, Bufferin, CAMA, Ecotrin, Empirin, Measurin, Momentum, Pabirin, Persistin, St. Joseph Aspirin.

Other aspirin-like pain relievers which may not interact as harshly as aspirin are:

> Arthralgen, Arthropan, Calurin, Disalcid, Dolobid, Magan, Mobidin, Pabalate, Salrin, Uracel, Uromide.

ALCOHOL....ASTHMA DRUGS (THEOPHYLLINE FAMILY)

THE EFFECT OF THE ASTHMA DRUG MAY BE DECREASED. Asthma drugs open lung air passages and make breathing easier in asthmatics. RESULT: The asthma episode may not be relieved properly. Theophylline-type asthma drug brand names are:

> Accurbron, Amesec, Asbron G, Brondecon, Bronkodyl, Choledyl, Dilor, Elixicon, Elixophyllin, LaBID, Lufyllin, Marax, Mudrane, Quibron, Quibron-T, Respbid, Slo-Phyllin, Somophyllin, Somophyllin-T, Sustaire, Tedral SA, Theobid, Theodur, Theolair, Theophyl, Theovent.

ALCOHOL....CHLORAL HYDRATE (Noctec, Somnos)

THIS COMBINATION MAY CAUSE A REACTION SIMILAR TO THAT CAUSED BY DISULFIRAM. Disulfiram

(Antabuse) is the drug given to alcoholics to discourage them from drinking. RESULT: dizziness, shortness of breath, flushing, headache, heart palpitations. Also, since both drugs are central nervous system depressants, excessive depression may occur with associated symptoms: drowsiness, dizziness, loss of muscle coordination and mental alertness; in severe cases, failure of blood circulation and breathing functions causing coma and death. Chloral hydrate is used as a sedative or sleeping pill.

ALCOHOL....DIABETES DRUGS

THE EFFECT OF THE DIABETES DRUG MAY BE INCREASED. RESULT: Alcohol may cause unpredictable changes in the blood sugar level with the most serious effect being a dangerous *fall* in the blood sugar level with associated symptoms of hypoglycemia (low blood sugar): nervousness, faintness, weakness, sweating, confusion, tachycardia (rapid heart beat), heart beat irregularities, loss of coordination, visual disturbances; also, an acute reaction may occur similar to that when an alcoholic on the anti-alcoholic drug disulfiram (Antabuse) ingests alcohol: dizziness, shortness of breath, flushing, headache, heart palpitations. NOTE: Limiting alcohol to small amounts (especially if taken with food) will probably prevent this interaction. Diabetes drug brand names are:

Diabinese, Dymelor, Orinase, Tolinase, Insulin.

ALCOHOL....DISULFIRAM (Antabuse)

THIS COMBINATION MAY CAUSE THE "DISULFIRAM REACTION." Disulfiram is the drug given to alcoholics to discourage them from drinking. RESULT: dizziness, shortness of breath, flushing, headache, chest pain, blurred vision, nausea.

ALCOHOL....GUANETHIDINE (Esimil, Ismelin)

THIS COMBINATION MAY CAUSE THE BLOOD PRESSURE TO DROP TOO LOW. RESULT: Postural hypotension (sudden drop in blood pressure when changing positions, especially when rising after sitting or lying down) with associated symptoms: dizziness, weakness, faintness; a severe drop in blood pressure may cause seizures or shock. Limiting alcohol ingestion to small amounts minimizes this interaction.

ALCOHOL....ISONIAZID (INH, Niconyl, Nydrazid)

THIS COMBINATION MAY CAUSE LIVER DAMAGE. This interaction is most significant to those who drink large amounts of alcohol. However, chronic alcohol use even in moderate amounts may decrease the effect of isoniazid. Isoniazid is used to treat tuberculosis.

ALCOHOL....METRONIDAZOLE (Flagyl, Metryl, Satric)

THIS COMBINATION MAY CAUSE A REACTION SIMILAR TO THAT CAUSED BY DISULFIRAM. Disulfiram (Antabuse) is the drug given to alcoholics to discourage them from drinking. RESULT: dizziness, shortness of breath, flushing, headache, heart palpitations. Metronidazole is prescribed for trichomonas vaginalis, a type of vaginitis.

ALCOHOL....RIFAMPIN (Rifadin, Rimactane)

THIS COMBINATION MAY CAUSE LIVER DAMAGE. This interaction is most significant to those who drink large amounts of alcohol. However, chronic alcohol use even in moderate amounts may decrease the effect of rifampin. Rifampin is used to treat tuberculosis and may be given to suspected meningitis carriers.

ALCOHOL....TRICLOFOS (Triclos)

THIS COMBINATION MAY CAUSE A REACTION SIMILAR TO THAT CAUSED BY DISULFIRAM. Disulfiram (Antabuse) is the drug given to alcoholics to discourage them from drinking. RESULT: dizziness, shortness of breath, flushing, headache, heart palpitations. Also, since both drugs are central nervous system depressants, excessive depression may occur with associated symptoms: drowsiness, dizziness, loss of muscle coordination and mental alertness; in severe cases, failure of blood circulation and breathing functions causing coma and death. Triclofos is used as a sedative or sleeping pill.

VITAMIN ↔ DRUG INTERACTIONS

VITAMIN C....ANTICOAGULANTS

THE EFFECT OF THE ANTICOAGULANT MAY BE DECREASED. Anticoagulants are used to thin the blood and prevent it from clotting. RESULT: The anticoagulant might not be as effective as it should be. Warfarin in the Coumadin brand name is the most widely used anticoagulant. Anticoagulant brand names are:

Athrombin-K, Coufarin, Coumadin, dicumarol, Hedulin, Miradon, Panwarfin.

VITAMIN C....ASPIRIN

RESULT:
A. The effect of vitamin C is decreased.
B. High doses of vitamin C (over 2000 mg a day) can raise aspirin blood levels to toxic concentrations.

VITAMIN C....BARBITURATES

RESULT: POSSIBLE PROLONGED DURATION OF BARBITURATE EFFECTS. Barbiturates are used as sedatives or sleeping pills. Barbiturate brand names are:

phenobarbital, Alurate, Amytal, Butisol, Buticap, Carbrital, Eskabarb, Lotusate, Luminal, Mebaral, Nembutal, Seconal, Sedadrops, Solfoton, Tuinal.

VITAMIN C....BIRTH CONTROL PILLS (oral contraceptives)

RESULT: POSSIBLE INCREASED RISK OF PREGNANCY if large doses of vitamin C (1000 mg or more daily) are taken irregularly—due to a "rebound" lowering of the birth control pill's hormonal ingredients when the vitamin is stopped. Breakthrough bleeding is a sign of a possible interaction. NOTE: Taking vitamin C in the 250-500 mg range probably minimizes this interaction. Birth control pill brand names are:

Brevicon, Demulen, Enovid, Loestrin, Lo-Ovral, Micronor, Modicon, Nor-Q.D., Nordette, Norinyl, Norlestrin, Ortho-Novum, Ovcon, Ovral, Ovrette, Ovulen.

VITAMIN C....QUINIDINE

RESULT: POSSIBLE PROLONGED DURATION OF QUINIDINE EFFECTS. Quinidine is used to restore irregular heartbeats to normal rhythm. Quinidine brand names are:

Cardioquin, Duraquin, Quinaglute Dura-Tabs, Quinidex Extentabs, Quinora.

VITAMIN C....QUININE (Coco-Quinine, Quinamm, Quine)

RESULT: POSSIBLE PROLONGED DURATION OF QUININE EFFECTS. Quinine is a nonprescription drug used for malaria and for nighttime leg cramps.

VITAMIN C....PRIMIDONE (Mysolone)

RESULT: POSSIBLE PROLONGED DURATION OF PRIMIDONE EFFECTS. Primidone is an anticonvulsant used to prevent seizures in disorders such as epilepsy.

VITAMIN C....URINE GLUCOSE TESTS

RESULT: POSSIBLE FALSE TEST RESULTS in measuring urine sugar level in diabetics.

VITAMIN B₂ (RIBOFLAVIN)....BORIC ACID

THIS COMBINATION MAY CAUSE A LOSS OF VITAMIN B_2 FROM THE BODY. RESULT: Possible vitamin deficiency. Boric acid sources: mouth washes, skin ointments, hemorrhoidal suppositories.

VITAMIN B₆ (PYRIDOXINE)....BIRTH CONTROL PILLS

THIS COMBINATION MAY CAUSE LOSS OF VITAMIN B_6 FROM THE BODY. RESULT: Possible vitamin deficiency. Take a vitamin B_6 supplement. Birth control pill brand names are:

Brevicon, Demulen, Enovid, Loestrin, Lo-Ovral, Micronor, Modicon, Nor-Q.D., Nordette, Norinyl, Norlestrin, Ortho-Novum, Ovcon, Ovral, Ovrette, Ovulen.

VITAMIN B₆ (PYRIDOXINE)....ESTROGENS (female hormones)

THIS COMBINATION MAY CAUSE LOSS OF VITAMIN B_6 FROM THE BODY. RESULT: Possible vitamin deficiency. Take a vitamin B_6 supplement. Estrogen brand names are:

Amen, Aygestin, DES, Estinyl, Estrace, Estratab, Estrovis, Feminone, Menest, Menrium, Milprem, Norlutate, Norlutin, Ogen, PMB, Premarin, Provera, Tace.

VITAMIN B₆ (PYRIDOXINE)....HYDRALAZINE (Apresoline)

THIS COMBINATION MAY CAUSE LOSS OF VITAMIN B₆ FROM THE BODY. RESULT: Possible vitamin deficiency. Take a vitamin B₆ supplement. Hydralazine is used to treat high blood pressure.

VITAMIN B₆ (PYRIDOXINE)....ISONIAZID

THIS COMBINATION MAY CAUSE LOSS OF VITAMIN B₆ FROM THE BODY. RESULT: Possible vitamin deficiency. Take a vitamin B₆ supplement. Isoniazid is used to treat tuberculosis. Isoniazid brand names are:

INH, Niconyl, Nydrazid, Triniad, Uniad.

VITAMIN B₆ (PYRIDOXINE)....LEVODOPA (Dopar, Larodopa, Sinemet)

THE EFFECT OF LEVODOPA MAY BE DECREASED. Levodopa is used to control the tremors of Parkinson's disease. RESULT: The condition may not be controlled properly. NOTE: Taking Levodopa in the Sinemet brand minimizes this interaction.

VITAMIN B₁₂....POTASSIUM CHLORIDE

RESULT: THE EFFECT OF VITAMIN B₁₂ MAY BE DECREASED. Potassium supplements are often prescribed for high blood pressure patients taking diuretics, most of which cause the body to lose potassium. Potassium chloride supplement brand names are:

Kaochlor, Kaon-Cl, Kato, Kay Ciel, K-Lor, Klorvess, K-Lyte, Slow-K.

NOTE: Salt substitutes used by those on low salt (sodium chloride) diets also contain potassium chloride:

Adolph's Salt Substitute, Morton Salt Substitute, Neocurtasal, NoSalt, Nu-Salt.

FOLIC ACID (VITAMIN B₉)....BARBITURATES

THIS COMBINATION MAY CAUSE LOSS OF FOLIC ACID FROM THE BODY. RESULT: Possible folic acid deficiency. Take a folic acid supplement. Barbiturates are used as sedatives or sleeping pills. Barbiturate brand names are:

phenobarbital, Alurate, Amytal, Butisol, Buticap, Carbrital, Eskabarb, Lotusate, Luminal, Mebaral, Nembutal, Seconal, Sedadrops, Solfoton, Tuinal.

FOLIC ACID (VITAMIN B₉)....BIRTH CONTROL PILLS (oral contraceptives)

THIS COMBINATION MAY CAUSE LOSS OF FOLIC ACID FROM THE BODY. RESULT: Possible folic acid deficiency. Take a folic acid supplement. Birth control pill brand names are:

Brevicon, Demulen, Enovid, Loestrin, Lo-Ovral, Micronor, Modicon, Nor-Q.D., Nordette, Norinyl, Norlestrin, Ortho-Novum, Ovcon, Ovral, Ovrette, Ovulen.

FOLIC ACID (VITAMIN B₉)....ESTROGENS (female hormones)

THIS COMBINATION MAY CAUSE LOSS OF FOLIC ACID FROM THE BODY. RESULT: Possible folic acid deficiency. Take a folic acid supplement. Estrogen brand names are:

Amen, Aygestin, DES, Estinyl, Estrace, Estratab, Estrovis, Feminone, Menest, Menrium, Milprem, Norlutate, Norlutin, Ogen, PMB, Premarin, Provera, Tace.

FOLIC ACID (VITAMIN B₉)....PHENYTOIN (Dilantin)

THIS COMBINATION MAY CAUSE LOSS OF FOLIC ACID FROM THE BODY. RESULT: Possible folic acid deficiency. Take a folic acid supplement, but not too much—large amounts of folic acid may decrease the effect of phenytoin. Phenytoin is an anticonvulsant used to control seizures in disorders such as epilepsy. Other interacting phenytoin-like drugs are Mesantoin and Peganone.

FOLIC ACID (VITAMIN B₉)....PRIMIDONE (Mysoline)

THIS COMBINATION MAY CAUSE LOSS OF FOLIC ACID FROM THE BODY. RESULT: Possible folic acid deficiency. Take a folic acid supplement. Primidone is an anticonvulsant used to control seizures in disorders such as epilepsy.

FOLIC ACID (VITAMIN B₉)
....SULFASALAZINE (Azulfidine)

THIS COMBINATION MAY CAUSE LOSS OF FOLIC ACID FROM THE BODY. RESULT: Possible folic acid deficiency. Take a folic acid supplement. Sulfasalazine is used to treat ulcerative colitis.

VITAMINS A,D,E,K....MINERAL OIL (laxative)

RESULT: DECREASED VITAMIN ABSORPTION.

VITAMINS A AND D....CHOLESTYRAMINE (Cuemid, Questran)

RESULT: DECREASED VITAMIN A AND D ABSORPTION. Cholestyramine is used in patients with elevated cholesterol blood levels.

VITAMIN D....PHENYTOIN (Dilantin)

RESULT: DECREASED VITAMIN D EFFECT. Phenytoin is an anticonvulsant used to control seizures in disorders such as epilepsy. Other interacting phenytoin-like drugs are Mesantoin and Peganone.

VITAMIN E....ANTICOAGULANTS

THE EFFECT OF THE ANTICOAGULANT MAY BE INCREASED. Anticoagulants are used to thin the blood and prevent it from clotting. RESULT: Increased risk of hemorrhage. Warfarin in the Coumadin brand name is the most widely used anticoagulant. Anticoagulant brand names are:

Athrombin-K, Coufarin, Coumadin, dicumarol, Hedulin, Miradon, Panwarfin.

VITAMIN K....ANTICOAGULANTS

THE EFFECT OF THE ANTICOAGULANT MAY BE DECREASED. Anticoagulants are used to thin the blood and prevent it from clotting. Vitamin K enhances the clotting effect of the blood. RESULT: The blood may clot despite anticoagulant treatment. Those on anticoagulant therapy should avoid foods high in vitamin K: liver, leafy vegetables (asparagus, broccoli, Brussels sprouts, cabbage, cauliflower, kale, lettuce, peas, spinach, turnip greens, watercress). Supplemental vitamin K is prescription-only. Warfarin in the Coumadin brand name is the most widely used anticoagulant. Anticoagulant brand names are:

Athrombin-K, Coufarin, Coumadin, dicumarol, Hedulin, Miradon, Panwarfin.

VITAMINS A AND B_1 (THIAMINE)....ANTACIDS (Maalox, Mylanta, etc.)

RESULT: DECREASED VITAMIN ABSORPTION.

IRON....ANTACIDS (Maalox, Mylanta, etc.)

RESULT: DECREASED IRON ABSORPTION.

IRON, CALCIUM, ZINC....TETRACYCLINE ANTIBIOTICS

THE EFFECT OF TETRACYCLINE MAY BE DECREASED. Tetracycline is an antibiotic used to combat infection. RESULT: The infection may not be controlled properly. NOTE: For tetracycline brand names, see the *Infection* chapter.

VITAMIN ↔ VITAMIN INTERACTIONS

VITAMIN A....VITAMIN C and VITAMIN E

RESULT: Increased vitamin A activity.

VITAMIN B_{12}....VITAMIN C

RESULT: Decreased vitamin B_{12} activity.

VITAMIN C....IRON

RESULT: Increased iron absorption.

VITAMIN E....VITAMIN C

RESULT: Increased vitamin E activity.

VITAMIN E....IRON

RESULT: Decreased vitamin E activity.

Index

333